CARDIAC IMAGING SECRETS

CARDIAC IMAGING SECRETS

Neil J. Weissman, MD
Associate Professor of Medicine
Georgetown University Medical College
Director, Cardiac Ultrasound and Ultrasound Core Laboratories
Cardiovascular Research Institute
Washington Hospital Center
Washington, District of Columbia

Gabriel A. Adelmann, MD
Fellow in Advanced Echocardiography
Washington Hospital Center
Washington, District of Columbia
Currently, Tel Aviv University Medical School
The Tel Aviv Medical Center
The Procardia/Maccabi Cardiology Center
Tel Aviv, Israel

HANLEY & BELFUS
An Affiliate of Elsevier

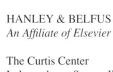

HANLEY & BELFUS
An Affiliate of Elsevier

The Curtis Center
Independence Square West
Philadelphia, Pennsylvania 19106

Note to the reader: Although the techniques, ideas, and information in this book have been carefully reviewed for correctness, neither the authors nor the publisher can accept any legal responsibility for any errors of ommissions that may be made. Neither the authors nor the publisher makes any guarantee, expressed or implied, with respect to the material contained herein.

Library of Congress Control Number: 2003107488

CARDIAC IMAGING SECRETS   **ISBN 1-56053-515-6**

Printed in the United States of America

Last digit is the print number: 9 8 7 6 5 4 3 2 1

DEDICATION

For Nancy and David, with love
—NJW

For little Alec and Samantha, the next Adelmanns
—GAA

CONTENTS

CONTRIBUTORS

Gabriel A. Adelmann, M.D.
Tel Aviv University Medical School, Tel Aviv Medical Center, Procardia/Maccabi Cardiology Center, Tel Aviv, Israel

Andrew E. Ajani, MBBS, FRACP, FJFICM
Senior Lecturer, Cardiology Department, Royal Melbourne Hospital, Melbourne, Victoria, Australia

Ernest K. Amegashie, M.D.
Assistant Professor, Division of Cardiology, Department of Medicine, Howard University College of Medicine; Howard University Hospital, Washington, District of Columbia

Matthew R. Brewer, M.D.
Department of Radiology, University of Vermont College of Medicine, Burlington, Vermont

David R. Buck, M.D.
Clinical Assistant Professor, Howard University College of Medicine; Senior Attending Radiologist, Department of Interventional Radiology, Washington Hospital Center, Washington, District of Columbia

Ellen M. Burton, R.N., B.S.N., CCRC
Cardiovascular Research Institute, Washington Hospital Center, Washington, District of Columbia

Marco T. Castagna, M.D.
Assistant Physician, Department of Cardiology, Hospital Mater Dei, Belo Horizonte, Brazil

Manuel D. Cerqueira, M.D.
Professor of Medicine and Radiology, Department of Medicine, Georgetown University School of Medicine, Washington, District of Columbia

Evagoras Economides, M.A., B.M., B.Ch.
Chief, Noninvasive Cardiology, Beebe Medical Center; Cardiologist, Cardiology Consultants, P.A., Lewes, Delaware

Shmuel Fuchs, M.D.
Director, Catheterization Laboratory, Rabin Medical Center, Campus Golda-Hasharon, Petach-Tikua, Israel

Anthon R. Fuisz, M.D.
Director, Cardiac Magnetic Resonance Imaging, Department of Medicine, Washington Hospital Center, Washington, District of Columbia

Steven A. Goldstein, M.D., FACC
Division of Cardiology, Washington Hospital Center, Washington, District of Columbia

Curtis E. Green, M.D.
Professor, Department of Radiology, University of Vermont College of Medicine; Director of General Radiology, Medical Center Hospital of Vermont, Burlington, Vermont

Luis Gruberg, M.D.
Director, Clinical Research, Division of Invasive Cardiology, Rambam Medical Center, Haifa, Israel

Kenneth Horton, RDCS, RCVT
Ultrasound Core Laboratory, Washington Hospital Center, Washington, District of Columbia

Benjamin Kleiber, M.D.
Washington Hospital Center, Washington, District of Columbia

Jun-ichi Kotani, M.D.
Intravascular Ultrasound Core Laboratory, Cardiovascular Research Institute, Washington Hospital Center, Washington, District of Columbia

Joseph Lindsay, M.D.
Professor, Division of Cardiology, Department of Internal Medicine, George Washington University School of Medicine; Director, Section of Cardiology, Washington Hospital Center, Washington, District of Columbia

Dorothea McAreavey, M.D., FACC
Director, Critical Care Medicine Fellowship Program, Department of Critical Care Medicine, Clinical Center, National Institutes of Health, Bethesda, Maryland

Michael A. Peterson, M.D.
Clinical Fellow, Division of Cardiovascular Diseases, Mayo Clinic, Rochester, Minnesota

Abraham Rothman, M.D.
Professor, Department of Pediatrics, University of California, San Diego, School of Medicine; Co-Director, Division of Cardiology, Children's Hospital, San Diego, California

Rina Sternlieb, M.D.
Senior Physician, Division of Geriatrics, Department of Internal Medicine, Tel Aviv School of Medicine, Tel Aviv Medical Center, Tel Aviv, Israel

Jonathan G. Tall, CNMT, CCRC
Director of Operations, Ultrasound Core Laboratories, Washington Hospital Center, Washington, District of Columbia

M. Therese Tupas-Habib, B.S., RDCS
Washington Hospital Center, Washington, District of Columbia

Neil J. Weissman, M.D.
Associate Professor of Medicine, Georgetown University Medical College; Director, Echocardiography and Ultrasound Core Laboratories, Cardiovascular Research Institute, Washington Hospital Center, Washington, District of Columbia

PREFACE

The advent of clinical radiology not only provided new avenues of patient investigation, but revolutionized medical thinking, ushering in the modern era of patient care. As a result, the 20th century witnessed an unprecedented development of imaging technologies, some of them (CT, contrast angiography) based on the principles of classic radiology, and others (MRI, nuclear medicine, ultrasound techniques) totally innovative. This technologic proliferation has proven a formidable challenge for the practicing physician. What test to use in which patient? How to interpret the results? Can therapeutic intervention be indicated based on the images obtained by the first test, or is another test needed for confirmation? How can the information essential for patient management be obtained in the most cost-effective way? These are just a few of the common questions facing today's medical care professional.

Cardiac Imaging Secrets provides a comprehensive review of the current methods of cardiac structural and functional evaluation in the normal and pathologic setting. The book's thirteen chapters discuss echocardiography, cardiac catheterization, nuclear cardiology, cardiac radiology, CT, MRI, and intravascular ultrasound (IVUS) with respect to their physical foundations and their application in the diagnosis and follow-up of patients with heart disease. Special chapters are dedicated to the latest developments in the field, cost-effectiveness issues, and the discussion of epidemiologic principles relevant to optimal use of cardiac imaging techniques.

The book is appropriate for a wide target audience, including medical students in senior years, radiologists, cardiology fellows, cardiologists preparing for recertification examinations, and general practitioners wishing to expand their knowledge in the rapidly evolving field of cardiac imaging. As the popular adage has it, "you see what you recognize, and you recognize what you know." We hope this book will prove a useful companion on the journey from image inspection to problem recognition, medical knowledge, and, ultimately, better patient care.

Neil J. Weissman, MD
Gabriel A. Adelmann, MD

ACKNOWLEDGMENTS

Gabriel Adelmann wishes to acknowledge Dr. Stephen Goldstein, the mentor and friend without whom this book would not have been possible; Dr. Pamela Sears-Rogan, for the countless hours of teaching that have forever enriched my understanding of echocardiography; Dr. Joseph Lindsay, Jr., for his general guidance during my fellowship at the Washington Hospital Center, and for his encouragement and support with this project; Drs. Anthon Fuisz and David Buck, for their editorial assistance with the MRI and, respectively, radiology sections; Kenneth Horton, Jonathan Tall, and Therese Tupas-Habib, for their professional expertise, willingness to help, and sense of humor—their share in the making of this book is much greater than the mere contribution to a few chapters; David Greer, for his inexhaustible technical resourcefulness, which provided solutions when none seemed possible; Annalisa Rowe, for expert secretarial help; Ellen Burton, for her friendship and encouragement; the technicians and associated lab personnel at the WHC who performed the diagnostic studies from which the images of this book have been taken; and the whole team of the WHC echocardiography lab, with whom I have spent 2 unforgettable years.

Neil Weissman expresses appreciation to the wonderful team of physicians and professionals I get to work with every day (many of whom are listed above) and, most of all, to thank my wonderful wife Nancy and son David, who are my never-ending source of inspiration and love of life.

COLOR PLATES

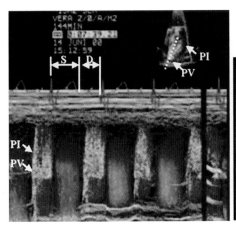

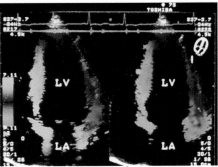

FIGURE 1. See Chapter 1, Figure 12 (page 20) for legend.

FIGURE 2. See Chapter 1, Figure 13 (page 21) for legend.

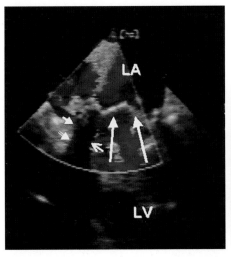

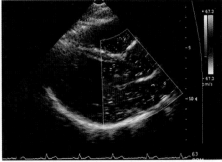

FIGURE 3. See Chapter 1, Figure 19 (page 25) for legend.

FIGURE 4. See Chapter 1, Figure 20 (page 26) for legend.

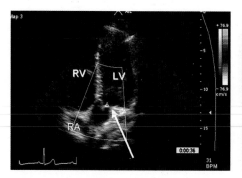

FIGURE 5. See Chapter 2, Figure 14 (page 67) for legend.

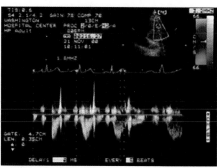

FIGURE 6. See Chapter 2, Figure 24A (page 74) for legend.

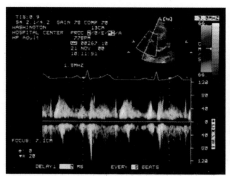

FIGURE 7. See Chapter 2, Figure 24B (page 74) for legend.

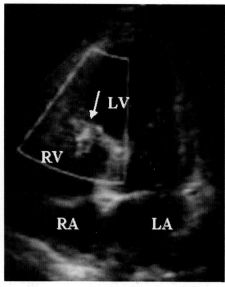

FIGURE 8. See Chapter 4, Figure 7 (page 124) for legend.

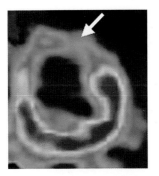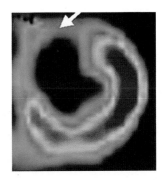

FIGURE 9. See Chapter 4, Figure 18B (page 152) for legend.

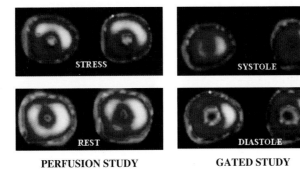

PERFUSION STUDY   **GATED STUDY**

FIGURE 10. See Chapter 4, Figure 24 (page 161) for legend.

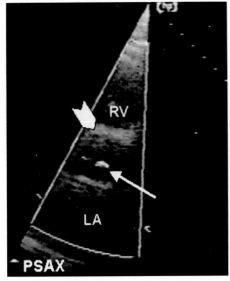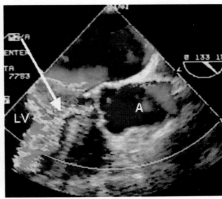

FIGURE 11. See Chapter 6, Figure 11A (page 210) for legend.

FIGURE 12. See Chapter 6, Figure 11B (page 210) for legend.

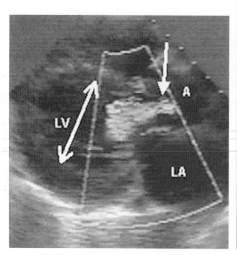

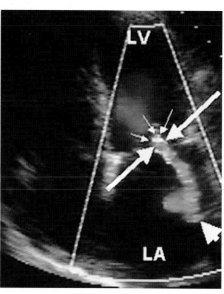

FIGURE 13. See Chapter 6, Figure 12 (page 212) for legend.

FIGURE 14. See Chapter 6, Figure 19A (page 222) for legend.

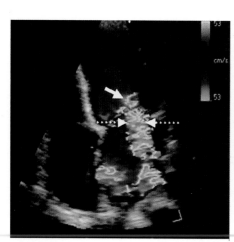

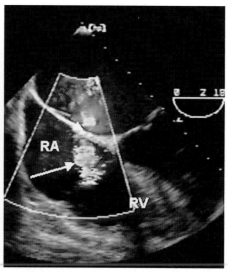

FIGURE 15. See Chapter 6, Figure 19B (page 222) for legend.

FIGURE 16. See Chapter 6, Figure 23 (page 232) for legend.

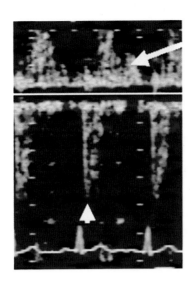

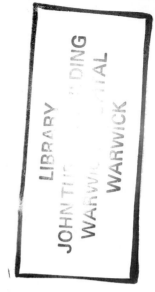

FIGURE 17. See Chapter 6, Figure 25 (page 235) for legend.

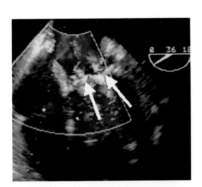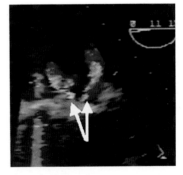

FIGURE 18. See Chapter 6, Figure 27 (page 236) for legend.

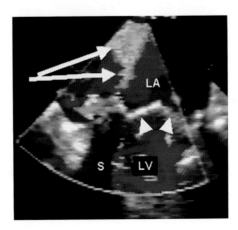

FIGURE 19. See Chapter 6, Figure 28 (page 237) for legend.

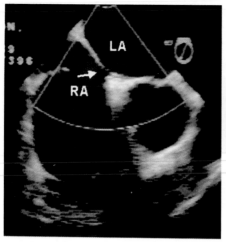

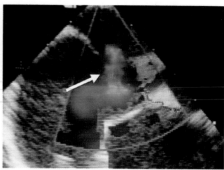

FIGURE 20. See Chapter 8, Figure 10A (page 286) for legend.

FIGURE 21. See Chapter 9, Figure 8B (page 312) for legend.

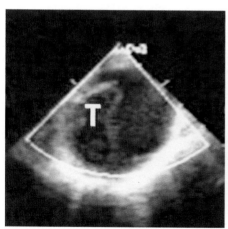

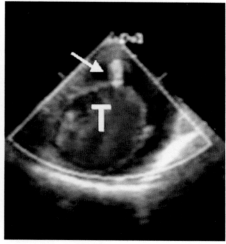

FIGURE 22. See Chapter 10, Figure 6C (page 333) for legend.

FIGURE 23. See Chapter 10, Figure 6D (page 333) for legend.

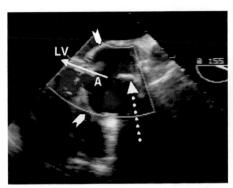 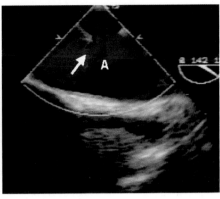

FIGURE 24. See Chapter 10, Figure 8 (page 334) for legend.

FIGURE 25. See Chapter 10, Figure 13 (page 339) for legend.

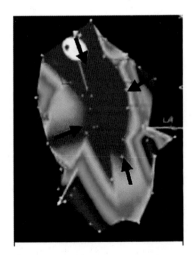 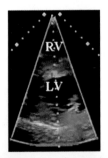

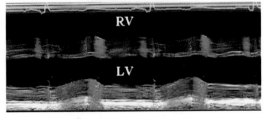

FIGURE 26. See Chapter 11, Figure 1 (page 355) for legend.

FIGURE 27. See Chapter 11, Figure 4 (page 361) for legend.

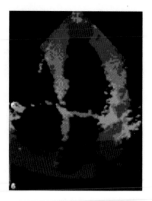
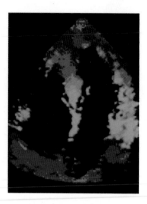

FIGURE 28. See Chapter 11, Figure 5 (page 362) for legend.

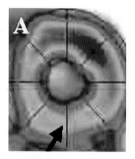
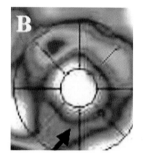

FIGURE 29. See Chapter 11, Figure 6 (page 364) for legend.

SHORT AXIS

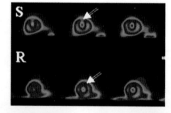

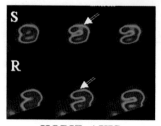
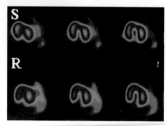

HORIZ. AXIS   **VERT. AXIS**

FIGURE 30. See Chapter 11, Figure 7 (page 365) for legend.

I. GENERAL PRINCIPLES

CARDIAC CATHETERIZATION

Gabriel Adelmann, M.D., Andrew E. Ajani, MBBS, FRACP,
Michael A. Peterson, M.D., and Benjamin Kleiber, M.D.

1. What are the main types of diagnostic procedures carried out in the cardiac catheterization laboratory (cath lab)?

The main diagnostic procedures performed in the cath lab are aimed at:

1. Defining cardiac **structure,** by means of angiographic procedures including:
   - The anatomy of the coronary arteries, by coronary angiography
   - The anatomy (size, shape, volume, mass) of the ventricles, by left and right ventriculography
   - The anatomy of the aorta and great vessels (e.g., aortography)
2. Defining cardiac **function,** including:
   - The function of the ventricles (ventriculography)
   - The function of the cardiac valves, by injecting contrast agents into the ventricles or the aorta (ventriculography, aortography) and by measuring the pressures in the ventricles and in the great arteries
   - Identification and quantification of cardiac shunt, characterization of the blood flow through the coronary arteries, and assessments at the level of the microcirculation, by special techniques

2. What are the main types of therapeutic procedures carried out in the cath lab?

Therapeutic procedures performed in the cath lab, also called percutaneous interventions (PCI), include:

- Balloon dilatation of coronary stenosis (percutaneous transcatheter coronary angioplasty [PTCA]), with or without stent deployment. Similar interventions may be performed on other arteries as well, such as the carotid or the renal arteries and even the aorta.
- Balloon dilatation of stenotic mitral valves, a procedure known as percutaneous transcatheter mitral valvuloplasty (PTMV)
- Repair of congenital cardiac anomalies (atrial septal defect [ASD], patent ductus arteriosus [PDA]) by deployment of different devices, such as coils and occluders
- Creation of an interatrial communication as the initial step in the treatment of certain congenital cardiac anomalies (the Rashkind procedure)
- Deployment of special therapeutic devices, such as the intraaortic balloon pump
- Special indications, some experimental, such as instillation of ethanol into one or more septal branches of the left anterior descending (LAD) artery in patients with hypertrophic obstructive cardiomyopathy (HOCM) (in order to produce controlled "shrinkage" [necrosis] of the hypertrophic portion of the interventricular septum) and lysis of blood clots in the right heart chambers or pulmonary artery by means of special catheters

3. What are stents?

Stents are synthetic cylinders of different lengths that can be inserted in coronary arteries to help them maintain their shape and dimensions after balloon dilatation.

4. What is coronary angiography?

This radiographic technique consists of coronary artery visualization by means of contrast agents injected directly into the coronaries. The contrast agents are injected through catheters inserted into the vascular system by puncturing a peripheral artery (most commonly the femoral artery) and advanced to the level of the coronary ostia. This procedure is generally complemented by injection of contrast into the left ventricle (left ventriculography); when necessary, contrast also can be injected in the aorta (aortogram) or in peripheral arteries (e.g., renal arteriogram, carotid arteriogram).

5. What is the purpose of coronary angiography?

- To establish the presence of coronary artery disease when noninvasive techniques cannot reasonably exclude this diagnosis
- To define the severity of coronary artery disease (the number and degree of coronary stenosis, measured in percent narrowing of the arterial lumen)
- To characterize the functional significance of an epicardial coronary stenosis (to what degree the capillary circulation is diminished by a stenosis in the larger portion of the artery)
- To provide information useful for the selection of the most appropriate therapeutic measures (e.g., conservative vs. interventional treatment, PCI vs. coronary artery bypass graft [CABG], the necessity for stent deployment and for special devices, such as rotational atherectomy [Rotablator, Scimed, Minneapolis, MN], intracoronary laser, atherectomy), and to assess the result of these interventions (coronary artery patency, graft patency)

6. What is the current role of coronary angiography in the diagnosis of coronary artery disease?

In current practice, coronary angiography remains the diagnostic gold standard for assessing coronary artery disease. Although magnetic resonance imaging (MRI) offers the promise of a noninvasive assessment of coronary artery disease, significant advances with this method are still necessary before it can become a viable alternative to coronary angiography. Additionally, noninvasive imaging methods are inherently not suited for interventional procedures.

7. What are the indications for coronary angiography?

The American Heart Association (AHA) guidelines for coronary angiography summarize the indications for this diagnostic modality. According to the strength of the recommendation for angiography, these indications are categorized as classes I, II, or III.

Class I includes conditions for which there is evidence or general agreement that this procedure is useful and effective. **Class II** includes two subclasses: **class IIa** (weight of evidence or opinion is in favor of usefulness or efficacy) and **class IIb** (usefulness or efficacy is less well established by evidence or opinion). **Class III** refers to conditions for which there is evidence or general agreement that the procedure is not useful or effective and in some cases may be harmful.

The Table summarizes the class I indications for coronary angiography. For additional information, the reader is referred to the AHA guidelines, which are accessible online (www.acp.org).

Class I Indications for Coronary Angiography

1. In patients with known or suspected CAD who are currently asymptomatic or have stable angina, angiography is indicated in the presence of:
   - Severe angina despite medical treatment
   - High-risk criteria on noninvasive testing regardless of anginal severity
   - Patients who have been successfully resuscitated from sudden cardiac death *or*
   - Have had sustained (> 30 seconds) monomorphic ventricular tachycardia *or*
   - Nonsustained (< 30 seconds) polymorphic ventricular tachycardia
2. In patients with nonspecific chest pain, angiography is indicated in the presence of high-risk findings on noninvasive testing.
3. In patients with unstable coronary syndromes, angiography is indicated in the presence of:
   - High or intermediate risk for adverse outcome in patients with unstable angina refractory to initial adequate medical therapy or recurrent symptoms after initial stabilization. Emergent catheterization is recommended in these patients
   - High risk for adverse outcome in patients with unstable angina. Urgent catheterization is recommended in these patients.
   - High- or intermediate-risk unstable angina that stabilizes after initial treatment
   - Initially low short term-risk unstable angina that is subsequently high risk on noninvasive testing
4. In patients with postrevascularization ischemia angiography is indicated in the presence of:
   - Suspected abrupt closure or subacute stent thrombosis after percutaneous revascularization

(continued)

Class I Indications for Coronary Angiography (Continued)

- Recurrent angina or high-risk criteria on noninvasive evaluation within 9 months of percutaneous revascularization

5. During the initial management of acute MI (MI suspected and ST elevation or bundle branch block [BBB] present), angiography is indicated.
    - When it is to be coupled with the intent to perform primary PTCA
    - As an alternative to thrombolytic therapy in patients who can undergo angioplasty of the infarct artery, if performed within 12 hours of the onset of symptoms or beyond 12 hours if ischemic symptoms persist (if performed within 90 minutes of tPA administration, by skilled personnel in an appropriate laboratory environment)
    - In patients who are within 36 hours of an acute ST elevation or Q wave or new left BBB MI who develop cardiogenic shock, are < 75 years of age, and in whom revascularization can be performed within 18 hours of the onset of shock

6. Early coronary angiography in acute MI (MI suspected but no ST segment elevation) is indicated:
    - In patients with persistent or recurrent (stuttering) episodes of symptomatic ischemia, spontaneous or induced, with or without associated ECG changes
    - In the presence of shock, severe pulmonary congestion, or continuing hypotension

7. Coronary angiography during the hospital management phase (patients with Q wave and non-Q wave infarction) is indicated:
    - In patients with spontaneous myocardial ischemia or myocardial ischemia provoked by minimal exertion during recovery from infarction
    - Before definitive therapy of a mechanical complication of infarction such as acute mitral regurgitation, ventricular septal defect, pseudoaneurysm, or LV aneurysm
    - In patients with persistent hemodynamic instability

8. Coronary angiography during the risk stratification phase (patients with all types of MI) is indicated in patients with ischemia at low levels of exercise with ECG changes ($\geq$ 1 mm ST segment depression or other predictors of adverse outcome) and/or imaging abnormalities.

9. For perioperative evaluation before (or after) noncardiac surgery, angiography is indicated in patients with suspected or known CAD, including those with:
    - Evidence for high risk of adverse outcome based on noninvasive test results
    - Angina unresponsive to adequate medical therapy
    - Unstable angina, particularly when facing intermediate- or high-risk noncardiac surgery
    - Equivocal noninvasive test result in a high clinical risk[†] patient undergoing high risk[*] surgery (level of evidence: C)

10. Recommendations for use of coronary angiography in patients with valvular heart disease include:
    - Before valve surgery or balloon valvotomy in an adult with chest discomfort, ischemia by noninvasive imaging, or both
    - Before valve surgery in an adult free of chest pain but of substantial age and/or with multiple risk factors for coronary disease
    - Infective endocarditis with evidence of coronary embolization

11. In patients with congenital heart disease, angiography is indicated:
    - Before surgical correction of congenital heart disease when chest discomfort or noninvasive evidence is suggestive of associated CAD
    - Before surgical correction of suspected congenital coronary anomalies such as congenital coronary artery stenosis, coronary arteriovenous fistula, and anomalous origin of left coronary artery
    - In patients with forms of congenital heart disease frequently associated with coronary artery anomalies that may complicate surgical management
    - Unexplained cardiac arrest in a young patient

---

[*]Cardiac risk according to type of noncardiac surgery. *High risk:* emergent major operations, aortic and major vascular, peripheral vascular, anticipated prolonged surgical procedures associated with large fluid shifts and/or blood loss; *intermediate risk:* carotid endarterectomy, major head and neck, intraperitoneal and/or intrathoracic, orthopedic surgery, prostate surgery; *low risk:* endoscopic procedures, superficial procedures, cataract surgery, breast surgery.

[†]Cardiac risk according to clinical predictors of perioperative death, MI, or CHF. *High clinical risk:* unstable angina, recent MI and evidence of important residual ischemic risk, decompensated CHF, high degree of atrioventricular block, symptomatic ventricular arrhythmias with known structural heart disease, severe symptomatic valvular heart disease, multiple intermediate risk markers such as prior MI, CHF, and diabetes; *intermediate clinical risk:* Canadian Cardiovascular Society (CCS) class I or II angina, prior MI by history or ECG, compensated or prior CHF, diabetes mellitus.

Adapted from Scanlon PJ, Faxon DP, Audet AM, et al: ACC/AHA guidelines for coronary angiography: A report of the American College of Cardiology/American Heart Association Task Force on Practice Guidelines (Committee on Coronary Angiography). J Am Coll Cardiol 33:1756–1824, 1999.

8. When is coronary angiography contraindicated?

Currently, the only absolute contraindication to cardiac catheterization is the refusal of a mentally competent patient. Relative contraindications are:

Unexplained fever	Digitalis toxicity
Untreated infection	Previous contrast dye allergy without steroid
Severe anemia with hemoglobin	pretreatment
< 8 gm/dl	Active stroke
Severe electrolyte imbalance	Decompensated heart failure (unless the
Severe active bleeding	procedure can be performed with the
Uncontrolled systemic hypertension	patient sitting up)

Of these relative contraindications, preexisting renal failure, particularly in a patient with diabetes, and a history of prior anaphylactic reaction to contrast medium are especially important.

9. What types of radiographic contrast agents are used?

The radiographic contrast agents can be classified into two groups:

1. **High-osmolality, ionic agents:** These are the conventional contrast agents that have been used for many years. High-osmolality agents have a series of adverse effects, including: (a) arrhythmia (most frequently, sinus arrest, atrioventricular block, or ventricular fibrillation); (b) myocardial depression and vasodilatation with potential aggravation of the coronary ischemia; (c) allergic reactions; and (d) renal insufficiency

2. **Low-osmolality, nonionic agents:** These newer agents do not cause rhythm disturbances or myocardial depression but can cause allergic reactions and renal insufficiency. In addition, they lack the calcium-chelating properties of the older agents and may be responsible for coronary thrombosis. A major drawback of these agents is their increased cost, which is up to 20 times higher than that of the high-osmolality agents.

10. What are the most common approaches for coronary angiography?

The femoral artery approach is by far the most common. In selected patients, the brachial or the radial artery may be used for vascular access.

11. Why is the femoral artery approach used most often?

The larger diameter of the femoral artery is associated with easy access and good compressibility.

12. What are the indications for coronary angiography by the brachial or radial artery approach?

This approach is indicated:

- In patients with severe **atherosclerotic disease of the iliac arteries and of the abdominal aorta** in whom fragments of atherosclerotic plaque may be dislodged while negotiating the guidewire or the catheter
- In patients with known or suspected **abdominal aortic aneurysm** (thrombus can be dislodged by the catheters or guidewires)
- In patients with known or suspected abdominal **aortic dissection**
- In patients with **ischemia of the lower limbs** in whom the decreases in femoral blood flow caused by the catheterization procedure itself or by the ensuing artery compression may cause acute leg ischemia
- In the rare patient in whom it is **difficult to palpate the femoral artery** (e.g., obese patients)

13. What are the main coronary angiography techniques?

Over the decades, several coronary angiography techniques have been proposed. Of these, two are in current use:

- **Judkins technique,** which uses a femoral approach with preformed "coronary-seeking" catheters, the shape of which allows them to easily negotiate the coronary ostia
- **Sones technique,** which uses the radial artery approach

14. What is quantitative coronary angiography (QCA)?

As the name indicates, this is a method of quantitative measurement of the coronary lumen as seen on angiography. This is done by tracing the lumen contour of the stenosis and of an adjacent unaffected segment. The dimensions of the coronary artery lumen at the site of the stenosis are then expressed as a percentage of the normal coronary lumen (Fig. 1). For instance, if half of the coronary artery lumen is obstructed, the severity of the coronary stenosis is 50%. QCA is the most commonly used method of coronary stenosis assessment and serves as a basis for management decisions in the cath lab (e.g., deciding whether a coronary intervention is indicated).

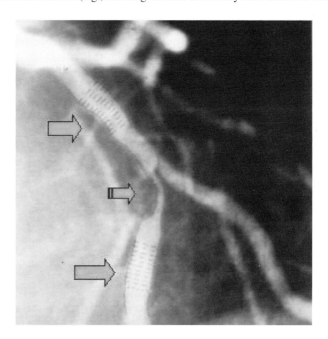

FIGURE 1. The QCA method. Normal coronary artery lumen proximal and distal to stenosis are shown by *large arrows,* stenotic lesion by the *small arrow.* By expressing the dimensions of the coronary artery lumen at the site of the stenosis as a percentage of the normal coronary lumen, a quantitative assessment of the stenosis is obtained.

15. What are the limitations of QCA?

1. **It is operator-dependent**. Although a computer can rapidly and accurately calculate the ratio of two coronary diameters and express it as a percentage, the actual lumen contour is generally traced or edited by a human operator (although some newer programs use special software for this task). Whatever the method applied, the accuracy of the QCA assessment is equal to that of the lumen tracing. The interventional cardiologist is treating an artery, not a number; therefore, whenever there is a discordance between the results of the QCA and the visual assessment of the coronary stenosis, QCA should be repeated or additional tests should be considered, such as intravascular ultrasound (IVUS) or invasive determinations of coronary blood flow or coronary reserve, by means of special catheters.

2. **It represents the analysis of a luminogram.** Therefore, QCA should be calculated from as many angles as possible. The lowest QCA (i.e., the most severe degree of stenosis) should serve as a basis for management decisions.

16. It is often stated that a coronary angiogram is, in fact, a *luminogram*. What is the meaning of this statement and why is it important?

When interpreting a coronary angiogram, what is actually visualized is not the artery in its entirety, but only that portion of the lumen that fills with contrast material. In other words, an angiogram is a depiction of the vessel lumen—that is, a luminogram. Although coronary stenosis generally can be visualized as a portion of the vessel lumen, which does not fill with contrast material, angiography can miss important atherosclerotic disease in several settings:

- **Diffuse concentric atherosclerotic disease,** which "coats" the inner aspect of the vessel wall
- **Positive remodeling of the artery,** which consists of arterial dilatation in response to atherosclerotic disease, with preservation of a normal vessel diameter
- **Stenotic segments masked by superimposed** normal segments of other coronary arteries

17. What are the advantages of IVUS compared with conventional angiography?

Although angiography depicts a silhouette of the coronary lumen, IVUS visualizes the vessel from a cross-sectional perspective, providing direct measurements of luminal dimensions, including minimum and maximum diameter and cross-sectional area. Additionally, IVUS enables characterization of atheroma size and plaque distribution and gives an insight into the composition of the plaque. These parameters are important for selection of the appropriate coronary interventions and for assessing the results of these interventions. For further detail regarding the place of IVUS in clinical practice, the reader is referred to Chapter 4.

18. When is IVUS indicated for validation of the QCA assessment of a coronary stenosis?

There are several class II indications (i.e., some authorities agree that the modality may be clinically useful) for IVUS in current practice:

- Evaluation of **lesion severity** in patients with suboptimal angiography results
- Assessment of the adequacy of coronary **stent deployment** and determination of the mechanism of **stent restenosis** (inadequate expansion versus neointimal proliferation)
- Preinterventional assessment of **lesion characteristics** as a means **to select an optimal revascularization device**
- Further evaluation of patients with characteristic anginal symptoms and a **positive functional study** with no focal stenoses or mild coronary artery disease (CAD) on angiography.
- Diagnosis and management of coronary disease **after cardiac transplantation**

19. True or false: Coronary angiography has a tendency to underestimate the severity of coronary stenosis?

True. Because of the inherent limitations of a luminogram, angiography may underestimate the severity of coronary stenosis. In some cases, this may lead to improper management decisions. For instance, hemodynamically significant stenosis may be missed, and areas of remaining stenosis after PCI may not be noticed, leading to subsequent vessel occlusion and development of an acute coronary syndrome.

20. What is the spatial resolution of coronary angiography?

The spatial resolution of coronary angiography is approximately 300 microns. This represents the smallest distance between two separate points that can be displayed separately on a coronary angiogram.

21. What are the main diagnostic inaccuracies that may occur when visualizing coronary arteries in the cath lab?

Inaccurate diagnosis of coronary artery disease may consist in either **underdiagnosis** (missing a stenosis altogether; underestimating its severity) or **overdiagnosis** (diagnosing a stenosis when in fact none is present; overestimating the severity of a true stenosis).

22. What segments of the coronary vasculature are most prone to inaccurate diagnosis of coronary stenosis?

Ostial lesions and side branches.

23. What are the most frequent causes of inaccurate diagnosis of coronary stenosis (the pitfalls of coronary angiography)?
- **Inadequate contrast opacification** (i.e., an inadequately small volume of contrast agent is injected into the coronary artery)
- **Branch superposition.** A uniplanar view of two distinct coronary artery branches can create the impression of a stenosis in one or both of them, at the site of superposition.
- **Superselective angiography.** In patients with a short left main coronary artery, the catheter may inadvertently be positioned at the ostium of the left anterior descending artery, creating the false impression of a total occlusion of the left circumflex artery.
- **Coronary vasospasm.** This functional cause of coronary flow decrease or interruption can usually be relieved by the administration of vasodilators (Fig. 2).
- The introduction of a **stiff guidewire through a tortuous coronary** artery. The solution to this problem consists of prompt withdrawal of the guidewire.
- **Improper recording of pressure curves**

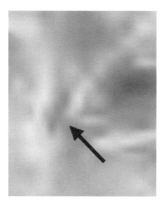 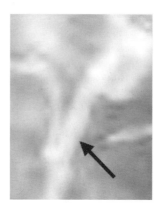

FIGURE 2. Pitfalls of angiography. Coronary vasospasm *(A)*, promptly remitted after intracoronary administration of nitroglycerin *(B)*. If the pharmacologic agent were not administered, a false diagnosis of long proximal RCA stenosis would have been made.

24. What principles are necessary to follow in order to avoid inaccurate diagnosis of CAD?
- Inject a **sufficient volume of contrast** material over a time interval long enough to allow optimal visualization of the coronary arteries but not long enough to create coronary ischemia. Keep in mind that, for the brief period of time that contrast fills a coronary artery, there is no adequate blood flow through that artery.
- Use **multiple angiographic views**.
- Ensure meticulous **calibration** of the measuring devices in the cath lab.

25. What are the main complications of coronary angiography?
The main complications of coronary angiography are related to the contrast agents, arterial puncture, and the course of the catheter through the great vessels (aorta, brachial artery, subclavian artery). The most frequent complications involved the vascular access site (in up to 1.5% of patients), followed by an arrhythmia (in up 2.5% of patients), and by stroke, anaphylaxis, and cholesterol embolism (around 0.1% of patients). Death occurs in < 0.1% of patients. An additional complication is represented by renal failure (contrast nephropathy), with an incidence highly dependent on the presence of specific risk factors (see question 28).

26. What are the manifestations of contrast-induced anaphylaxis?
The usual manifestations of anaphylaxis are bronchospasm, angioedema, urticaria, and hypotension.

27. Which patients are at a higher risk of allergic reaction to angiography contrast material?
This group includes patients with:
- Prior allergic reaction to contrast
- Prior history of atopic disorder
- Allergy to penicillin
- Allergy to seafood (which contains organic iodine)

28. What are the main risk factors for azotemia as a result of radiographic contrast agent exposure?

Preexisting renal failure	Intravascular volume depletion
Diabetes mellitus	Congestive heart failure
Older age	High contrast volume load

29. What are the prophylactic measures for contrast-induced nephropathy?
Contrast-induced nephropathy can be prevented by adequate hydration and by minimizing the amounts of contrast material used during the procedure. Preliminary reports indicate that using of acetylcysteine and fenoldopam (dopamine D1 receptor agonist) prior to angiography may prevent renal failure.

30. What is contrast ventriculography?
Contrast ventriculography is a catheterization technique consisting of intraventricular injection of contrast material for visualization of the shape, dimensions, and function of the ventricles and appreciation of coexistent mitral or tricuspid regurgitation.

31. How does contrast ventriculography correlate with other methods of assessment of left ventricle (LV) function?
Contrast ventriculography reflects the three-dimensional (3-D) complexity of the ventricle in a two-dimensional (2-D) image. This may lead to overestimation or, more frequently, underestimation of the LV function for a number of reasons:
- Different myocardial segments may be superimposed on the same image, with "obliteration" of the normal segments by superimposed abnormal ones.
- LV function is usually assessed from the right anterior oblique (RAO) view, which visualizes the anterior and inferior wall of the LV. These segments are most frequently affected by ischemic heart disease, and, consequently, assessing the LV function based on this view alone can be misleading.
- High-osmolality contrast agents have a myocardial depressant action.
- Contrast ventriculography is often performed under conditions of acute ischemia, when several segments may be hypokinetic, due to myocardial stunning (reversible contraction decrease caused by an episode of acute, transient ischemia). Although this does not, in fact, represent an underestimation of LV function (but rather its assessment under ischemic conditions), the ejection fraction obtained in this setting may not be representative of the everyday ventricular performance in that patient.

32. What is the single most important method for increasing the accuracy of left ventriculography?
The most important method for increasing the accuracy of LV function assessment by ventriculography is the use of at least two perpendicular imaging planes (biplanar ventriculography). This principle applies to any tomographic imaging method.

33. What is the role of contrast ventriculography in the era of high-accuracy noninvasive methods for LV function assessment?
Contrast ventriculography has several limitations but is simple, speedy, widely available, and, if performed in properly selected patients, safe. It allows an assessment of the impact of CAD on LV function and may demonstrate previously unsuspected cardiac pathology, such as valvular dysfunction or intracardiac shunt. These advantages explain the ongoing popularity of this method.

34. How is assessment of LV function by contrast ventriculography different from echocardiographic assessment (tomographic vs. silhouette method)?

As outlined above, contrast ventriculography is a typical tomographic method, displaying on a single plane the superimposed information originating from different LV segments, whereas echocardiography displays the information relevant to a specific "slice" of the LV. Of note, with both methods, it is essential to visualize the LV from more than a single angle to avoid under- or overestimation of LV function.

35. How is LV ejection fraction measured?

The ejection fraction is defined as that percentage of the end-diastolic LV blood volume expelled into the aorta in systole.

$$EF\ (\%) = (LVED - LVES) / LVED$$

where
    LVED is the LV end-diastolic
    LVES is the LV end-systolic

Thus, calculation of the ejection fraction is based on calculation of the LV end-systolic and end-diastolic volume. These can be determined in the cath lab by means of Simpson's method, in which the LV cavity is divided into a series of superimposed cylinders, visualized from two perpendicular projections. The individual volume of each cylinder is calculated based on its measured diameter and height, and the volumes are summated to obtain the volume of the LV in systole and diastole and to calculate the ejection fraction. A simplified (biplane) version relies on tracing the end-systolic and end-diastolic LV endocardial borders in two orthogonal planes.

36. Is it important to actually measure LV ejection fraction (as described in the previous question) in clinical practice?

The classic Simpson's method is generally reserved for research purposes, whereas the simplified method is routinely used. However, the visual assessment of LV function is generally sufficient for clinical purposes.

37. What are the pressure-volume loops of the LV and how are they affected by heart disease?

These loops are graphic displays of the pressure and volume of the LV. Because of the cyclical nature of these pressure changes, the actual graphic depiction of pressure against time has the aspect of a loop. Intraventricular pressure changes inversely with ventricular volume in the different phases of systole and diastole. Thus, it is possible to identify the intraventricular pressure at any given point in time. For example, an increase in LV pressure at end-diastole is very suggestive of LV dysfunction and will result in a position of the corresponding point on the diagram "higher" than in normal subjects (the loop is "shifted upwards"). After instituting appropriate therapy, this point will "descend" at or toward its normal position.

38. What are the indications for right contrast ventriculography?

Ventriculography is a much less often performed on the right ventricle (RV) than on the LV and is mainly indicated in patients with congenital heart disease, where it allows assessment of the cardiac and great vessel anatomy. For images illustrating right contrast ventriculography, the reader is referred to Chapter 9.

ECHOCARDIOGRAPHY

Gabriel Adelmann, M.D., Kenneth Horton, RDCS, Benjamin Kleiber, M.D., and Neil J. Weissman, M.D.

39. What is ultrasound and how are ultrasound waves characterized?

Ultrasound consists of sound waves with a frequency higher than those audible with the human ear. Sound waves are cyclical mechanical vibrations in a physical medium. They are characterized by:

- Frequency, measured in Hertz (Hz), the number of vibratory cycles per second
- Wavelength (λ), the distance between two consecutive peaks on the sound wave
- Amplitude (dB), the intensity or strength of the sound
- Velocity of propagation, the distance covered by sound in each second. The velocity of propagation is the product of frequency and wavelength. Sound travels 1540 m/sec in the human body (Fig. 3).

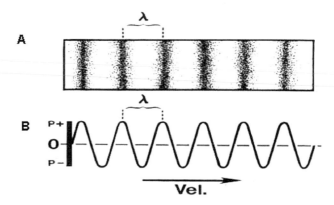

FIGURE 3. Ultrasound wave characteristics. (From Weyman AE: Principles and Practice of Echocardiography, 2nd ed. Philadelphia, Lippincott Williams & Wilkins, 1993, with permission.)

40. What are an ultrasound transducer and piezoelectric crystal?

An ultrasound transducer includes one or more piezoelectric crystals. A piezoelectric crystal is a material that expands when stimulated by electrical current. When exposed to an alternating electrical current, a piezoelectric crystal undergoes cycles of expansion and contraction, moving air next to the crystal and generating ultrasound waves. Alternatively, when the piezoelectric crystal is struck by ultrasound waves, the crystals change shape and generate electrical currents. The electric currents are electronically converted into an ultrasound image. The stronger the ultrasound wave, the stronger the electric signal produced and the brighter the image displayed.

41. How does an ultrasound transducer work?

Short bursts of ultrasound are produced by the transducer followed by periods during which the reflected echoes are received by the transducer. Because sound travels at a known speed, the time it takes for an ultrasound wave to travel (from the transducer, to the structure it is bounced off of, and back to the transducer) can be converted into distance. By determining the time it takes for ultrasound to bounce back, the ultrasound machine can display where the structure is located in relationship to the transducer. Because sound bounces off several structures at once, multiple structures can be displayed at once on the image.

42. List the main types of ultrasound transducer used in echocardiography and their respective applications.

Based on the echocardiographic approach used, several types of transducers can be distinguished:

- Transthoracic imaging and nonimaging transducers (emitted frequency of 2.5–3.5 MHz), which are handheld
- Transesophageal transducers (5.0–7.5 MHz) mounted at the end of a gastroscope
- Epicardial and vascular ultrasound transducers (7–10 MHz), which are smaller and lighter handheld transducers
- IVUS transducers (30–40 MHz) mounted at the end of a very small catheter (< 1 mm in diameter) and used during a cardiac catheterization

43. What are the main components of the ultrasound machine?

The ultrasound machine consists of an ultrasound transducer (see above), an image processing unit, and a display screen. An electrocardiogram (ECG) monitor is built into the ultrasound machine, and all echo labs should have a blood pressure cuff.

44. What is the importance of the ECG monitor in echocardiography?

The ECG is an essential component of any echo study. It allows correct timing of heart wall motion and blood flow (systolic vs. diastolic).

45. What is the importance of assessing blood pressure in echocardiography?

It is essential to record the blood pressure at least once during any echo study. Variations in the blood pressure (afterload) may affect the overall LV systolic function or left-sided valvular function. For example, a fixed deformity of the mitral valve may be associated with different degrees of mitral regurgitation under different degrees of afterload (blood pressure). If a patient is being followed with sequential echocardiograms to assess for change in mitral regurgitation, a change in blood pressure may be responsible for a change in the volume of regurgitation even without a progression of the mitral deformity. This is especially important for moderate degrees of regurgitation.

46. What are the different ways sound can interact with tissue as it travels through the body?

Sound can undergo reflection, scattering, refraction, and attenuation.

47. What is sound reflection?

Reflection, the fundamental principle required for ultrasound imaging, is the reversal of direction of the sound waves when they encounter a tissue with different physical properties. The absolute amount of ultrasound reflection at a given tissue–tissue interface is dependent on the differences in the two tissue properties (acoustic impedance; see question 48). However, the amount of reflected ultrasound ultimately detected by an ultrasound imaging transducer is dependent on the angle of the transducer relative to the reflected sound beam. Optimal reflection occurs when the angle between the beam and the reflecting interface is 90° so all the ultrasound "bounces back" directly to the transducer (Fig. 4). Thus, when performing an ultrasound study, it is essential to

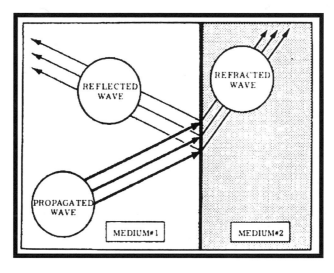

FIGURE 4. Reflection and refraction. (From Feigenbaum H: Echocardiography, 5th ed. Philadelphia, Lippincott Williams & Wilkins, 1994, with permission.)

angle the transducer as close as possible to 90° to the tissue of interest. Patience and experience in performing these fine angulations are essential components of the sonographer's skill and are major determinants of image quality.

48. What is acoustic impedance?

Impedance is defined as the product of tissue density and sound propagation speed. Because sound travels at essentially the same speed in all body tissues, the primary determinant of acoustic impedance (and therefore the main determinant of the magnitude of sound reflection) is tissue density. This is why when sound travels through the air and hits the hard rock of a canyon wall, it bounces off and echoes are produced.

49. What is sound scattering?

Unlike reflected sound, which propagates along a definite vector, scattered sound travels in all directions (Fig. 5). Thus, the amplitude of scattered signal that can return to a transducer is much lower than that of a reflected signal. Therefore, sound bouncing off of a smooth surface will have a stronger returning signal than sound bouncing off of a "rough" signal *if* the tissue is perpendicular to the transducer. However, if the tissue surface is not perpendicular to the transducer, then a smooth surface will reflect all of the ultrasound away from the transducer, whereas a rough surface, which scatters the signal in all directions, will still reflect some of the ultrasound back to the transducer. Luckily, most biologic tissues produce some scattering, allowing us to image tissues that are not perfectly perpendicular to the transducer.

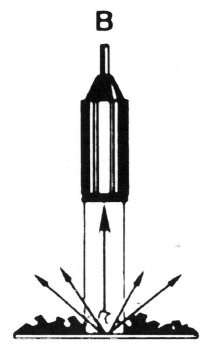

FIGURE 5. Sound scattering. B = ultrasound transducer, functioning both as an emitter and a receptor of ultrasound. (From Weyman AE: Principles and Practice of Echocardiography, 2nd ed. Philadelphia, Lippincott Williams & Wilkins, 1993, with permission.)

Different sound-scattering patterns may also be used for tissue characterization, although this application is still experimental.

50. What is sound refraction?

Refraction is a change in sound wave direction between two media with slightly different acoustic impedance. As opposed to reflected sound, refracted sound actually continues its "forward" propagation, albeit at an angle, as compared to its previous route (see Figure 5). Refraction can, in some cases, be responsible for ultrasound imaging artifacts.

51. What is sound wave attenuation?

Attenuation is the gradual loss of acoustic energy as sound waves travel through tissues (Fig. 6). Attenuation is caused by:

- **Sound reflection** and **scatter,** which depend on the impedance mismatch between adjacent tissues. For example, strong scatter and reflection are seen at the air–tissue interface because of the high acoustic impedance of air. To minimize attenuation from the transducer to the body, gel is placed on the transducer to obtain acoustic coupling. Additionally, recording ultrasound images after expiration minimizes the impact of air on study quality.
- **Conversion of sound waves to heat,** which is directly proportional to wavelength. The higher the ultrasound frequency, the greater the attenuation and the lower the depth of penetration.

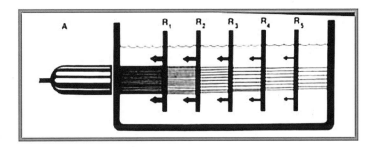

FIGURE 6. Attenuation. On its course through the patient's body, the sound beam encounters different tissues, which can be regarded as a series of reflectors placed "in parallel." Some of the energy of the incident ultrasound waves is retained by each of these layers (attenuation), so that the layers situated farther away from the transducer receive a smaller amount of incident ultrasound and, therefore, generate weaker echoes. (From Weyman AE: Principles and Practice of Echocardiography, 2nd ed. Philadelphia, Lippincott Williams & Wilkins, 1993, with permission.)

52. What is sound wave penetration?

Penetration is the depth to which sound can travel through a particular medium. At a certain depth, all the sound is reflected, scattered, or converted to heat (i.e., attenuated) and there is no sound energy left. Sound wave penetration is inversely related to attenuation.

53. What is image resolution?

Image resolution, which refers to how fine or blurry the image appears, is defined as the smallest resolvable distance between two points. Thus, if the distance between two reflectors that can be individually distinguished is very small, there will be a lot of detail in the image. If the resolvable distance is large, there will not be a lot of detail.

54. What is the relationship between image resolution and wavelength?

There is an inverse relationship between image resolution and sound wavelength. Smaller wavelengths can distinguish two objects that are closer to each other. Image resolution (distance between two resolvable points) is theoretically equivalent to 1–2 wavelengths. Thus, the smaller the wavelength, the finer the image resolution.

55. What is the relationship between image resolution and transducer frequency?

Because there is an inverse relationship between transducer frequency and wavelength (higher frequencies have smaller wavelengths), there is a direct relationship between higher frequency and higher resolution. A typical transthoracic transducer (2.5 MHz) will have a lower resolution than a transesophageal transducer (5 MHz), which will have a much lower resolution than an intravascular ultrasound transducer (25–40 MHz).

56. If higher frequency transducers have higher resolution, why not use the highest frequency transducer all the time?

There is a trade-off between image resolution (higher with higher frequency transducers) and sound penetration (deeper with lower frequency transducers). Longer wavelengths (lower frequency transducers) can go around particles in the medium, not bounce off of them and therefore travel farther. A practical example of this is how the higher frequency of a jet engine is the predominant sound when standing next to an airplane (i.e., a whine), but lower frequency sounds become predominant once that jet engine is far away on the runway (i.e., roar).

Therefore, it is only in situations where the distance between the transducer and the heart is very small, such as transesophageal or intravascular echocardiography that we can use high-frequency transducers to maximize image resolution. During routine transthoracic echo, we need lower frequency transducers to penetrate the chest wall to the heart. The Table illustrates examples of the relationship between transducer frequency, resolution, and penetration.

IMAGING MODE	TRANSDUCER FREQUENCY	RESOLUTION	PENETRATION DEPTH
Transthoracic echo	2.5–3.5 MHz	Approx. 2–3 mm	15 cm
Transesophageal echo	5.0–7.0 MHz	Approx. 1–2 mm	10 cm
Intravascular ultrasound	30–40 MHz	Approx. 0.1 mm	< 1 cm

57. What is A-mode echocardiography?

A-mode (amplitude-mode) echocardiography was the first diagnostic ultrasound modality used in cardiology. In A-mode echocardiography, the amplitude of reflected ultrasound is displayed on an oscilloscope screen. This modality is of historical interest only.

58. What is M-mode echocardiography? What are its clinical uses?

M-mode (motion) echocardiography evolved from the A-mode technique. First, the reflected sound signal was displayed as a point with varying brightness that correlated with the strength of the reflected ultrasound signal (B-mode). Then, the points representing different structures that the sound is reflecting off of were displayed on paper moving at a set speed. The horizontal axis of the paper displays time, and the vertical axis displays the distance from the transducer to the object reflecting ultrasound. This depiction is based on a gray scale, where dark lines correspond to a higher amplitude of reflected sound and light lines correspond to lower reflected amplitudes. For each given point in time, it is possible to observe the position and the amplitude of sound reflection corresponding to all the structures along the interrogation axis. Figure 7A shows an M-mode through the mitral valve.

M-mode echocardiography has the **advantage** of a very high temporal resolution, which allows precise assessment of the timing and extent of cardiac wall and valve motion. The **downside** of M-mode is that it displays only a linear section through the heart (i.e., as if you were assessing the interfaces of the heart that would be encountered if a laser went through it). This makes it relatively difficult for many to have an integrated mental image of the three-dimensional complexity of the heart structures. Figure 7B is a typical sweep of the heart from the left ventricle to the aorta. This is not intuitively obvious to the untrained eye.

M-mode echocardiography is best viewed as an adjunct to 2-D studies. Its current uses include:
- Measurement of cardiac chamber thickness and diameter, because the M-mode allows precise timing of the measurements to end-systole and end-diastole
- Demonstration of some abnormalities of myocardial and valvular motion that may otherwise go undetected by 2-D echocardiography (e.g., systolic anterior motion of the mitral valve [SAM] in patients with HOCM).
- Correct timing of systolic and diastolic flow through the heart chambers and valves when used in conjunction with color Doppler (see question 71)

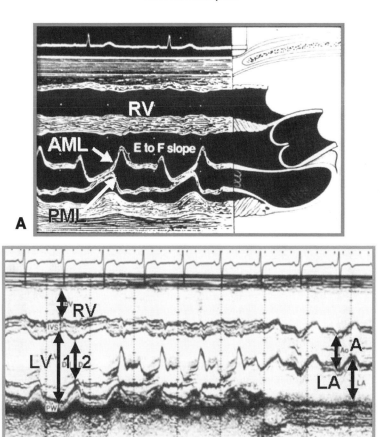

FIGURE 7. *A,* M-mode echo at the level of the mitral valve. The M-shaped lines represent the two mitral valve leaflets as they open in diastole and close in systole. The two peaks are termed, in order, E and F, and the slope of the segment between them gives information about the structural and functional status of the mitral valve. RV = right ventricle; AML = anterior mitral leaflet; PML = posterior mitral leaflet. *B,* M-mode echo sweep from the left ventricle to the aorta. The double-headed arrow in the RV shows the RV diameter, and the two double-headed arrows in the LV show the end-systolic and end-diastolic diameter of this chamber. Note that, along the strip, the different anatomic structures displayed gradually change. Thus, the transducer is not simply placed and kept at the same spot on the patient's chest, but rather is angulated to intercept the cardiac structures through different angles. This particular technique is called an *M-mode sweep.* RV = right ventricle; LV = left ventricle; LA = left atrium; A = aorta.

59. What is 2-D echocardiography?

As its name implies, this modality allows real-time display of 2-D section planes through the heart. Two-dimensional echo images are generated by sweeping the tomographic plane of interest along a series of scan lines. The greater the number of scan lines, the better the image resolution. However, the time needed for processing the information in each frame increases proportionally to the number of scan lines employed. In other words, the higher the spatial resolution, the lower the ability to "update" the image (lower temporal resolution). Conventional 2-D echocardiography uses a frame rate of at least 30 frames per second (similar to other video imaging) and, more recently, up to 80–100 frames per second.

The obvious **advantage** of 2-D echocardiography is the real-time visualization of cardiac structures. Two-dimensional imaging used in conjunction with Doppler is the current echocardiographic method of choice for the assessment of the myocardium, pericardium, heart valves, and blood flow (Fig. 8).

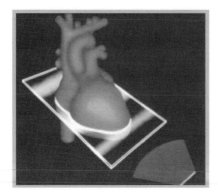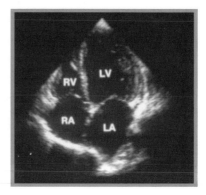

FIGURE 8. Two-dimensional echo image of the heart (apical four-chamber view).

60. What is the Doppler effect? What is Doppler echocardiography?

When a source of sound approaches a detecting system (e.g., ultrasound transducer, human ear, radar), its frequency is higher than when it moves away from the detecting system. Even though the physicist Christian Doppler described this phenomenon when inspired by astronomical observations, many everyday occurrences can illustrate this phenomenon. The classic example is the whistle of a train. As the train approaches the station, its whistle is higher-pitched. and when it leaves the station, the sound of the whistle is lower-pitched. This change in frequency is due to the sound waves being pushed together or drawn apart as the train moves toward or away from the listener, respectively (Fig. 9). By knowing the frequency of the sound emitted by the mobile source, the speed of motion of the emitter can be calculated based on the detected change in sound frequency (Doppler shift).

Doppler echocardiography allows assessment of the velocity and direction of blood flow, based on the Doppler shift of ultrasound emitted by a transducer. Because the frequency of the emitted ultrasound from the transducer is known, and the frequency of the received ultrasound back to the transducer can be determined, the frequency shift from emitted to received ultrasound can be calculated. Using mathematical calculations, the direction (higher or lower frequency) and the speed of the blood that the sound bounced off of can be determined. The Doppler study is an integral part of any echocardiographic procedure. It allows determination of normal or abnormal flow through the heart and heart valves.

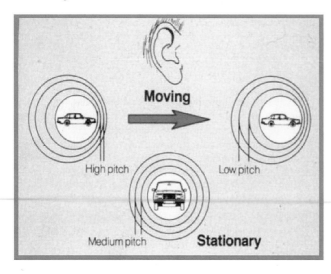

FIGURE 9. The Doppler effect.

61. What are the different types of Doppler echocardiography currently available?

Pulsed wave (PW) Doppler
Continuous wave (CW) Doppler
Color Doppler
Tissue Doppler

62. What is pulsed wave (PW) Doppler ultrasound? What are its clinical uses?

PW Doppler uses bursts of ultrasound sent out and analyzed at predetermined time intervals that correspond with a set distance from the transducer. The Doppler shift of the reflected ultrasound signal allows the calculation of the velocity of blood flow at that location in the heart. This analysis is performed on a small volume of blood (sample volume) at a given depth. The sample volume can be adjusted by a control on the echo machine. The typical sample volume diameter is 5–10 mm.

The main **advantage** of this method is that it allows determination of blood flow velocity at a specified location. However the waiting time between bursts of ultrasound limits the maximum flow velocity that can be detected. (As an analogy, think of a movie of a revolving wheel. To properly visualize the wheel motion, the frame rate of the camera must be at least double the rotation frequency of the wheel.)

The main **clinical use** of PW Doppler is to assess flow velocity at a specified depth. (e.g., differentiate midventricular flow obstruction of hypertrophic cardiomyopathy from valvular aortic stenosis).

63. What is signal aliasing?

Signal aliasing occurs when the blood velocity exceeds the measuring limit of the pulse Doppler and the signal "wraps" around the baseline, making it difficult to establish the direction of flow (Fig. 10). In the analogy of the moving wheel in question 62, if the frame rate of the camera is less than the rotation frequency of the wheel, the wheel will be depicted as spinning backwards!

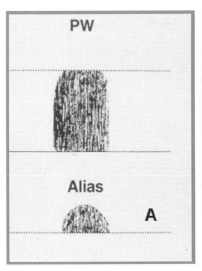
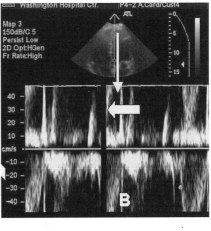

FIGURE 10. Signal aliasing on spectral Doppler (PW). Signal aliasing on a Doppler tracing consists of signal display in a "wrap-around" fashion on both sides of the baseline. *A,* In this PW study of the LVOT, the Doppler signal below the baseline is "cut off" at the point of aliasing velocity and is superimposed on the other side of the baseline *(arrow). B,* An echo Doppler study through the left ventricular outflow tract. Because the modality being used is PW Doppler, some of the signal will alias, i.e., wrap around and be displayed in a physiologically incorrect orientation. Therefore, although the "true velocity" is that depicted below the baseline as the flow is away from the transducer in this position, all the supplementary areas of flow above the baseline do not represent real blood flow, but rather represent the aliasing artifact.

64. What is the Nyquist limit?

The Nyquist limit is the highest detectable Doppler shift for a given PW system (by analogy, the highest frequency of wheel rotation that can still be recorded as "forward motion" by a given camera, with a given frame rate). If the Nyquist limit is exceeded, signal aliasing will occur. Aliasing of the PW signal typically occurs at a velocity of approximately 2 m/sec, which corresponds to a gradient of 16 mmHg.

65. What is continuous wave (CW) Doppler ultrasound? What are its clinical uses?

CW Doppler is the simultaneous use of ultrasound emission and reception. By continuously emitting and receiving ultrasound and listening for the direction and extent of Doppler shift of the frequency, CW can record high-velocity blood flow well above 2 m/sec. Unfortunately, the primary **drawback** is that, by simultaneously recording signals from the whole length of the ultrasound beam, it is not possible to determine the location along the length of the beam that is causing the Doppler shift. Thus, CW Doppler indicates the highest flow velocity along the interrogation axis but does not allow the localization of the highest velocity blood flow. For instance, if an increased velocity is registered along the left ventricular outflow tract (LVOT), it is not possible to accurately determine if the high velocity (high gradient) is localized to the LVOT (hypertrophic cardiomyopathy) or the aortic valve (aortic stenosis). Although the shape of the Doppler tracing can suggest the valvular or subvalvular site of flow obstruction, the exact site of velocity "step-up" along the LVOT will have to be located by means of PW or color Doppler. Therefore, PW and CW are used in a complementary fashion to, respectively, localize and quantify the highest velocity (gradient).

66. When should I use CW, and when should I use PW Doppler?

CW Doppler displays the highest flow velocity along the interrogation axis, whereas PW represents flow velocity at a given site along the axis. CW Doppler is the modality of choice for high-velocity blood flows, whereas PW allows the "isolation" of a low-velocity flow from other flows occurring along the same axis. Thus, in aortic stenosis, a CW Doppler through the LVOT depicts transvalvular aortic flow, because the flow across the aortic valve has the highest velocity. However, if there is associated subvalvular obstruction to flow, selective assessment of the LVOT flow requires PW Doppler. In other instances, two blood flow velocities occurring along the same axis can be of the same order of magnitude, and CW would superimpose both flows (e.g., transmitral and pulmonary vein flow on an apical four-chamber view). Using PW Doppler in this case will allow individual characterization of these flows.

67. What is color Doppler imaging? How is it different from other Doppler modalities?

Color Doppler imaging is a simultaneous PW mapping of multiple regions of interest superimposed on a 2-D echo image. The recorded velocities are depicted in a conventional color scale, where flow toward the transducer is depicted in red and flow directed away from the transducer is blue. Higher velocities are depicted in lighter color hues and lower velocities are represented by darker hues. These color-encoded signals are superimposed on a 2-D image. Thus, although based on the general principles of Doppler echocardiography, a color study is an "anatomically intuitive" depiction of blood blow through the heart chambers and valves.

68. What are the clinical uses of color Doppler?
- Identification and semiquantitative visual assessment of valvular regurgitation
- Assessment of pathologic intracardiac flows, such as those caused by shunts, subaortic stenosis, fistulas, or myocardial rupture
- Assessment of pathologic intra- and extracardiac flows in patients with congenital heart disease and for follow-up after surgery
- Assessment of pathologic flows in the great arteries, such as aortic dissection or coarctation or PDA
- Guiding PW or CW Doppler measurements (e.g., color Doppler identification of the area

of subaortic stenosis in hypertrophic cardiomyopathy, followed by spectral pulse and continuous Doppler studies to perform quantitative assessments of the velocity and gradient)

69. What is harmonic imaging?

The echoes reflected at the interface between two different tissues are actually a mix of several wave frequencies, including:

- A main (fundamental) frequency, which is the frequency of the ultrasound emitted by the transducer (i.e., if the ultrasound from the transducer has a frequency of 2.5 MHz, then the fundamental reflected frequency will be 2.5 MHz)
- Additional frequencies, termed *harmonics,* are multiples of the fundamental frequency (i.e., if the emitted ultrasound has a frequency of 2.5 MHz, then the second harmonic frequency would be 5 MHz)

Echocardiography has classically used fundamental imaging, based on detection of fundamental reflected frequencies (i.e., 2.5 MHz for an emitted ultrasound of 2.5 MHz). As its name implies, harmonic imaging uses the detection of the second harmonic-reflected signals to improve image formation.

The use of this application for better endocardial border delineation is called *tissue harmonics.* Although, for the most part the interaction of tissues with ultrasound is linear (e.g., incident ultrasound of 2.5 MHz will result in reflected echoes of 2.5 MHz), there is a small, but detectable nonlinear component of tissue-ultrasound interaction (5 MHz echoes for a 2.5-MHz incident ultrasound). The intensity of tissue-generated harmonic echoes depends on:

- The depth of imaging: as opposed to fundamental frequencies, which get weaker with increasing depth, harmonic frequencies become stronger at greater imaging depth
- The intensity of incident ultrasound: the stronger the ultrasound, the stronger the harmonics

Thus, harmonic imaging will provide a better image resolution in difficult echo subjects, such as overweight patients (Fig. 11).

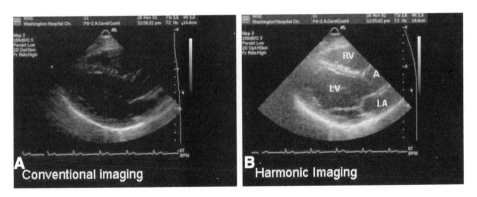

FIGURE 11. Fundamental *(A)* and harmonic images *(B).* Harmonic imaging allows better endocardial definition and reduces artifact, thus enhancing image quality.

Contrast echocardiography was the first to use harmonic imaging. Contrast is used to image the blood pool in the heart cavities and in the myocardium. Because the main objective of contrast echo is to accurately detect the contrast bubbles and distinguish them from the surrounding myocardium, harmonic imaging is used because contrast bubbles have a nonlinear interaction with ultrasound, resulting in a higher proportion of second harmonics. It is possible to filter out these second harmonics and thus separate the two types of echoes—those from the myocardium and those from the contrast. This will eventually allow the detection of contrast as it propagates into the myocardium and noninvasive ultrasound assessment of myocardial blood flow.

70. In view of the superior quality of harmonic imaging, is there any place today for conventional 2-D imaging?

Most new echo machines have harmonic imaging, and many studies done on these machines use only harmonics. Nonetheless, there will probably still be an important place for fundamental imaging because harmonics tend to make images more black and white with loss of different tissue textures and display even normal heart valves as appearing thick. In a patient with excellent echocardiographic images, fundamental imaging may be preferable to harmonic imaging.

71. What is color M-mode echocardiography? What are its clinical uses?

Color Doppler displays are usually superimposed on 2-D echo images. Although sufficient in most clinical situations, this conventional color Doppler display may be insufficient to establish with certainty the timing of a given blood flow. For instance, a brief "flicker" of color in the LVOT adjacent to the aortic valve can be either systolic (and thus physiologic) or diastolic (representing aortic regurgitation). If the duration of this flow is very brief or if the patient is tachycardic, it can be difficult to distinguish between these two possibilities. Due to its excellent temporal resolution (much higher than that of 2-D echo), M-mode echo is ideally suited for clarifying this question. Color M-mode echo superimposes the color Doppler data onto the M-mode. This allows clear delineation of systolic versus diastolic flow along with its precise location (Fig. 12).

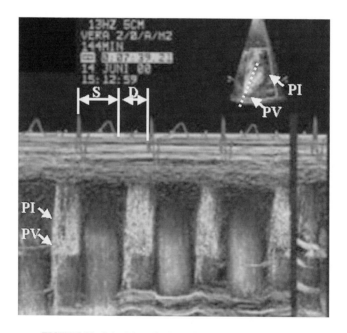

FIGURE 12. Color M-mode. (*See also* Color Plates, Figure 1.)

72. What is tissue Doppler? What are its clinical uses?

As its name implies, this is yet another application of Doppler technology. Whereas conventional Doppler systems are set up to detect the high-velocity motion (m/sec) characteristic of blood flow, tissue Doppler is set up to detect low velocities (cm/sec) typical for myocardial wall motion. Thus, tissue Doppler is the application of the Doppler principle (detecting the velocity of movement) to the tissue.

Among other applications, tissue Doppler (sometimes called *tissue Doppler imaging* [TDI] or *Doppler tissue imaging* [DTI]) has been shown to be useful in assessing left ventricular sys-

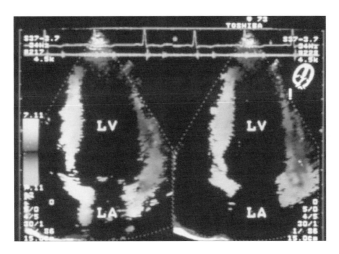

FIGURE 13. Tissue Doppler. Apical four-chamber view using color Doppler M-mode allows display of the heart in its anatomic complexity, as revealed by the regular 2-D study, but with substantial additional information about the amplitude and direction of motion of the myocardium itself. Segments depicted in red or yellow represent motion toward the transducer, whereas areas depicted in shades of blue or green represent those segments that move away from the transducer (*see* Color Plates, Figure 2). By the simultaneous inscription of an ECG, it is possible to analyze the behavior of each myocardial segment during the several faces of systole and diastole and thus characterize normal and pathologic situations.

tolic and diastolic function and in distinguishing restrictive cardiomyopathy from constrictive pericarditis. Despite the interesting insights it offers, tissue Doppler remains in development for clinical applications (Fig. 13).

73. What is 3-D imaging? What are its current uses?

Three-dimensional echocardiography displays the cardiac structures in all their spatial complexity. Obviously, this is achieved by using different shades of gray and the pictorial laws of perspective to suggest depth, because the images are displayed on a regular 2-D screen (3-D imaging is not yet a hologram!).

There are two basic technologies for obtaining the 3-D images:

1. Reconstruction of nonsimultaneous 2-D images, obtained from different windows but aligned using a fixed reference or true spatial registration

2. Using a transducer that emits and receives images in 3-D volumes ("real-time 3-D")

74. How might 3-D echo be used in the future?

The 3-D approach is expected to have an important role in the future for imaging complex structures such as congenital heart defects or determining true volumes of heart chambers with complex geometry (such as the right ventricle); it also has the potential to be far more accurate at the assessment of left ventricular mass. Nonetheless, 3-D echo remains investigational and in development for clinical applications.

75. What is intravascular ultrasound (IVUS)? What are its clinical uses?

In IVUS, a miniature ultrasound transducer is attached to the tip of a catheter that is inserted into vascular structures to image the vessel from the inside out. The close contact of the transducer with the vessel wall allows the use of high-frequency ultrasound (10–40 MHz), which allows excellent definition (spatial resolution) of the vessel anatomy and pathology (e.g., atherosclerosis). It is used to guide and assess the success of percutaneous interventions (e.g., stent deployment). See Chapter 5 for more details.

76. What are the main imaging controls available on contemporary echocardiography machines?

Imaging controls are technical parameters pertaining to the emitted ultrasound and to its electronic processing of the received signal. Imaging controls are essential for optimizing the image and producing high-quality, diagnostic ultrasound images.

Some of the most important imaging controls include:

- **Gain** — defined as the degree of brightness with which a given signal intensity is displayed. This control is similar to the volume dial on a radio. A high gain setting will result in a brighter image, just as increasing the volume on the radio set will produce a louder sound. It may be necessary to increase the gain when the existing image settings do not allow proper visualization of the heart structures (just as one might increase the volume in order to hear better a remote radio station for which there is poor reception) or when the echo is performed in a space where the brightness of surrounding light competes with that on the echo screen such as in the operating room (increasing the volume in order to better hear a radio program on a noisy highway).
- **Time-gain compensation (TGC)** — allows differential adjustment of gain along the axis of the transducer and makes it possible to selectively increase the gain from the area farthest from the transducer (Fig. 14).

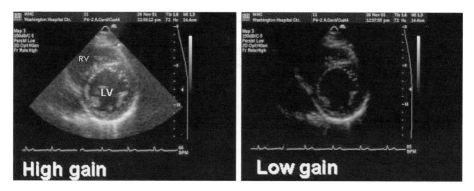

FIGURE 14. High gain (*left*) vs. low gain (*right*) images. An increased image gain results in a "brighter" image.

- **Depth** — allows optimal display of an area of interest on the screen. The standard depth displays all of the heart structures from the transducer (Fig. 15).
- **Gray scale (dynamic range)** — represents the gradation of shades of gray that compose the echocardiographic image. In other words, the gray scale regulates the amount of contrast between the lightest and the darkest areas of the echo image. An amplitude range of diagnostic echoes between a and b decibels can be displayed in n or $10 \times n$ shades of gray, resulting in a either a grainy or a "smooth" image. This control is similar to the setting regulating the number of colors displayed on your computer screen: choosing a 256-color display results in a much better image than a 16-color display (Fig. 16)!
- **Power output (mechanical index [MI])** — controls the total energy delivered by the ultrasound emitter and is especially important in contrast echocardiography (a method using microbubbles for imaging the blood pool; a high power output will destroy the bubbles, whereas lower output will cause the bubbles to resonate).

77. What are image artifacts? How are they different from imaging pitfalls?

Artifacts are images generated by the ultrasound machine and do not correspond to a real cardiac structure or blood flow. Imaging artifacts may preclude visualization of existing struc-

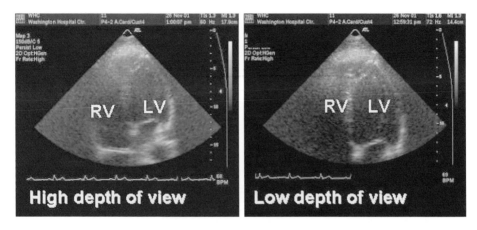

FIGURE 15. High (*left*) vs. low (*right*) depth images. Adjusting depth allows optimal display of the area of interest on the screen. For instance, a deep transgastric view on a transesophageal echocardiogram requires a much greater depth of imaging than the midesophageal view.

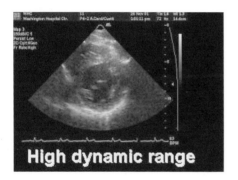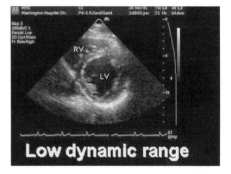

FIGURE 16. Low (*left*) vs. high (*right*) gray scale. Gray scale (dynamic range) regulates the amount of contrast between the lightest and the darkest areas of the echo image.

tures, distort the appearance or dimensions of an existing structure, or display a pseudostructure where in fact none exists.

Pitfalls are the misinterpretation of a real structure for another.

78. What are the main imaging artifacts encountered in echocardiography?

Shadowing results when no ultrasound can penetrate through a structure, creating a dark (shadowed) area beyond the reflective plane. Typical ultrasound shadowing is produced by bone, mechanic valve prostheses, pacemaker wires, and other intracardiac devices. When shadowing occurs, an alternative echocardiographic window or an alternative technique (transesophageal echocardiography) may be necessary.

Reverberation occurs when ultrasound waves are reflected back and forth between two strong reflectors before returning to the transducer and appear as irregular, dense lines extending into the far field. Reverberations commonly occur in patients with prosthetic heart valves, pacemaker wires, or other intracardiac devices. The bones (e.g., ribs) are an additional common source of reverberation (Fig. 17).

Beam-width artifact results from projection of all the structures included in the 3-D profile of the ultrasound beam within a single tomographic plane. Side lobe artifacts are strong reflectors

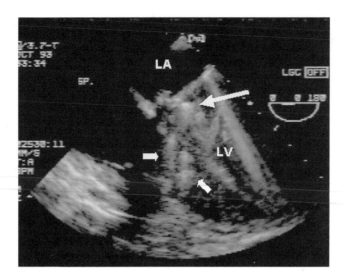

FIGURE 17. Reverberation artifact. Reverberations *(thick arrows)* appear on this TEE image as irregular, dense lines extending into the far field; they prevent accurate interpretation of the ultrasound image. Prosthetic valve *(thin arrow);* left atrium (LA); left ventricle (LV).

at the edge of a wide beam, which may be displayed as if they belonged to the center of the beam. This may result in visualization of certain cardiac structures at sites different from their true anatomic location (e.g., aortic valve appears to be in the left atrium).

Lateral resolution artifact causes a point target to be displayed as a line. Thus, prosthetic valve struts or a calcified mass may appear much longer or wider than it really is. Decreasing the gain may correct this artifact.

Refraction is the deviation of the ultrasound signal from its straight path when it crosses the border between different tissues. This is a rare occurrence with contemporary machines.

79. What are some of the most important clues indicating that a visualized "structure" might in fact be an artifact?

Artifact typically:

- Are visualized in a single imaging plane and "disappear" with transducer angulation or placement of the transducer in a different location
- Do not respect anatomic borders or locations (e.g., aortic valve appearing in the left atrium)
- Are exceedingly bright or, on the contrary, perceived as "cones of shadow"

As a general rule, echocardiographic diagnosis should never be based on a single view or imaging plane. Critical judgment is an integral part of any imaging test; conversely, a high-quality imaging study represents much more than just the collection of a standard set of views.

80. What are the main artifacts of CW and PW Doppler ultrasound?

Frequently seen artifacts of Doppler ultrasound include

- **Velocity underestimation** due to nonparallel beam alignment. The transducer should be parallel to the direction of blood flow; blood flow should never be assessed if its long axis is more than 30° away from the ultrasound beam.
- **Aliasing,** seen with pulse Doppler
- **Mirror image artifact,** consisting of a second, fainter Doppler tracing on the opposite side of the baseline from the "real" Doppler curve—i.e., directed in a nonphysiologic direction (e.g., toward the apex, in a systolic CW Doppler recording of the LVOT) (Fig. 18)

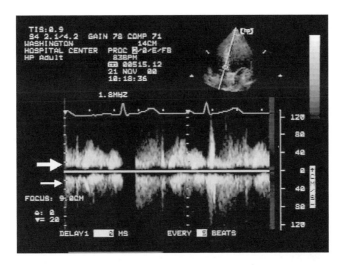

FIGURE 18. The Doppler mirror image artifact. A second Doppler tracing can appear as a mirror image of the "real" Doppler curve, on the opposite side of the baseline. True tricuspid flow *(thick arrow)*; mirror image flow *(thin arrow)*.

- **Electronic artifacts,** which may be caused by the echo machine or by other electronic equipment (e.g., in the ICU)
- **Shadowing** of part of the Doppler tracing by strong reflectors, such as mechanical prosthetic valves

81. What are the main artifacts associated with color Doppler imaging?
- **Electronic interference** (colored bands superimposed on the image)
- **Shadowing** by strong reflectors (resulting in entire image sectors being obscured) (Fig. 19)

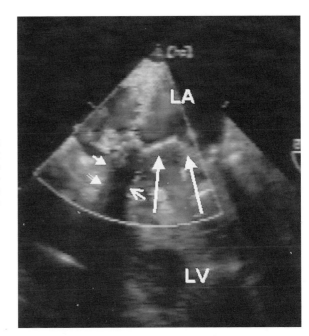

FIGURE 19. Shadowing artifact on color Doppler. In this color Doppler study of a patient with a St. Jude prosthetic mitral valve *(large arrows),* shadowing obscures entire image sectors *(small arrows). (See also* Color Plates, Figure 3.)

- Color **aliasing.** The aliasing artifact can be of diagnostic value. Thus, many pathologic flows are turbulent (mosaic color) rather than laminar (pure color). In addition, it is possible to quantitate mitral regurgitation based on color flow aliasing (the proximal isovelocity surface area [PISA] method).
- **Ghosting** (brief flashes of color not respecting anatomic boundaries and caused by the presence of strong reflectors)
- **Background noise** (uniform color speckling of the whole image, when the gain setting is too high) (Fig. 20)

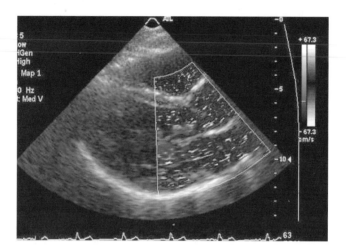

FIGURE 20. Background noise artifact on color Doppler, seen as uniform color speckling of the whole image when the color gain is set too high. (*See also* Color Plates, Figure 4.)

- **Gain-dependent flow area underestimation.** For instance, if the gain is too low, the displayed area of a mitral regurgitant flow may appear smaller than it really is. Maximizing the gain to a level just below that of background noise helps solve this problem.

82. What are the main biologic effects of ultrasound? Discuss diagnostic ultrasound safety.

There is no evidence to indicate adverse effects of diagnostic ultrasound. Neither the thermal effects (tissue heating) nor the ultrasound-induced cavitation (creation of new gas-filled bubbles or induction of vibration in gas-filled bodies) is sufficiently strong to exert a deleterious action in vivo.

MAGNETIC RESONANCE IMAGING

Anthon R. Fuisz, M.D., and Gabriel Adelmann, M.D.

83. What is the physical basis of magnetic resonance imaging (MRI)?

Similar to other noninvasive imaging techniques, MRI is based on the interaction of an emitted signal with the patient's tissues and on recording the "modified" signal exiting the patient's body. Complex electronic processing of these exiting signals results in an image display on a monitor. In the case of MRI,

- The **emitted signals** are electromagnetic waves generated by the movement of electrical current through the coils of a magnet.

- The electromagnetic waves **interact** with the patient's hydrogen nuclei, making them resonate to varying degrees.
- The **exiting signal** is represented by the electromagnetic waves generated by the differential resonance of the hydrogen nuclei in the patient's body.

84. What are the main determinants of electromagnetic wave modification after interaction with the patient's body?

The degree of resonance elicited in different hydrogen nuclei depends on (1) the physical properties of the tissue to which the hydrogen nuclei belong and (2) the settings of the magnet. By modifying the settings of the magnet, it is possible to modulate the resonance of the hydrogen nuclei in a fashion that allows it to localize the resonating nuclei in space.

85. What is the Fourier transform and what is its importance for MRI imaging?

The MRI processing system receives a "single" waveform of electromagnetic energy from the patient's body. In order to obtain a two-dimensional image of the patient's anatomy, it is essential to separate this waveform into its different components, which originated from different points in space. This will allow it to distinguish between these different points in space, that is, to create an interpretable image. This separation is achieved by means of the Fourier transformation.

The Fourier transform is a system of highly complex mathematical equations that, in essence, decompose a waveform into different frequencies (the inverse operation, the summing of these different frequencies, would yield the original frequency). This separation in the frequency domain is subsequently translated into spatial separation. Combining the spatial information obtained along the orthogonal axes results in the final image displayed on the MRI screen.

86. What is the k-space and what is its relevance to MRI imaging?

As mentioned in the previous question, an essential component of signal processing by an MRI imaging system is the combining of the information obtained from the three different orthogonal axes into one final image. For convenience, these axes are termed x, y (for the transverse axes), and z (for the longitudinal axis). K-space is nothing more than the special matrix in which MRI signals are arranged prior to their processing by Fourier transform.

87. What is the difference among the terms MRI, NMR, and MRA?

MRI (magnetic resonance imaging) is synonymous with **NMR** (nuclear magnetic resonance). **MRA** is magnetic resonance angiography, the technical variant of MRI that selectively visualizes blood flow, while suppressing signals originating from all other structures. By taking advantage of the specific blood flow direction and velocity, it is possible to individually visualize arteries and veins.

88. Explain the most frequently used MRI terms.

- **Magnetic field** is a form of energy produced by the MRI magnet and results from the motion of the electrons in the electrical current coursing through the coils. The magnetic field of an MR imaging system is more than 10,000 times stronger than the Earth's magnetic field.
- **Coil** is the fundamental component of the MRI magnet. Electrical current coursing through the coils is responsible for the generation of the MRI magnetic field. Conversely, reception of electromagnetic waves generates electrical current that courses through the coils. Thus, the coils function as both emitters and receptors of electromagnetic waves.
- **Radiofrequency energy** is the type of energy used by the MR imaging system and is composed of waves that are in the radiofrequency wavelength.
- **Field strength** is the amount of energy carried by the electromagnetic field generated by the MR magnet. Generally, higher field strength results in brighter MR images.
- **Resonance** is the vibration of hydrogen nuclei (protons) that results from their interaction with a magnetic field.

- **Spin echo and gradient echo** are fundamental MRI acquisition techniques (see questions 92 and 93).
- **T1 and T2** are fundamental properties of the electromagnetic waves generated by the patient's body (see question 94).
- **X, y, and z gradients** are the differences in electromagnetic field intensity along the three orthogonal axes.
- **Voxel** is a unit of volume within the patient's body,
- **Pixel** is a discrete point on an MR image. Each pixel is the graphical representation of a corresponding voxel.
- **Signal intensity** is the intensity of the electromagnetic signal emitted by a voxel of tissue and characterized by a specific degree of brightness of the corresponding pixel.

89. If higher field strength results in better MR images, why ever use lower field strength imaging systems?

One of the main challenges of MRI is its lack of portability and the necessity to place the patient in a narrow magnetic device. These shortcomings are addressed by the so-called open MRI systems, which can use only lower strength magnetic fields. However, this comes at the price of a somewhat lower image quality (blurry images).

90. Similar to x-ray or computed tomography (CT) images, MR images are displayed in shades of gray, varying between pure white and pure black. Do these shades indicate the density of the different tissues, as in x-ray or CT images?

No. Unlike CT or "classic" radiography, where different colors represent different tissue densities, the shades of gray in MRI represent the interplay of the emitted electromagnetic field and the physical properties of the tissues being studied. Basically, the same structure can be displayed as either black or white, depending on:
- The use of the spin echo vs. gradient echo technique (see question 93)
- The use of T1- vs. T2 -weighted images (see question 98)

91. The different shades of gray on an MR image have a different significance than in the case of an x-ray or CT image (see previous question). How is this reflected in MRI terminology?

Whereas in x-ray techniques a white (bright) image is referred to as a *density* (reflecting the physical mechanism of image generation), in MRI, image brightness is referred to as *intensity*. Thus, a pathologic structure can be hyper-, iso-, or hypointense compared to the surrounding tissues.

92. What is the difference between the spin echo and gradient echo techniques?

These are the two basic techniques of MR imaging. The underlying physical mechanisms are beyond the scope of this text, but it can be briefly stated that:
- **Spin echo** depicts blood as being black (in general, hydrogen-poor substances are also depicted in black by this technique).
- **Gradient echo** depicts blood as being white (in general, hydrogen-rich substances are also depicted in white by this technique).

93. Practically, when should I use spin echo and when should I use gradient echo imaging?

Spin echo imaging is ideal for morphologic studies (e.g., the detection of congenital cardiac malformations). Spin echo images are generally displayed as "still frames."

Gradient echo imaging is the modality of choice for functional assessments (in cardiac MRI, assessment of the ventricular ejection fraction, perfusion studies, viability studies).

94. What is the difference between T1- and T2-weighted images?

The electromagnetic field emitted by the resonant hydrogen nuclei in the tissues being imaged can be characterized by different physical parameters, including T1 and T2. A detailed explanation of the physical meaning of these parameters is beyond the scope of this text, but it can be briefly stated that:

- An MR imaging system may selectively display the T1 or the T2 "population" of electromagnetic waves emitted by the patient's body, or display both populations equally.
- Depending on the T1-weighted, T2-weighted, or T1–T2 balanced nature of the MR imaging, the same structures may be displayed as either white or black.

95. What color are structures displayed in white on a T1-weighted image?
In white: fat, subacute hemorrhage, gadolinium (MR contrast agent)
In black: water

96. What structures are displayed in white on a T2-weighted image?
In white: water
In black: calcium, gas, chronic hemorrhage, mature fibrous tissue

97. Why is it important to remember the color in which water is displayed on T1 and T2 imaging?
Most pathologic processes are characterized by the presence of edema, that is, an increased water content (bright on T2 images, dark on T1 images).

98. Practically, when should I use T1-weighted imaging? T2-weighted imaging?
In general practice, T1 imaging is most commonly used. The addition of T2 imaging is necessary in select circumstances, such as identification of certain types of cardiac tumors (e.g., cardiac pheochromocytoma). Combined T1 and T2 imaging can be viewed as an MRI *tissue characterization* method, which can be used in certain circumstances.

99. What are the main advantages and disadvantages of MRI over CT and echocardiography?

FEATURE	MRI	CT	ECHOCARDIOGRAPHY
Use of ionizing radiation	No	Yes	No
Dependence on optimal imaging windows	No	No	Yes
Availability	Variable	Wide	Wide
Cost	Relatively expensive	Cheaper	Cheapest noninvasive technique
Portability	No	No	Yes
Imaging of the great vessels	Excellent	Excellent	Limited to the thoracic aorta and pulmonary artery
Evaluation of soft tissue	Excellent	Good	Generally inferior to the other techniques
Ability to distinguish between fat, blood, and water	Excellent	Fair	Limited
Multiplanar imaging ability	Yes	No	Yes, but limited views using TTE
Use for initial patient evaluation	Limited	Yes	Usual procedure of choice
Duration	30–60 minutes	A few minutes	Approximately 15 minutes
Use in claustrophobic patients	Usually not possible	Usually possible	Not an issue

TTE = transthoracic echocardiography.

100. What are the main artifacts in MR imaging?
Overall, the artifacts encountered in MRI have a relatively smaller importance than in the setting of other imaging modalities. MR artifacts can be:

- **Motion-related.** Patient motion during acquisition sequences can create an **unintended** (e.g., cardiac motion) or **intended** (e.g., breathing or wiggling) blurring ("ghosting") of the image.

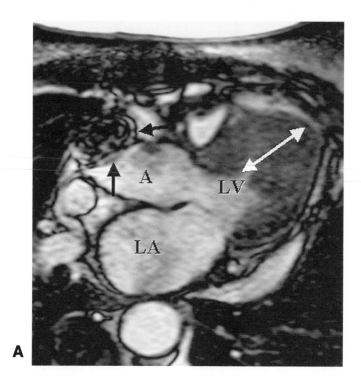

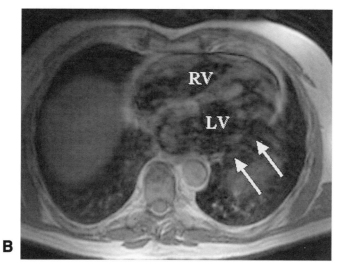

FIGURE 21. *A*, Example of an incorrect cut through the left ventricle, leading to a foreshortened view. Note the metallic artifact in the aorta (*arrows*), resulting from a bypass graft marker. *B*, Artifact produced by inadequate cardiac gating. Note that the left ventricular lateral wall is not visualized on this overall poor quality image. (*continued*)

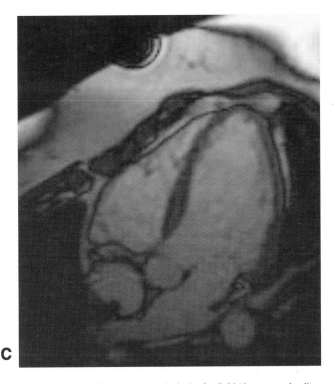

FIGURE 21. (*continued*) *C,* Drop-off in image intensity in the far-field (the greater the distance from the electromagnetic coil, the fainter the image).

- **Chemical-related.** Artifacts are caused by the physical-chemical properties of structures present in the magnetic field. For instance, certain metallic objects such as stents and sternal wires lead to areas of absent signal because of an effective magnetic shielding property of the metal (Fig. 21A). This loss of signal is rarely an issue clinically, unless the clinical question pertains to tissues directly adjacent (within a few millimeters) to the metallic object.
- **Off-axis imaging of the heart.** This leads to the acquisition of foreshortened images (*see* Figure 21A)
- **Gating artifacts.** For a discussion of ECG gating, the reader is referred to question 107) (Fig. 21B)
- **Far-field artifact.** Image intensity of organs situated at a greater distance from the electromagnetic coil is reduced (Fig. 21C)
- **"Phase-wrap" artifact.** A part of the body is wrapped into the image of another part of the body.

101. What are the main safety issues for MRI?
The main safety issue in the context of MRI is the possibility that the strong magnetic field should draw ferromagnetic objects toward the magnet, a potential hazard to the patient or to the other persons present in the MR lab. Additionally, metallic objects (medical devices or fragments that made their way accidentally into the patient's body, such as bullets or metallic shards) may be displaced by a strong magnetic field.

102. What are the main non–life-threatening adverse effects of MRI?
 Minor but potentially unpleasant adverse effects include:
- Intolerance by claustrophobic patients
- Metallic taste
- Dizziness and disorientation (more frequently seen with the newer generation, high–field-strength imaging systems)
- Muscle twitching. This adverse effect is not related to the field intensity, but rather to the rapid rate of electromagnetic amplitude switch, characteristic of newer imaging systems. Muscle twitching is very rare in clinical practice.

103. When is MRI contraindicated?
 MRI is contraindicated in patients with:
- Ferromagnetic aneurysm clips
- Known metallic fragments in the eyes or other vital areas
- Implanted devices not known to be MR safe, such as Swan-Ganz catheters, certain types of Foley catheters, implantable defibrillators, and early Starr-Edwards (ball-in-cage) valves
- Patients with pacemakers

 Sternal wires, most prosthetic valves (with the exception noted above), and cardiac stents are not contraindicated in MRI studies. The Web site www.mrisafe.com maintains a list of items that are compatible or incompatible with MRI studies.
 If in doubt, consult with the physician responsible for the study.

104. Is MRI safe in pregnant women?
 Although this has not been definitely proven, MRI may be associated with potential fetal damage caused by (1) the electromagnetic radiation itself or (2) the MRI contrast agent, gadolinium, which readily crosses the placenta.
 Like all imaging modalities, benefit to the mother and fetus need to be weighed against the potential risk.

105. Mention some of the current practical applications of cardiovascular MRI.
- Accurate measurement of cardiac chambers size and volume
- Assessment of global and segmental left and right ventricular function
- Detection and quantification of intra- and extracardiac shunts
- Structural and functional assessment of stenotic and regurgitant valves
- Detection of congenital heart anomalies and follow-up corrective surgery
- Assessment of intracardiac masses
- Assessment of myocardial viability
- Assessment of the proximal portion of the coronary arteries
- As a substitute for echocardiography in patients with inadequate windows for standard functional assessment and for dobutamine stress testing

106. Does my hospital need a special MRI to perform cardiac studies or is the "general" MRI adequate?
 It depends on the question you're asking. For **left and right ventricular ejection fraction (LVEF/RVEF)** and **morphology assessments,** most existing imaging systems are adequate, provided they possess the necessary software. For **visualization** of the coronary arteries and for perfusion studies, dedicated hardware is necessary.
 It is essential to keep in mind that most cardiac MR techniques are still in their development phase. Substantial expertise and dedicated training are necessary for their practical application.

107. What is ECG gating?
 Electromagnetic waves acquired in several heart cycles are "pooled" for obtaining the final MRI image. Using the ECG as a guide for timing of systole and diastole, the heart cycle is divided

into several slots, that correspond to the different phases of the heart cycle. Information acquired at a given point in time is placed in the corresponding slot, where it can be pooled together with information obtained from the same part of systole or diastole, acquired during other heart cycles. If ECG gating were not used when imaging the heart, the cardiac motion in the thorax during systole and diastole would result in superimposition of images from different parts of the cardiac cycle (when the heart has different positions in the thorax), which would produce an illegible image. Importantly, ECG gating is not necessary when imaging structures that are more or less static, such as the aorta or the great vessels.

108. What field strength is used in cardiac MRI?

Generally, cardiac MRI systems use high-strength electromagnetic fields, which are able to generate high-quality images.

109. What is the role of contrast administration in cardiac MRI?

- Visualization of the aorta and the great arteries (MRA)
- Assessment of coronary perfusion
- Assessment of viability
- Assessing the degree of vascularity of cardiac tumors
- Assessment of myocarditis (specific patterns of contrast enhancement have been demonstrated)

110. Are contrast agents useful for visualization of the coronary arteries?

Although it is tempting to infer that MR coronary **angiography** would benefit from administration of contrast agents, similar to other forms of MRA, this is, in fact, not the case. The currently available MRA contrast agents are not blood pool agents; that is, they diffuse into the peripheral tissues. Although this is not a concern regarding the aorta and the great vessels, it does preclude the use of contrast agents for visualization of the coronary arteries where contrast diffusion would obscure the boundaries between the coronaries and the myocardium.

Direct visualization of the coronary arteries should not be confused with the functional assessment of coronary flow (perfusion studies), where the use of contrast agents is essential.

111. Name a few frequent settings when the use of contrast agents for MRI visualization of heart structures is *not* helpful.

- Visualization of the coronary arteries (see above)
- Functional assessment of the ventricles (LVEF and RVEF)
- MRI assessment of heart valves
- MRI assessment of the pericardium

112. MRI has an excellent capacity to distinguish between flowing blood and the surrounding structures. Why, then, use contrast for MRA in the first place?

The use of contrast agents improves the signal-to-noise visualization of blood and reduces the duration of an MRA study, as compared to the no-contrast technique.

113. How is the use of contrast different in MRA and in classic (invasive) angiography?

X-rays cannot distinguish the arterial lumen from the arterial wall. Visualization of the arterial lumen is only possible if contrast agents are used. Thus, contrast agents are essential for x-ray angiography. In contrast, MRA has the intrinsic ability to distinguish the vessel lumen from the vessel wall, based on the specific physical properties of flowing blood. However, in the interest of expediency, contrast agents can be used.

114. What is the typical slice thickness in MR cardiac imaging?

The usual slice thickness used in clinical MRI studies is 8–10 mm, but most imaging systems are capable of providing even thinner slices, if required.

115. What is a phase velocity map?

This is an MR technique of assessing blood flow direction and velocity by gray-scale encoding. In Figure 22, the ascending aorta is depicted in white, and the descending aorta, in which the blood flows in a different direction and at a different velocity, is depicted in dark gray.

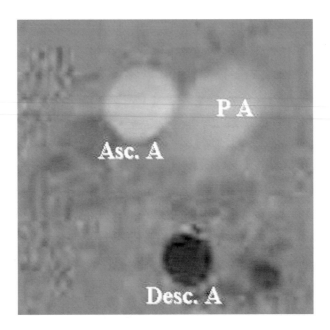

FIGURE 22. Phase velocity map. Asc. A = ascending aorta; Desc. A = descending aorta; PA = pulmonary artery.

NUCLEAR MEDICINE

Manuel D. Cerqueira, M.D., Gabriel Adelmann, M.D., and Evagoras Economides, M.A., B.M., B.Ch.

116. What is radioactivity?

Radioactivity is the process whereby a substance emits energy in the form of particles, called *photons*.

117. What is a radionuclide?

In all physical systems, there is a tendency toward stability (expressed in a higher degree of entropy). In the case of a radionuclide, this stability is reached by getting rid of part of the excess energy of the compound. A radionuclide is an unstable atom that emits radioactivity in the form of atomic particles, photons, or both. These emitted photons are imaged by a *gamma camera,* a special radiation detector. The original, unstable radionuclide is called the *parent,* whereas the more stable one (resulting from particle or photon emission) is the *daughter.*

118. How can radioactivity be used for cardiac imaging?

Radioactive decay of special molecules that can be imaged to assess perfusion and function forms the basis of nuclear cardiology, an exciting and clinically important method of diagnosis and management of patients with suspected or proven heart disease. Nuclear cardiology is based on the intravenous injection of special radioactive substances that selectively accumulate in the heart to define the myocardial cavity. The emitted radiation is then detected by the gamma camera, giving important information about the blood flow to the heart muscle and the contractility of the heart.

119. What is a radioactive tracer, and how is it different from a radionuclide?

Radionuclides may be used for diagnostic purposes either by themselves or attached to special molecules that are responsible for selective accumulation in targets. A *radioactive tracer* is any substance used for diagnostic purposes in the nuclear medicine lab, whether it includes an organ-specific molecule or not. The term *tracer* simply means that this substance follows (traces) the blood flow into the myocardium, which is the object of nuclear cardiology perfusion studies.

120. What kinds of radioactivity are used for diagnostic purposes in the nuclear lab?

Nuclear cardiology is based on two types of radioactivity:

1. The **direct** emission of single photons by the injected radionuclide, which is then detected by the gamma camera. In this case, the photons are emitted one at a time by the radionuclide during decay and are detected one at a time by the camera (single-proton techniques).

2. The emission of special atomic particles, called *positrons,* which have to first interact with an electron in order to emit photons (**indirect** emission of photons). The collision of a positron and an electron results in the emission of two high-energy photons with an energy of 511 keV. These two photons travel along the same axis but in opposite directions at 180° and are simultaneously detected by gamma camera elements that face each other. This diagnostic method is called positron emission tomography (PET).

121. Besides assessment of myocardial perfusion and function, what other questions can be assessed using nuclear cardiology studies?

Other clinically relevant parameters that can be assessed in the nuclear cardiology lab include:

Diastolic LV function   Myocardial innervation
Systolic and diastolic function of the RV   Intracardiac shunts
Myocardial metabolism

Note that many of these studies are rarely performed in clinical practice, most currently being of research interest only.

122. Once they are injected intravenously, what happens to radioactive perfusion tracers?

The radioactive tracers pass through the RA and RV and enter the pulmonary circulation and the left-sided heart chambers. They are then ejected by the LV through the aorta into the coronary arteries and reach the capillary bed of the myocardium, provided this is not damaged. From the capillary bed, myocardial cells take up the radiotracers in proportion to myocardial blood flow. These radiotracers have the highest extraction during this first pass through the heart. They remain in the circulation and make subsequent passes through the myocardium for additional extraction. If images are taken every 25–50 msec during this passage through the heart, the ejection fraction can be measured separately for the right and left ventricles and abnormal circulation of blood caused by shunts can be detected. Thus, it is possible to distinguish two separate phases of the radiotracer's course through the patient's body:

- Its passage through the heart chambers (allowing measurement of the systolic function of the ventricles) (see question 123)
- Its passage through the microcirculation and subsequent cellular uptake allowing measurement of myocardial blood flow (see Chapter 4)

123. Why would one want to follow the passage of a radiotracer through the cardiac chambers?

By following the progress of a radiotracer through the heart chambers, and by measuring the radioactivity emitted by the tracer-charged intracardiac blood pool in systole versus diastole, one can assess the LV ejection fraction. In fact, current technology not only allows identification of decreases in the systolic function of the LV, but also can pinpoint the responsible hypo-, a-, or dyskinetic segments. This technique, termed *nuclear angiography,* is discussed in detail in Chapter 4.

124. Why would one want to follow the progress of a radiotracer through the capillary microcirculation and its ultimate uptake (or lack thereof) by the myocardial cells?

The delivery of radiotracers to the capillary microcirculation shows the integrity of the myocardial capillaries, whereas cellular uptake of the tracer is dependent on the structural and functional integrity of the myocardial cells. Ischemic heart disease generally affects in parallel the integrity of the myocardial microcirculation and that of the myocytes. Thus, these two components (microcirculation and myocytes) are assessed simultaneously in the nuclear lab by the so-called nuclear myocardial perfusion studies.

125. What is the appearance of a myocardial segment with preserved microcirculation on a nuclear study?

The radioactivity emitted by the tracer present in the myocardial cells of well-perfused segments is translated into *intense (high) uptake* areas, as opposed to scarred myocardial segments, depicted as *absent or diminished uptake* areas. These areas of absent or decreased uptake are termed *perfusion defects.*

126. What techniques can be used for gamma camera radionuclide imaging of the heart?

There are three basic techniques for radionuclide imaging of the heart, classified based on the type of radionuclides they are able to image. Planar and single photon emission computed tomography (SPECT) imaging are used for detecting conventional single photon radionuclides, such as thallium-201 (Tl-201) and the technetium 99m (Tc-99m) perfusion agents, whereas PET is used for detecting dual-photon radionuclides such as rubidium 82 or fluorine 18 fluorodeoxyglucose.

1. **Planar imaging** is a 2-D imaging technique in which the heart is imaged in two planes by a gamma camera, and all the structures contained within that plane are superimposed on each other (similar to the conventional x-ray technology). In order to see all the walls of the heart, multiple planes must be imaged. The most frequently used views include the anterior, the 45° left anterior oblique, and the left lateral view. This was the only available method of nuclear imaging of the heart until the mid 1980s, but is not widely used today.

2. **SPECT** technique uses a rotating gamma camera with one or more heads to acquire 32–64 individual planar images of the heart. These individual planar images are used to reconstruct the heart in a 3-D or tomographic format. This is the currently preferred method of imaging.

3. **PET** is less widely available but can be used with cyclotron-produced radioisotopes for imaging perfusion and myocardial viability.

127. What are the most frequently asked clinical questions regarding myocardial perfusion that can be assessed by nuclear cardiology?

- Diagnosis of obstructive coronary disease in patients with chest pain ("Does this patient have flow-limiting coronary artery stenosis?")
- Prognosis or outcome in patients with known coronary artery disease ("I know this patient has coronary artery disease, but what is the risk of nonfatal myocardial infarction or cardiac death?")
- Assessment of myocardial viability in a patient with chronic left ventricular dysfunction and known coronary artery disease ("If I refer my patient for coronary artery bypass grafting or PTCI, will the hypo- or akinetic myocardial segment regain function?")

128. During acquisition of myocardial perfusion studies, there may be spatial overlap of adjacent walls and temporal blurring of the images due to movement of the heart during contraction. What is the significance of this spatial overlap and temporal blurring?

Spatial overlap is associated with planar perfusion imaging. In this technique, radioactivity originating from different depths in one of the heart walls overlaps with the adjacent segments on that particular view. For instance, one does not see separately the basal, mid-, and apical levels of the anterior wall, but rather one "average anterior wall" on the final planar image. SPECT overcomes this limitation by allowing imaging of myocardial radioactivity at discrete levels of the heart.

The motion of the heart causes temporal blurring during acquisition of perfusion images. Studies are routinely acquired for hundreds to thousands of individual heartbeats, and the resulting borders of the endocardium on the final images are a composite average of the moving radioactivity. This does not deter one from obtaining accurate information on myocardial perfusion, because with perfusion studies one is not interested in the endocardial border motion but rather in the patterns of radionuclide uptake by the myocardium. For assessment of the ejection fraction, precise distinction between the position of the endocardium at end-systole and end-diastole is essential and is achieved by means of ECG gating. ECG gating allows 8 or 16 individual images or time frames to be acquired for each heartbeat, and corresponding frames from each beat are summed, so that the temporal motion of the heart can be captured. (As an analogy, imagine a camera recording of a running athlete processed so that each step the athlete takes is "decomposed" into different stages (e.g., lifting of the right leg, placing the right foot on the ground, lifting of the left leg), with similar stages from different steps being pooled together. What would result is an "average step," representative of that athlete's locomotory mechanics. Of course, the more "segments" into which the motion is decomposed, the clearer the images.

129. If perfusion images are acquired using ECG gating, how accurate is the assessment of global and regional left ventricular function?

Global and regional assessment of function is very accurate from the ECG gated perfusion images. It has been compared and shown to have a high correlation relative to equilibrium radionuclide angiography (so called multiple gated acquisition [MUGA] studies), first pass studies, quantitative echocardiography, and contrast ventriculography and cardiac MRI.

130. What characteristics of radiotracer uptake by the myocardium are important for the diagnosis of coronary artery disease and the differentiation between normal, ischemic, and infracted myocardium?

All studies require two separate imaging sessions: one at rest and one following exercise or pharmacologic stress. Characteristic patterns are present for each of the three types of myocardium:

1. **Normal** myocardium — uniform radiotracer uptake at rest and following stress
2. **Ischemic** myocardium — normal radiotracer uptake at rest and absent or diminished following stress
3. **Infarcted** myocardium — diminished or absent radiotracer at rest and stress

131. Can other imaging modalities provide information on myocardial perfusion similar to radionuclide perfusion studies?

Yes. **Contrast echocardiography** is a relatively new technology that enables visualization of the myocardial blood pool, based on the reflection of ultrasound on the surface of injected "bubbles" (echocardiographic contrast agents). **Cardiac catheterization** can demonstrate myocardial perfusion based on a specific "ground-glass" appearance of the normally perfused myocardium (the so-called myocardial blush). **MRI** can provide assessment of myocardial flow and of myocytes integrity, using special contrast agents.

132. What is the place of non-nuclear diagnostic methods in the assessment of myocardial perfusion?

At present, none of these methods can replace in a reliable and cost-effective manner the nuclear perfusion studies. Many of these methods are not available for routine clinical use.

Contrast echocardiography has been envisioned as a serious contender in this setting. The main potential advantage is the possibility of a comprehensive cardiac evaluation, in a cost-effective manner, under a wide spectrum of clinical conditions (ranging from outpatients, to the hospitalized, and even to critically ill patients). However, despite extremely active research, contrast echocardiography has not yet been conclusively proven to be a reliable alternative to nuclear medicine.

The proponents of **cardiac MRI** state that this method will provide, in the foreseeable future, a "one-stop shopping" for cardiac evaluation, including structural data on the heart chambers, valves, and vessels and functional data about intracardiac and intramyocardial blood flow and myocardial metabolism. The main problems with cardiac MRI are its high cost, reduced availability, and reduced applicability in unstable or critically ill patients. Additionally, currently MRI cannot be performed in the setting of diagnostic or interventional procedures.

Myocardial blush, identified by **cardiac catheterization,** offers valuable additional information regarding the degree of microcirculation damage caused by an epicardial coronary artery stenosis. However, the sensitivity and specificity of this method are still insufficiently documented. Attempts at quantitative techniques have not been successful.

Gamma Cameras

133. What is a gamma camera and how does it work?

The gamma or "scintillation" camera allows imaging of the radiation emitted by the radioisotope carried by the bloodstream in the heart chambers and that retained in the myocardium. The main components of the camera are as follows:

- The **collimator** is equivalent to a focus instrument, that lets past only radiation perpendicular to the plane of the scintillation detector. It consists of lead-lined holes perpendicular to the face of the gamma camera, similar to a sieve. Radioactive decay occurs in all directions (360°), and imaging without a collimator produces a "blob" of radioactivity without any spatial resolution. The collimator eliminates the radiation scattered from the patient's body at different angles and only accepts photons that are completely parallel to the lead walls. This process is essential, because scattered radiation can provide inaccurate information about the location of the emitting tracer.
- The **scintillation detector** is a special crystal that converts and amplifies the gamma radiation emitted by the radiotracer in the patient's body to light photons.
- The **photocathode** converts the photons to electrons.
- **Photomultiplier tubes** amplify the electrons into a detectable electrical current.
- The **electronic processor** generates images based on the intensity and spatial distribution of the electrical signals.

Nuclear cameras have one to three heads. The acquisition time decreases proportionally with the number of heads.

134. Why is it important to shorten the acquisition time in a nuclear cardiology study?

The acquisition of nuclear cardiology images takes approximately 10 minutes for each planer image and anywhere from 15 to 30 minutes for a SPECT study. The longer the acquisition time, the higher the total number of photons or counts. Higher counts improve image quality. Unfortunately, if studies take too long to acquire, patients are likely to move during the acquisition. This motion creates artifacts that limit the accuracy of the studies.

135. What are the different types of gamma cameras used in nuclear cardiology?

Three types of cameras are currently used in nuclear cardiology.

1. The **Anger camera,** described above, has a long track record of successful utilization.

2. The **multicrystal (multidetector) camera** has many small individual crystals attached directly to a single photomultiplier tube. This allows acquisition of very high count rates so that adequate images can be acquired at temporal resolution of 25–50 msec. These cameras are most useful in first-pass imaging, where very fast acquisition of images is essential to measure blood flow through the heart chambers in a very rapid temporal sequence. They cannot be used for acquiring perfusion information because they have very poor spatial resolution. For this reason they are no longer being manufactured.

3. The **positron camera,** used in PET, is composed of crystals arranged in a ring around the patient and only register a signal if two photons strike opposite crystals simultaneously (coincidence counting). They are becoming more widely available due to their important application in the field of oncology.

Artifacts

136. What are the main causes of artifact in nuclear cardiology?
Attenuation, patient motion, and image processing.

137. What is attenuation?
Attenuation is one of the fundamental problems of all the imaging techniques. It represents energy loss, as the particles emitted by the heart (e.g., ultrasound echoes, photons) interact with body tissue on their way to the external detecting device (e.g., ultrasound transducer, photon camera). In the case of radionuclide imaging, attenuation results from absorption of photon energy by the tissues between the heart and the camera.

138. How does attenuation affect nuclear cardiology studies?
In the absence of attenuation, myocardium with normal blood flow would have a uniform and homogenous intensity. However, tissue overlying the heart causes some of the emitted photons to lose energy and be reoriented in proportion to the distance and the density of the tissue through which they travel. Thus, dense tissue, such as bone, has a higher attenuation coefficient and causes a greater loss of photon energy than air in the lung and soft tissue. This means that the final images do not directly measure the total amount of radiotracer that is retained in the myocardium, but rather the total uptake minus the amount lost due to attenuation.

139. What are the main tissue types responsible for the attenuation seen in nuclear cardiology studies?
Breast attenuation in female patients and attenuation caused by the chest wall in male patients are most commonly encountered in the nuclear lab. Additional organs that can cause attenuation include the arms, diaphragm, abdominal organs, and excess body fat (obesity). Figures 23A and B show a breast attenuation artifact, which can be differentiated by ECG-gated SPECT: Figure 23C demonstrates the imaging artifact produced by a large hernia.

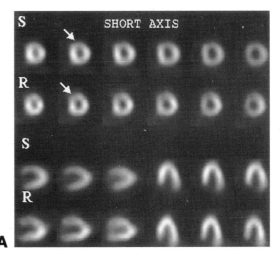

FIGURE 23. *A,* SPECT study in an obese female patient with large breasts. The *arrows* indicate an area of apparent anterior perfusion defect, present both at stress (*S*) and rest (*R*). This may be due to an old myocardial infarction or to breast attenuation. If the nuclear cardiologist does not confidently establish this distinction, the referring physician gains no real additional knowledge from the nuclear study and may unnecessarily refer the patient for cardiac catheterization. The differentiation of this finding (artifact vs. true perfusion defect) can be demonstrated using attenuation correction software or by gated SPECT. (*continued*)

A

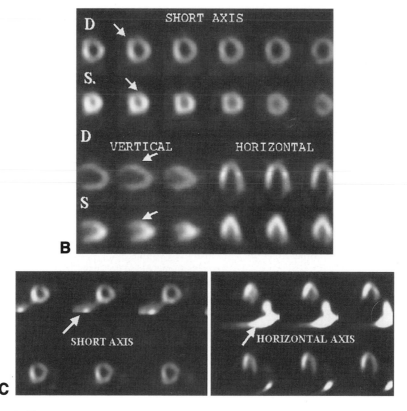

FIGURE 23. (*continued*) *B,* Selected end diastolic (*D*) and end systolic (*S*) rows of images of the gated SPECT study in the same patient shows normal motion and thickening of the anterior wall (in systole, the endocardial border of this segment has a normal inward excursion and increases in intensity, *arrows),* and demonstrates that the apparent perfusion defect is actually a breast attenuation artifact in an overweight female patient. *C,* Extracardiac uptake of a Tc-99m radiotracer excreted into the duodenum and with retrograde flow into the stomach and into a hernia extending into the chest. This not only causes attenuation but also adds counts during the acquisition.

140. What are the main elements that influence attenuation?

The degree to which the radioactivity emitted by a myocardial segment is attenuated depends on:

- The type of extracardiac tissues overlay that segment (e.g., bone vs. soft tissue)
- The type of radionuclide used. Lower energy photons are more easily attenuated then higher energy photons. Therefore, attenuation has a higher impact on thallium- than on technetium-based perfusion tracers.

141. Can attenuation artifact be corrected?

Although several attenuation correction algorithms have been developed and are available, the final role of attenuation correction has not been determined. PET attenuation correction is performed routinely for all acquisitions and is accurate. Some of the problems with SPECT attenuation correction systems include:

- High cost
- Not always reimbursable by insurance companies
- The tendency of eliminating true perfusion defects, resulting in false-negative studies
- Failure to correct for scattered radiation, causing counts to be added inappropriately

142. What is motion artifact and how does it impact the quality of a nuclear study?

Simply stated, a nuclear image affected by motion artifact is blurry (Fig. 24). When a family photograph is blurry because the subjects could not hold still, you can often tell who is who on the final image but you cannot distinguish the fine features of that person's face or body. Similarly, a blurry nuclear scan will not be able to demonstrate clearly the details regarding the tracer uptake by the various myocardial segments. Unlike a family picture, which is a single snapshot image, a SPECT image actually represents the summation of multiple images acquired during systole and diastole. In this process, radioactivity originating from a certain location in the patient's body on one of the individual pictures is malpositioned during the process of image reconstruction. The basic assumption that must be met for accurate imaging is that an organ is in the same location throughout the entire acquisition.

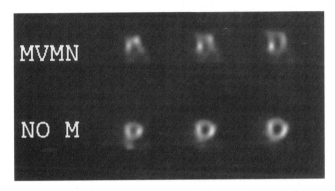

FIGURE 24. Motion artifact (short axis views from a SPECT perfusion study). Note the "blurry," distorted shape of the LV during patient motion (MVMN). Occasionally, motion artifact is more subtle and may result in incorrect interpretation of the nuclear study.

143. What findings suggest that a defect in a perfusion scan may in fact be an artifact?

A perfusion defect is likely to be an artifact if it extends outside the normal distribution of coronary topography, it corresponds to an area of attenuation, and there is patient motion observed during the acquisition. An apparent perfusion defect that disappears when the patient's position is changed (e.g., prone vs. supine imaging) is most probably an artifact, much like what happens when an echocardiographic "mass" suddenly "disappears" on slight transducer angulations.

Safety Issues in the Nuclear Lab

144. What is the safety profile of the currently used diagnostic radionuclides?

Most of the data on radiation risk originates from the atomic bombs in Hiroshima and Nagasaki and from nuclear reactor accidents. The doses and isotope half-lives and energy used in diagnostic nuclear cardiology pose a low risk to the patient. The risk is greater to nuclear medicine personnel who are in contact with radiation on a daily basis. It is advised that radiation exposure be limited to levels as low as reasonably achievable. The gonads and eye lenses seem to be the organs that are most sensitive to the effect of radiation.

145. How can radiation exposure be monitored and minimized?

Radiation exposure is monitored using film badges and dosimeters. Frequent monitoring of the nuclear cardiology laboratory is required, with some parameters being checked daily and others checked weekly. A good rule of thumb for ensuring safety in the nuclear lab is summarized by the acronym ALARA; that is, exposure radiation should be kept *a*s *l*ow *a*s *r*easonably *a*chievable. This is attained by minimizing the time of exposure to radiation and maximizing the distance and utilizing shielding between the source of radiation and the handler.

CHEST X-RAY

David R. Buck, M.D., Gabriel Adelmann, M.D., and Curtis E. Green, M.D.

146. What are x-rays?
X-rays are a form of electromagnetic radiation composed of particles of energy called *photons*.

147. How can x-rays be used for imaging the heart?
X-rays generated by a special tube (the x-ray tube) propagate through the part of the patient's body that is to be imaged. On their course through the different tissues, x-rays lose part of their energy; the energy loss is proportional to the density of the tissues. Thus, dense tissues (such as bones) block most of the x-rays, whereas air (in organs such as the lungs) does not interfere with the progress of x-rays as they traverse the body.

X-rays entering the patient's body are relatively uniform but those x-rays exiting the body vary widely because of the interaction with tissues of different densities. After leaving the body, the x-rays interact with a photographic film to produce different degrees of photochemical reaction on the surface of the film. This is the physical basis of x-ray use for clinical imaging. Newer systems allow digital capture of the image for picture archiving and communication system (PACS).

148. What are the main types of tissue that can be distinguished radiologically based on their different densities?
Five basic densities can be differentiated radiologically. In order of density, these are:
1. Air
2. Fat
3. Water (including blood and soft tissues)
4. Bone (and calcifications)
5. Metal

149. What are the limitations of cardiac imaging by classic radiology?
The thorax is composed of adjacent tissues with widely different densities (soft tissues, bones, lung tissue, myocardium, and blood-filled cardiac cavities). The different densities allow differentiation of these structures. For example, the heart shadow can be distinguished from the surrounding pulmonary air. However, the diagnostic ability of classic radiography is limited whenever it becomes necessary:
- To distinguish between two adjacent tissues of similar density (e.g., separating the myocardial shadow from a surrounding pericardial effusion)
- To identify low-contrast internal structures (e.g., identifying a noncalcified intracardiac tumor from the surrounding myocardium and blood)

In these cases, other imaging modalities (echocardiography, CT scan, MRI) should be used.

150. What is the significance of the white color and the black color on a radiologic image?
Areas of the film impacted by more x-rays appear as black, and, conversely, areas impacted by less x-rays are depicted as white. In other words, high densities (e.g., bone and metal) result in more attenuation and appear as whiter areas, whereas low densities (e.g., air) result in less attenuation and appear as blacker areas. For a discussion of attenuation, the reader is referred to questions 154 and 155.

151. What are the main components of an x-ray machine?
The x-ray machine has the following main components
- An **x-ray tube,** responsible for the emission of the diagnostic x-rays
- An **image receptor,** consisting of phosphorus adjacent to radiographic film (in the case of plain film radiography), a **digital detector** (in PACS, also known as *digital radiology*), or a **fluoroscopic screen** and **video camera** (in fluoroscopy)

The most important current cardiac application of fluoroscopy is the contrast-based technique for imaging the blood vessels. These techniques are commonly designated as *angiography*. The most important angiographic technique used in cardiology is cardiac catheterization, which is discussed in the Cardiac Catheterization section of this chapter (see question 4). The remainder of this chapter deals exclusively with static x-ray imaging (radiography).

152. What are the main physical phenomena that influence the formation of a radiographic image?

    Penetration
    Attenuation
    Geometric effects (magnification)

153. What is x-ray penetration?

Penetration is the distance that x-rays can progress through a tissue before they lose all their energy. The degree of penetration depends on:

- The initial energy of the x-rays—Generally, the higher a photon's energy, the greater the penetration. However, higher energy photons produce a higher percentage of forward scattering (see question 155), which diminishes tissue contrast.
- The dimensions of the patient's body (obese vs. normal weight)
- The density of the tissues through which the x-rays are coursing—The higher the density, the less the penetration. For example, an equal increase in chest anteroposterior [AP] diameter may be due to more subcutaneous fat or increased lung size due to chronic obstructive pulmonary disease (COPD).

154. What is attenuation?

Attenuation is the exact opposite of penetration. Attenuation is caused by the loss of energy of x-rays as they course through a tissue. The greater the energy loss, the greater the attenuation.

155. How does tissue attenuate x-rays?

The following phenomena are responsible for x-ray attenuation by tissue:

- **Scattering** is a change in the direction of propagation of x-rays as they bounce off tissue. A scattered photon may end up propagating backward, forward, or sideways compared to its initial direction. This is the predominant mechanism of x-ray attenuation seen in clinical practice.
- **Absorption** is the transmission of energy to the tissue.

156. How do penetration and attenuation affect the formation of the radiographic image?

Penetration is the fundamental physical phenomenon governing the formation of radiographic images. As mentioned above, differential penetration of x-rays through adjacent tissues allows one to distinguish between these tissues on the radiographic film. In order to achieve this, photon energy should be:

- **Sufficiently strong** to allow x-rays to exit the tissues and to impact the radiographic film ("soft" or low energy photons deposit all their energy in the tissue, which means none of it reaches the film and no image is created)
- **Not excessively strong,** so as not to create a level of forward scattering that would result in a misty (fogged or white-out) image
- **Appropriate to the tissue of interest**. A lower average energy depicts calcium from soft tissue, whereas a higher average energy better depicts nodules from air-filled lung tissue.
- **Within the linear range of the detector**. Too few or too many photons result in reduced contrast.

157. What is the consequence of suboptimal penetration (i.e., too low or too high) on an x-ray?

- An under-penetrated film is too white. In other words, there is an overall low degree of photochemical reaction on the radiographic film as a result of too little x-ray energy. This is

generally due to inadequately selected x-ray characteristics in a specific patient and is often seen in obese people.
- An over-penetrated film is too black; that is, there is excessive x-ray energy relative to the patient's dimensions.

158. What is image magnification, what are its determinants, and how does it impact the final image quality?

Image magnification is the degree of enlargement of the image of an organ, compared to the true anatomic dimensions of that organ. Magnification leads to overestimation of the size of an object (it measures larger on the film than its real size). Magnification results from:
- **Distance of the body part from the detector**. X-rays have a divergent course between the emission source and the radiographic film. Thus, the farther an object is from the image detecting system, the greater the magnification. Placing the detector against the body on the surface nearest the object of interest minimizes magnification.
- **Distance of the source from the detector**. Increasing the distance from the source to the detector reduces magnification.

The application of magnifying techniques can increase image resolution in a fluoroscopic or digital-based system by placing the image of the object across a larger portion of the detector (resulting in a larger number of picture elements [pixels]). Magnification techniques do, however, result in larger radiation doses.

159. What are the main terms used to describe image quality in diagnostic radiology?

The main parameters of image quality are **contrast, resolution,** and **noise**. A high-quality radiologic image has a high resolution, an optimal degree of contrast, and a minimal degree of background noise.

160. What is contrast?

In diagnostic radiology, the concept of contrast has two meanings:
1. **Subject contrast** refers to the degree of contrast inherent in the imaged object. It is independent of imaging system and technique.
2. **Image contrast** refers to the difference in brightness as displayed in the radiographic image. Within certain limits, a higher contrast can result in higher image quality. Image contrast is determined by the technical parameters of the exposure and the imaging system.

161. What is image resolution?

Resolution refers to the image sharpness and is defined as the smallest distance between two individual points that can still be individually detected on the final image. The higher the resolution, the sharper the image appears.

162. What is the definition of *noise* in diagnostic radiology?

Noise represents random fluctuations in the brightness of the radiographic image and can obscure true differences or artificially display differences when in fact none exist. High-quality images have a low level of background noise.

163. What are the main types of x-ray imaging used in clinical practice ?

1. Static x-ray imaging (radiography)
2. Dynamic x-ray imaging, consisting of imaging loops displaying the motion of tissues or contrast agents in real time (fluoroscopy)

164. Name some common clinical indications of chest radiography.

Radiography is indicated whenever a static image of the heart and lungs is sufficient for obtaining the necessary information. Common indications for cardiac radiography include:

- Assessment of the degree of congestion in the pulmonary circulation (a valuable indicator concerning the presence or absence of congestive heart failure)
- Gross assessment of the heart dimensions
- Gross assessment of the thoracic aorta
- Gross assessment for pulmonary masses

165. What is the current role of radiography in the diagnosis of heart disease?

Despite the widespread use of newer imaging techniques, chest radiography is the most frequently used and least costly modality for imaging the heart. Practically every patient, as well as most healthy subjects, has had at least one chest x-ray examination in his or her life. Radiography may be used:

- For initial patient evaluation (e.g., a patient presenting to the emergency room with dyspnea)
- For patient follow-up (e.g., assessing the response to diuretic therapy in a dyspneic patient with pulmonary congestion on the initial chest x-ray study)
- As an adjunct to more sophisticated imaging techniques. Thus, a patient presenting with an acute myocardial infarction and pulmonary edema will usually undergo an echocardiographic examination on admission to the hospital, followed by serial in-hospital radiologic follow-up.

166. What are the main cardiologic indications of fluoroscopy?

Fluoroscopy is performed whenever dynamic imaging is necessary for establishing the diagnosis. In other words, fluoroscopy demonstrates the *changes* in a given area of interest over time. This technique can be used:

- Without the administration of contrast substance (i.e., fluoroscopy of a mechanical valvular prosthesis to assess for "rocking" caused by dehiscence or to assess prosthetic leaflet motion)
- With intra-arterial administration of a contrast substance. (These techniques are commonly referred to as *angiography*. The currently used angiographic techniques are discussed in detail in the Cardiac Catheterization section of this chapter.)

167. What is the current role of fluoroscopy in the diagnosis of heart disease?

Contrast-based fluoroscopy techniques (cardiac catheterization, left ventriculography) are the most frequently used diagnostic and therapeutic techniques in current cardiology practice.

168. What are the most frequently used radiologic views of the heart (the most commonly used angles between the patient's body and the radiologic imaging system)?

- The frontal view, either posteroanterior (PA; front against film) or AP (back against film)
- The lateral view
- Oblique views, representing intermediary positions between the frontal and the lateral views

169. What are the main technical characteristics of a good-quality x-ray image?

- An optimal degree of penetration is needed so that spine and lung detail is visible behind the heart and diaphragm.
- It is performed at the end of inspiration when the lungs are expanded (Fig. 25A and B).
- In case of a frontal film, the patient is not rotated (i.e., the clavicular heads are positioned on either side of the midline), allowing a consistent assessment of the dimensions of the heart.
- The scapulae are outside the lung fields (Fig. 25C and D).
- A short exposure time is needed to minimize cardiac motion.

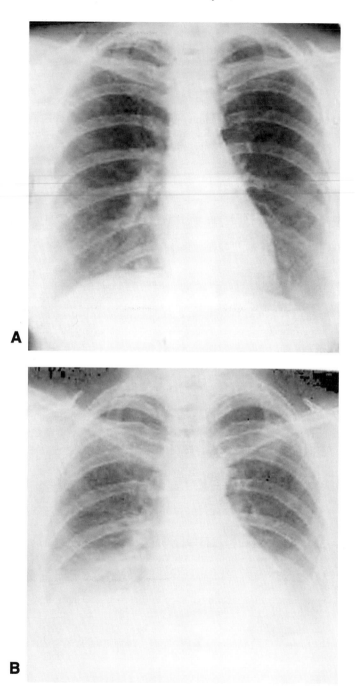

FIGURE 25. *A*, Chest x-ray at end-inspiration. *B*, Chest x-ray performed without deep inspiration. Note that the cardiac borders are less clearly delineated than in *A* and there is apparent cardiomegaly (the cardiac shadow is enlarged, as compared to the previous figure). (*continued*)

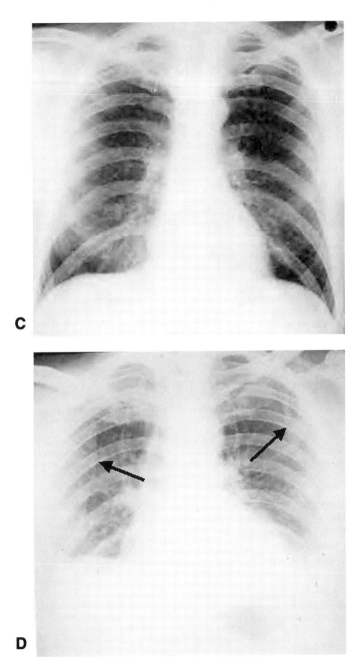

FIGURE 25. (*continued*) *C*, Good quality chest x-ray, where the scapulae are not seen in the lung fields. *D*, Poor quality chest x-ray, where the scapulae are seen protruding into the lung fields *(arrows)*.

170. What are the differences between an anteroposterior (AP) and a posteroanterior (PA) frontal chest radiograph?

AP and PA refer to the direction the x-ray beam passes through the patient.

A **PA** chest radiograph is taken with the x-ray tube behind the patient and the film cassette against the patient's anterior chest wall. This is the preferred technique for obtaining frontal chest x-rays. The patient ideally must be able to stand and press his or her chest against the radiographic cassette.

An **AP** chest radiograph is taken with the x-ray tube in front of the patient and the film cassette placed behind the patient. This technique is used for patients who are unable to stand. The cassette is placed on the bed or chair under or behind the patient's back.

171. How are the images obtained by the PA and AP techniques different?

X-rays are generated from a point source and diverge as they travel through the patient's body. The shorter the distance between the heart and the film cassette, the lower the magnification and the more accurate the final image. Because the heart has an anterior position in the thorax, the PA technique will result in a smaller distance between the heart and the film cassette. Conversely, the AP technique has a greater distance between the heart and film and will cause greater magnification of the heart and apparent widening of the mediastinum. This is very important because cardiomegaly is often a significant concern in the differential diagnosis of a critically ill patient.

172. What are the main sources of personnel x-ray exposure?

The main source of personnel exposure in the field of cardiology is the x-ray energy scattered out of the patient's body in the cath lab. This exposure is especially high during angiographic cases involving repeated imaging and time-consuming angioplasty procedures.

173. What are the main types of biologic effects of diagnostic x-rays?

1. **Deterministic** effects occur after a certain threshold dose has been exceeded. These effects include skin erythema, epilation, and cataracts. These events are seen with accidents from uncontrolled personnel exposure to high levels of radiation or prolonged fluoroscopic procedures in the same position.

2. **Probabilistic** effects do not have a threshold dose; the probability for such effect is proportional to the total exposure to radiation. These effects include cancer induction (seen in the exposed personnel) and genetic abnormalities (seen in their offspring). Probabilistic effects represent the main safety concern in the x-ray diagnostic laboratory.

174. What are the main protective measures against the potentially deleterious effects of x-rays?

As in the case of nuclear medicine personnel, the personnel working in the radiology department should apply the ALARA principle (see question 145). This can be accomplished through the following measures:

- **Time**—Minimize the duration of fluoroscopy as much as possible.
- **Distance**—Keep operators and assisting personnel as far from the portion of the patient undergoing fluoroscopy as practical.
- **Shielding**—Use protective garments (lead aprons and glasses) and shields (movable partitions and/or floating shields) between the patient and operators.
- **Monitoring radiation exposure**—Use special radiation detecting badges and rings to provide information about the total dose of radiation to which an operator has been exposed. Monthly radiation-exposure monitoring of those with occupational exposure to radiation is mandatory. Limits for monthly, quarterly, annual, and lifetime allowed doses to the eyes, trunk, and hands are available.

2. THE NORMAL HEART

CARDIAC CATHETERIZATION

Luis Gruberg, M.D., Benjamin Kleiber, M.D., Andrew E. Ajani, MBBS, FRACP, and Gabriel Adelmann, M.D.

1. Describe the angiographic appearance of the normal coronary arteries.

A normal coronary artery is well-opacified, running its course without any interruptions or significant *local* decreases in diameter and gradually tapering off. The normal coronary arteries have a variable number of branches, generally with a smaller diameter than that of the main artery.

2. Name the main angiographic views used for visualization of normal coronary arteries.

Left anterior oblique (LAO), right anterior oblique (RAO), and anteroposterior (AP), all with different cranial and caudal angulations.

3. What is the angiographic appearance of a stenotic coronary artery?

The angiographic description of a coronary stenosis is based on the following characteristics:
- **Position** along the course of the artery (ostial, proximal, mid, distal artery stenosis, stenosis at the point of arterial bifurcation)
- **Native versus in-stent** stenosis
- **Length** (focal versus diffuse)
- Degree of **symmetry** (concentric or eccentric lesions)
- **Borders** (well defined or hazy)
- Presence or absence of **calcification**
- Presence or absence of coronary **thrombus** (generally expressed as haziness of the arterial lumen)

4. Describe the general angiographic appearance of a normal left ventricle (LV).

Shape: The normal ventricle is an ovoid from the RAO view and a circle from the LAO view. The normal LV contour is regular, without any segmental distortion or outpouching.

Thickness: This can be assessed as the thickness of tissue between the radioopaque contrast material inside the ventricular cavity and the radiotransparent lung tissue on the exterior border.

Systolic function: Systolic function refers to the degree of endocardial excursion toward the central axis of the LV in systole; in the normal ventricle, this degree of excursion (contraction) is equal in all the myocardial segments.

5. What is the preferred angiographic view for assessing the LV function?

The 30° RAO projection. The 60° LAO view also is used occasionally if a more detailed assessment is warranted.

6. List the myocardial segments best visualized from the RAO view.
- Anterior wall
- Apex
- Inferior wall (Fig. 1)

7. Which cardiac valve can be assessed best from the RAO view?

The mitral valve. This is the preferred view for demonstration of mitral regurgitation.

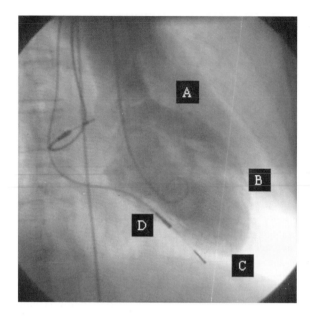

FIGURE 1. LV segments from RAO—anterobasal (A); anterolateral (B); apical (C); and inferior (D).

8. List the myocardial segments best visualized from the LAO view.
- Interventricular septum (IVS)
- Lateral wall
- Posterior wall

9. Which cardiac valve can be assessed best from the LAO view?
The aortic valve. This is the preferred view for demonstration of aortic regurgitation.

10. List the LV abnormalities most commonly seen in the catheterization laboratory (cath lab).
LV **structural** abnormalities
- Chamber dilation
- Abnormal chamber shape (e.g., spherical ventricle in the case of extreme systolic dysfunction, aneurysmal after a myocardial infarction, apex obliteration in apical hypertrophic cardiomyopathy)
- Ventricular wall thinning
- Ventricular rupture (involving the LV, the right ventricle [RV], or the IVS)
- Different pathologic or man-made intracavitary or intramural structures, such as thrombus, tumor, pacemaker wires, and catheters

LV **functional** abnormalities
- Hypokinesis
- Akinesis
- Dyskinesis

11. What are the characteristics of normal heart valves, as shown in the cath lab?
The normal heart valves may be seen as thin, mobile structures within the contrast-opacified ventricles. Normally functioning heart valves do not allow regurgitation of contrast material.

12. What are the characteristics of the normal pericardium, as assessed in the cath lab?
Structure: The normal pericardium is not visible on either fluoroscopy or ventriculography. If there are abnormal pericardial calcifications, these are recognized easily on fluoroscopy.

Function: The normal intrapericardial pressure is lower than that in the right heart cavities (< 5 mmHg). An increased intrapericardial pressure is seen in patients with a chronic or acute pericardial effusion. Because of the availability of other, more easily obtainable diagnostic modalities (echocardiography) in these patients, intrapericardial pressures are not measured routinely in clinical practice.

13. How are intracardiac pressure tracings obtained in the cath lab?

Precise intracardiac pressure tracings are obtained using catheters with pressure sensors at their tip. These catheters can be introduced into the heart chambers, the great arteries, or the pericardium.

14. What is the diagnostic importance of intracardiac pressure tracings?

Pressure tracings are used for:
- Calculation of pressure gradients across a heart valve, by simultaneously measuring the pressure in the two heart chambers separated by that valve
- Calculation of intracavitary pressure gradients, using the same principle (e.g., intracavitary pressure gradient in the LV, in patients with hypertrophic obstructive cardiomyopathy)
- Determination of valve area, by means of Gorlin's formula
- Measurement of intrapericardial pressures

15. Which of the parameters mentioned in question 14 can be measured at the bedside and do not require taking the patient to the cath lab?

Generally, procedures that require cannulation of the veins (right heart catheterization) can be performed at the patient bedside (measuring right-sided pressures), whereas left heart catheterization, coronary catheterization, and aortography generally are done in the cath lab.

16. Name two common procedures that can be carried out at the patient bedside and require cannulation of the patient's arteries.

1. Insertion of an arterial line for direct pressure systemic blood pressure monitoring
2. Insertion of an intra-aortic counterpulsation device (balloon pump) in emergent/urgent situations

17. What is a Swan-Ganz catheter, and what is its clinical purpose?

The Swan-Ganz catheter is a device used for right heart catheterization. It generally is inserted through the subclavian or internal jugular vein and the pressure transducer at the tip of the catheter is placed sequentially in the right atrium (RA), RV, and pulmonary artery, and "wedged" into a pulmonary artery branch.

18. Practically, what are the main elements of information obtained by means of a Swan-Ganz catheter?

Swan-Ganz catheters allow measurement of the pressures in the **RA, RV,** and **pulmonary artery** and **pulmonary capillary wedge pressure** (PCWP).

19. What is the correct position of the tip of a Swan-Ganz catheter?

The tip (with the balloon down) should be located in the right or left main pulmonary artery or in one of their major lobar branches. This position can be ascertained easily in the cath lab (by fluoroscopy) or at the patient's bedside (by chest radiography).

20. How can the PCWP be measured by means of a Swan-Ganz catheter?

The tip of the catheter is advanced into a branch of the pulmonary artery, and its communication with the lumen of the pulmonary artery is interrupted by inflation of a special balloon. With the balloon inflated, the pressure transducer measures the pressure in the pulmonary capillary arteries instead of the pressures in the pulmonary artery.

21. What is the significance of the PCWP?

The PCWP is a reflection of the pressure in the left atrium (LA). It is possible to obtain a measurement referring to the **left** cardiac chambers by introducing a catheter into the **right** cardiac chambers.

22. What are the normal PCWP values, and what is the significance of increases in this measurement?

The PCWP reflects the pressure in the LA and has normal values < 10 mmHg. The PCWP is increased whenever the LA pressure increases. Two common clinical conditions that increase LA pressure include LV failure with increased LV end-diastolic pressure and mitral stenosis.

23. Practically, when should I consider obtaining a PCWP measurement in my patients?

- To establish whether or not a dyspneic syndrome in a patient is due to pulmonary congestion from LV failure or from a primary lung abnormality (which may increase pulmonary artery, RV, and RA pressure but should not increase PCWP)
- To assess the response of LV failure to therapy (e.g., diuretic therapy to reduce pulmonary congestion)

24. How can the cardiac output be measured by means of a Swan-Ganz catheter?

Determination of the cardiac output using the Swan-Ganz catheter is based on the **thermo-dilution principle.** When a bolus of cold saline is injected into the proximal port of the catheter, it produces a minor, but detectable, decrease in local blood temperature. The higher the cardiac output, the faster this temperature decrease propagates distally (between the proximal port of the catheter into which the saline is injected and the temperature detector at the tip of the catheter). Computer software can calculate the cardiac output based on these parameters. Practically, a set of three to four measurements of cardiac output are carried out and averaged. Meticulous technique is required for accurate results. If a cardiac output measurement differs from the rest of the measurements by > 0.5 L/min, that specific measurement generally is excluded.

25. Explain the significance of increased RA pressures, as detected by a Swan-Ganz catheter.

The RA pressure reflects the central venous pressure (CVP), and is increased in cases of:

- Increased RV end-diastolic pressure (RV failure, most frequently resulting from LV failure; this is the most frequent cause of increased RA pressure, also referred to as *increased CVP*)
- Tricuspid stenosis (infrequent)
- Pericardial pathology (tamponade or constriction)

26. Explain the significance of increased RV pressure.

Increased RV pressure may be secondary to:

- Increased afterload (pulmonary hypertension), which may be primary or (more frequently) secondary to LV failure or pulmonary disease
- Increased preload, resulting from tricuspid regurgitation or left-to-right shunt
- Decreased RV contractility (RV infarction or cardiomyopathy)

27. Explain the significance of an increased CVP, in the absence of an increased PCWP.

This combination of findings indicates that the hemodynamic problem originates "behind" the LA (i.e., in the pulmonary arterial circulation or the RV itself). The clinical settings include:

- Chronic obstructive pulmonary disease or other hypoxic lung disorders
- Primary pulmonary hypertension
- Pulmonary embolism
- RV infarction or cardiomyopathy
- Tricuspid stenosis

28. Name the main epicardial coronary arteries.
- The left coronary system, including the left main coronary artery (LMCA), which takes off from the aorta at the level of the left sinus of Valsalva and bifurcates into the left anterior descending artery (LAD) and the left circumflex artery (LCx)
- The right coronary system, represented by the right coronary artery (RCA), originating from the aorta at the level of the right sinus of Valsalva

29. What are the angiographic characteristics of the normal LMCA?
The LMCA arises from the upper portion of the left aortic coronary sinus, passes behind the RV outflow tract, and extends over a distance of ≤ 10 mm. This artery has a diameter of 4–6 mm. Rarely, the LMCA is absent, and the LAD and LCx have separate aortic ostia.

30. List the preferred angiographic views for assessing the LMCA.
1. The **ostium** is seen best from the anteroposterior (AP) projection.
2. The **main course of the artery** is seen best from the RAO caudal projection.
3. The **bifurcation** of the LMCA into the LAD and LCx is seen best from the LAO caudal projection, also called *spider view* (Fig. 2)

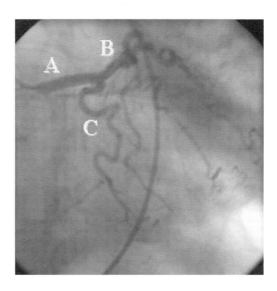

FIGURE 2. LMCA from the LAO caudal projection ("spider view"). The figure shows the LMCA bifurcation (A) into the LAD (B) and the LCx (C).

31. Name a useful clinical maneuver that allows better imaging of the LMCA in overweight patients.
Forced expiration accentuates the horizontal position of the heart in overweight patients and allows for a better imaging of the vessel.

32. What are the angiographic characteristics of the LAD?
The LAD passes down the anterior interventricular groove toward the apex of the heart. The **septal** branches originate from the LAD at a 90° angle and perfuse the IVS. The **diagonal** branches of the LAD pass over the anterolateral aspect of the heart and are present in 99% of patients and supply the anterior and lateral segments of the myocardium.

33. List the main branches of the LAD.
Proximal LAD—between the LAD ostium and the emergence of the first diagonal branch

Mid LAD—comprising approximately 50% of the rest of the artery (the mid LAD is often referred to as the segment between the first two large diagonal arteries)

Distal LAD—including the rest of the artery

Figure 3 illustrates a patient with a normal left coronary system (normal LMCA, LAD, and LCx).

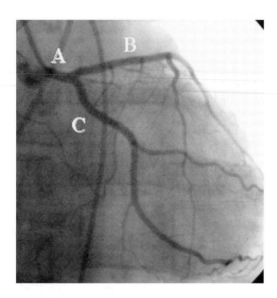

FIGURE 3. Normal left coronary system, LAO view. LMCA (A); LAD (B); LCx (C).

34. What are the best views for assessing the LAD coronary artery?

1. The **ostium and the proximal portion** of the LAD are seen well from any of the following **caudal** projections: RAO, AP, or LAO.

2. The **mid and distal portions** of the artery are seen best from the following **cranial** projections: RAO, left lateral, or AP.

3. The **diagonal branches** are assessed best from the following **cranial** views: LAO or RAO.

35. Describe the angiographic characteristics of the LCx.

The LCx originates at the bifurcation of the LMCA and passes down the left atrioventricular (AV) groove (see Figure 3). The LCx gives rise to several oblique marginal branches, which supply the lateral wall of the LV and, in patients with a dominant left circulation, the inferior portion of the IVS. The LCx generally is divided into a proximal and a distal segment, separated by the takeoff of the first marginal branch. Frequently a diminutive LCx gives rise to a large first marginal, which carries the bulk of the blood flow to the myocardium.

36. What are the preferred angiographic views for assessing the LCx?

1. The **ostium and the proximal segment** are seen best from the following caudal views: LAO, RAO, or posteroanterior.

2. The **midportion** is seen best from the RAO caudal view.

3. The **distal portion** is seen best the RAO cranial views, especially in subjects with a left dominant system, in whom the left posterior descending coronary artery (PDA) originates from the LCx.

4. The **marginal branches** are seen best from either the RAO or the LAO caudal (spider) views.

37. What is the ramus medianus, and what is the optimal view for its visualization in the catheterization laboratory?

Occasionally, there is a third artery originating from the LMCA, called the *ramus medianus* (Latin for "mid branch"), running a course similar to that of the first marginal branch from the LCx. The best view to assess the ramus medianus is the AP caudal projection.

38. Describe the angiographic characteristics of the RCA.

The RCA originates from the right sinus of Valsalva, at a point slightly caudal to the origin of the LMCA. It passes down the right AV groove toward the crux. The RCA generally is divided into three portions (proximal, mid, and distal), which correspond to the two horizontal portions and one vertical portion of the artery (Fig. 4). The RCA gives rise to:

- **Acute marginal branches** (these supply the RV free wall)
- **Conus branch,** which supplies blood to the RV outflow tract

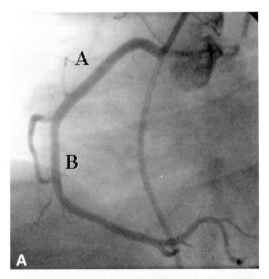

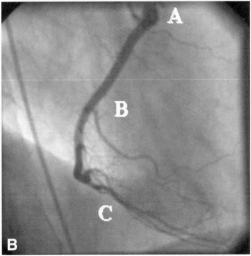

FIGURE 4. *A,* Normal RCA (LAO view). The standard left anterior oblique (LAO) view is very useful for assessing the proximal (A) and mid portions (B) of the right coronary artery (RCA). *B,* Normal RCA (RAO view). Proximal segment (A); mid segment (B); distal segment (C). (*continued*)

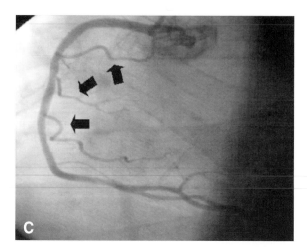

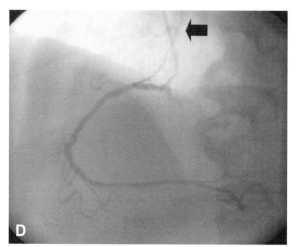

FIGURE 4. (*continued*) *C,* Acute marginal branches (*arrows*). LAO view of the RCA. *D,* The conus branch (*arrow*). LAO view of the RCA. *E,* The posterolateral branch (*arrow*) originating from the RCA in a patient with a right dominant circulation.

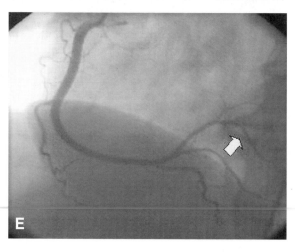

- **AV node artery**
- **Sinus node artery** (in 60% of cases; in the remainder of cases, the sinus node artery originates from the LCx)
- **Posterolateral branch,** in patients with a right dominant circulation

39. What are the preferred angiographic views for assessing the RCA?
- **LAO,** for the proximal and mid portions of the artery
- **RAO,** for the distal portion
- **Left lateral,** for the mid portion

40. What is coronary dominance, and what is its importance?
The vessel that gives rise to the PDA and supplies blood to the inferior portion of the IVS is considered dominant. The two coronary arteries that can give rise to the PDA are the RCA and the LCx. Because of the greater extent of supplied myocardium, coronary disease in a dominant artery is significantly more important than that occurring in a nondominant vessel.

41. What percentage of the general population has a right dominant circulation?
Approximately 85%. In this case, the LCx provides branches to the lateral free wall of the LV but does not reach the cardiac crux (Fig. 5).

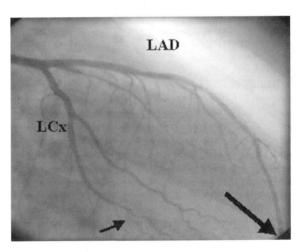
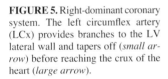

FIGURE 5. Right-dominant coronary system. The left circumflex artery (LCx) provides branches to the LV lateral wall and tapers off (*small arrow*) before reaching the crux of the heart (*large arrow*).

42. What percentage of the general population has a left dominant circulation?
In about 8% of subjects, the LCx provides blood supply to the PDA, the posterolateral LV branch, and the AV nodal artery. In these patients, the RCA supplies blood only to the RA and the RV and generally has limited clinical importance (Fig. 6).

43. What is considered a balanced-dominant circulation?
In approximately 7% of subjects, the blood supply to the inferior portion of the IVS is provided equally by the RCA and the LCx, with the RCA giving rise to the PDA and the LCx giving rise to the posterolateral and to a branch that supplies the IVS. This type of circulation is called *balanced-dominant.*

44. What are the most common coronary artery anomalies?
The RCA and the LMCA normally arise from the coronary ostia, located in the central part of right and left aortic sinus of Valsalva. In 1–2% of patients, there are anatomic variations termed *coronary anomalies.* The coronary anomalies include:

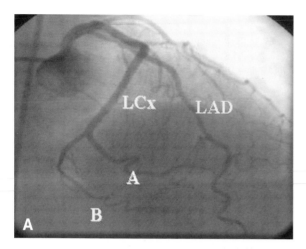

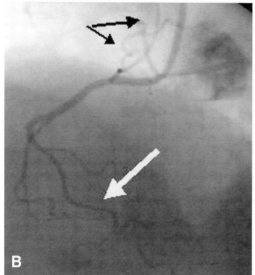

FIGURE 6. *A,* Left-dominant coronary system. The left circumflex artery (LCx) supplies the posterior descending artery (A) and the posterolateral artery (B); LAD-left anterior descending artery. *B,* Left-dominant coronary system. RCA supplies blood only to the right atrium (*black arrows*) and right ventricle (*white arrow*).

1. The origin of the LAD and the LCx from separate ostia, rather than as branches from the LMCA bifurcation. This is the most common anomalous coronary artery origin.

2. The origin of the LCx from the RCA or from the right sinus of Valsalva. This is the second most common anomaly, in regard to the origin of the coronary arteries (Fig. 7).

3. High origin of the RCA and a left coronary artery originating from the right aortic sinus of Valsalva.

4. Coronary artery fistula, most often from the RCA into the RV. These fistulas are often asymptomatic, but may be associated with ischemia, endocarditis, high-output heart failure, or rupture; this is the most common coronary anomaly.

45. Discuss the clinical importance of the coronary anomalies.

The possibility of **mistaking** separate coronary ostia for evidence of ostium occlusion of one of the coronaries (e.g., the mistaken diagnosis of an occluded LCx when this artery does not opacify on injection of contrast material through what is supposed to be the ostium of the LMCA,

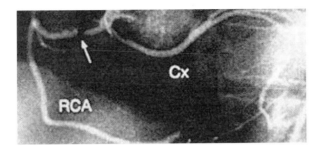

FIGURE 7. Anomalous origin of the left circumflex artery (Cx) from the ostium of the right coronary artery (RCA). The arrow indicates the common ostium of the two arteries.

but is in fact the separate ostium of the LAD) is perhaps the greatest practical importance of coronary anomalies. **Coronary ischemia** is seen in the infrequent patient in whom the LMCA originates from the PA an anomalous artery courses between the aorta and PA. **Sudden death** is seen in patients in whom the LMCA originates from the RCA or right sinus of Valsalva and subsequently travels between the aorta and the PA.

46. What is the preferred angiographic view used for assessing the aortic arch in the catheterization laboratory?

LAO projection (Fig. 8).

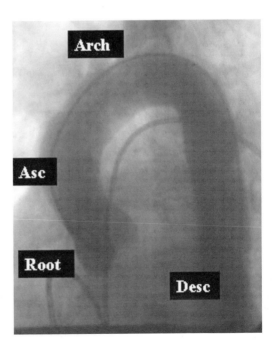

FIGURE 8. Aortography. The segments of the thoracic aorta from the LAO view.

47. Does coronary angiography have a role in the visualization of the RV?

Angiographic visualization of the RV (right ventriculography) is carried out infrequently in adults, owing to the complex three-dimensional (3-D) geometry of the RV; echocardiography and magnetic resonance imaging (MRI) are the imaging procedures of choice for this indication. Right ventriculography remains an important diagnostic tool in children with congenital heart disease, although MRI technology is assuming an increasing role in this setting.

48. What are the characteristics of the normal pulmonary artery as visualized in the catheterization laboratory?

The normal pulmonary artery is seen by direct injection of contrast material into the pulmonary artery through a central venous catheter. The main pulmonary artery divides into the left and the right pulmonary arteries, which subdivide further into smaller branches in the pulmonary parenchyma. The normal pulmonary artery does not show any filling defect and tapers smoothly toward its distal course.

ECHOCARDIOGRAPHY

Steven A. Goldstein, M.D., Gabriel Adelmann, M.D., Benjamin Kleiber, M.D., and Neil J. Weissman, M.D.

49. Summarize the main anatomic and functional data provided by echocardiography concerning the heart *chambers*.

Anatomic data
- Systolic and diastolic dimensions and shape of the atria and ventricles
- Systolic and diastolic myocardial wall thickness
- Presence of communication between the right and the left side of the heart (patent foramen ovale, atrial septal defect, ventricular septal defect)
- Presence and nature of intracardiac masses (thrombi; tumors; or man-made devices, such as lines, wires, and prosthetic valves)
- Information concerning the texture of the myocardium (normal versus infiltrated, calcified or scarred myocardium)
- Presence of pericardial effusion and effect of the effusion on ventricular function (see later)

Functional data
- Global and segmental function of the LV myocardium in systole and diastole
- Blood flow through the heart chambers

50. Summarize the main anatomic and functional data provided by echocardiography concerning the heart valves.

Anatomic data
- Thickness and motion of the valves
- Calcification of the valve leaflets or annulus
- Subvalvular apparatus (papillary muscles and chordae tendinae)
- Identification of valvular vegetation or abscess (or both) in patients with endocarditis
- Identification of valvular malformation in patients with congenital heart disease
- Assessment of prosthetic valves

Functional data
- Timing and completeness of valve opening and closure
- Velocity and direction of blood flow through the normal or prosthetic heart valves, allowing assessment of stenosis or regurgitation (or both)

51. Summarize the main anatomic and functional data provided by echocardiography concerning the large vessels of the heart and the coronary arteries.

Anatomic data
- Proximal ascending aorta (and, on transesophageal echocardiography [TEE], the aortic arch and part of the descending aorta), allowing diagnosis of atherosclerosis, calcification, dissection, intramural hematoma, aneurysm, coarctation, and extrinsic compression
- Main pulmonary artery and its main branches, allowing diagnosis of pulmonary hypertension and embolism and congenital abnormalities of the pulmonary vessels
- Pulmonary vein drainage into the LA

- Coronary sinus
- Anatomic variants of blood vessels, such as a persistent left superior vena cava (SVC)
- Ostia of the LMCA and the RCA
- Relationship between the great vessels and the two ventricles

Functional data (obtained by Doppler studies)
- Abnormal flow in patients with pathology of the aorta and great vessels
- Altered pulmonary blood flow in patients with pulmonary artery disease
- Pulmonary venous flow patterns, allowing indirect assessment of the severity of mitral regurgitation, LV compliance, and pericardial pathology (tamponade, constriction)
- Analysis of the hepatic venous flow patterns, allowing indirect assessment of the severity of tricuspid regurgitation and pericardial pathology

52. Summarize the main anatomic and functional data provided by echocardiography concerning the pericardium.

Anatomic data
- Pericardial effusion or thrombus
- Pericardial calcification

It is generally difficult to assess pericardial thickness by echocardiography.

Functional data are obtained indirectly, based on the analysis of mitral, tricuspid, pulmonary venous, and hepatic venous flow, and contribute to the diagnosis of pericardial tamponade and constrictive pericarditis.

53. Name the normal structure that can mimic an anterior pericardial effusion.

Pericardial fat often is seen in the parasternal long-axis view as an echo-free space anterior to the RV free wall and can mimic a pericardial effusion. True pericardial effusions tend to accumulate first posteriorly, however, owing to gravity. Pericardial fat also tends to have some small "echoes" within the fat (Fig. 9).

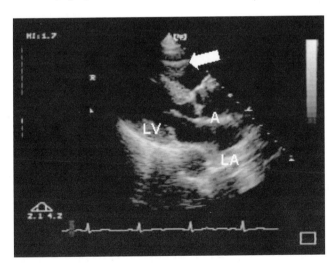

FIGURE 9. Epicardial fat. An isolated anterior echo-free space most frequently represents epicardial fat; LV = left ventricle, LA = left atrium, A = aorta.

54. What anatomic characteristic of the pericardium is the most difficult to evaluate by echocardiography?

Pericardial thickness is generally difficult to evaluate reliably by either transthoracic echocardiography (TTE) or TEE. MRI is a better imaging modality for assessing pericardial thickness.

55. What are normal echocardiographic dimensions of the left heart structures?

Selected Normal Echocardiographic Dimensions in Adults

	RANGE	RANGE INDEXED TO BSA	UPPER LIMIT OF NORMAL
Aorta			
Annulus diameter (cm)	1.4–2.6	1.3 ± 01 cm/m^2	< 1.6 cm/m^2 (men and women)
Diameter at leaflet tips (cm)	2.2–3.6	1.7 ± 0.2 cm/m^2	< 2.1 cm/m^2 (men and women)
Ascending aorta diamter (cm)	2.1–3.4	1.5 ± 0.2 cm/m^2	
Arch diameter (cm)	2.0–3.6		
Left Ventricle			
Short-axis dimension (cm)			
Diastole	3.5–6.0	2.3–3.1 cm/m^2	
Systole	2.1–4.0	1.4–2.1 cm/m^2	
Long-axis dimension (cm)			
Diastole	6.3–10.3	4.1–5.7 cm/m^2	
Systole	4.6–8.4		
End-diastolic volume (ml)			
Men	96–157	67 ± 9 ml	
Women	59–138	61 ± 13 ml	
End-systolic volume (ml)			
Men	33–68	27 ± 5 ml	
Women	18–65	26 ± 7 ml	
Ejection fraction (%)			
Men	0.59 ± 0.06		
Women	0.58 ± 0.07		
LV-wall thickness (cm) (end-diastolic)	0.6–1.1		Men ≤ 1.2 cm Women ≤ 1.1 cm
LV mass (g)			
Men	< 294 g	109 ± 20 g/m^2	< 143 g/m^2
Women	< 198 g	89 ± 15 g/m^2	< 102 g/m^2
Left Atrium			
Anterior-posterior dimension (cm) (PLAX)	2.3–4.5	1.6–2.4 cm/m^2	
Medial-lateral dimension (cm) (A4C)	2.5–4.5	1.6–2.4 cm/m^2	
Superior-inferior dimension (cm) (A4C)	3.4–6.1	2.3–3.5 cm/m^2	
Mitral Annulus			
End-diastole (cm)	2.7–0.4		
End systole (cm)	2.9–0.3		
Right Ventricle			
Wall thickness (cm)	0.2–0.5	0.2 ± 0.05 cm/m^2	
Minor dimension (cm)	2.2–4.4	1.0–2.8 cm/m^2	
Length			
Diastole (cm)	5.5–9.5	3.8–5.3 cm/m^2	
Systole (cm)	4.2–8.1		
Pulmonary Artery			
Annulus diameter (cm)	1.0–2.2		
Main PA (cm)	0.9–2.9		
Inferior Vena Cava Diameters (at RA juncion) (cm)	1.2–2.3		

BSA = body surface area; LV = left ventricle; PA = pulmonary artery; RA = right atrium.

References: Roman et al, AJC 1989 64:507; Schnittger et al, JACC 1983 2:934; Truiulzi et al, Echo 1984 1:403; Levy et al, AJC 1987 59:936; Pearlman et al, JACC 1988 12:1432; Pini et al, Circulation 1989 80:915; Erbel Dtsch Med Wschr 107:1872 (1982); Hahan et al, Z Kardiol 1982 71:445.

From Otto CM: Textbook of Clinical Echocardiography, 2nd ed. Philadelphia, W.B. Saunders, 2000, p 35, with permission.

56. At what level of the LV should the wall thickness and chamber diameter be measured in an echocardiographic study?

The LV thickness and LV cavity diameter (LV internal diameter) should be assessed at the tip of the mitral valve leaflets; this is usually done in the parasternal long-axis view measuring directly from the two-dimensional (2-D) image or with a 2-D–guided M-mode (Fig. 10).

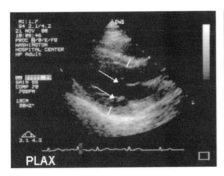
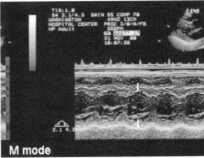

FIGURE 10. Demonstration of echo measurement of left ventricle thickness and diameter 2-D and M mode. LV thickness and chamber diameter should be assessed at the tip of the mitral valve leaflets (*arrows*). Thickness is assessed at the end of diastole, either on a 2-D or an M-mode tracing

57. Which cardiac structures are seen on the parasternal long-axis view?

Heart walls
RV free wall
IVS
LV posterior wall

Heart valves
Mitral valve
Aortic valve

Vessels
Aorta
Coronary sinus

This imaging plane also allows visualization of the anterior and posterior portions of the pericardial space, overlying and below the RV free wall and the LV posterior wall (Fig. 11).

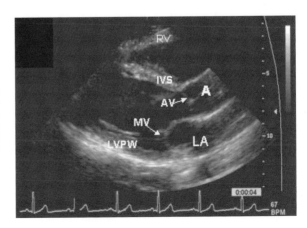

FIGURE 11. Parasternal long axis. LV = left ventricle, RV = right ventricle, LA = left atrium, A = aorta, IVS = interventricular septum, IVS = interventricular septum, MV = mitral valve, AV = aortic valve, LVPW = left ventricular posterior wall.

58. Is the parasternal long-axis view the appropriate view to visualize overall LV function?

The parasternal view is usually the first view obtained and gives an overall impression of LV function, but it does not visualize the LV apex, lateral wall, or true anterior wall. Occasionally a foreshortened (oblique) section through the anterolateral wall of the LV may be mistaken for the true apex.

59. Which papillary muscle can be visualized from the parasternal long-axis view, and why is this important?

Ideally the parasternal long-axis view would not display the papillary muscles. Many times, as the heart moves in and out of the imaging plane, the posteromedial papillary muscle comes into view. This muscle is "superimposed" on the posterior wall of the LV and may be mistaken for an ample movement, or contraction, of the posterior wall. This may lead to error in the assessment of the LV posterior wall thickness and motion. Thinning of the posterior myocardial wall after myocardial infarction can be missed if this wall is measured from the endocardial border of the papillary muscle.

60. How much of the aorta can be visualized from the parasternal long-axis view?

The first 3–4 cm of the ascending aorta may be seen anterior to the LA. This allows assessment of the aortic valve, sinuses of Valsalva, sinotubular junction, and proximal portion of the ascending aorta (see Figure 11).

61. Which cardiac structures can be imaged from the parasternal short-axis view?

The parasternal short-axis view can be obtained at multiple levels of the heart: at the level of the aortic valve, level of the mitral valve, mid papillary level, or the apex of the heart. The main short-axis cuts used in clinical practice and the respective cardiac structures visualized from each cut are as follows:

- At the level of the aortic valve: the aortic and the tricuspid valves the RV, the RA and LA, the interatrial septum, and the main pulmonary artery (MPA) (Fig. 12A)
- At the level of the mitral valve: mainly the mitral valve (Fig. 12B)
- At the mid papillary level: the LV and the RV (Fig. 12C)
- At the apex: the LV apex (Fig. 12D)

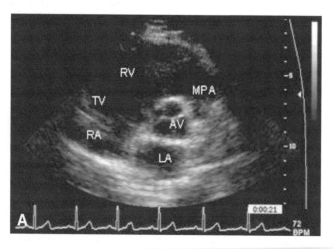

FIGURE 12. *A,* Parasternal short axis at the aortic valve level. LV = left ventricle, RV = right ventricle, TV = tricuspid valve, LA = left atrium, A = aorta, IVS = interventricular septum, MV = mitral valve, AV = aortic valve, MPA = main pulmonary artery. *B,* Parasternal short axis at the mitral valve level. RV = right ventricle, MV = mitral valve. *C,* Parasternal short axis at the mid-LV level. *D,* Parasternal short axis at the apex. LV = left ventricle.

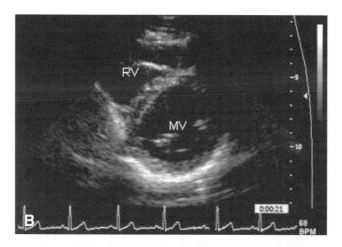

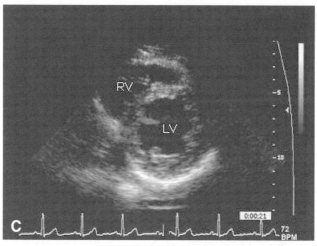

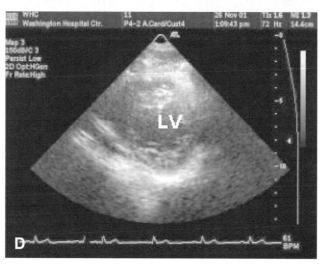

62. List the structures visualized from the apical four-chamber view.
    Heart walls
        RV free wall (Fig. 13)
        IVS
        LV lateral wall
        LV apex
    Heart valves
        Mitral valve
        Tricuspid valve
    Vessels
        Aorta (only if the transducer is angled anteriorly, to obtain a "5-chamber view")
        Pulmonary veins
        Coronary sinus (only if the transducer is angled posteriorly)

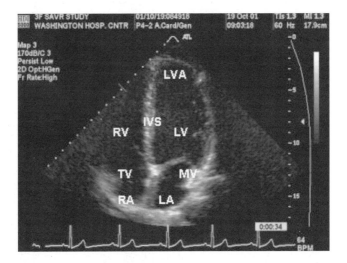

FIGURE 13. Apical four-chamber view. LV = left ventricle, LVA = LV apex, RV = right ventricle, TV = tricuspid valve, LA = left atrium, RA = right atrium, IVS = interventricular septum, MV = mitral valve, AV = aortic valve.

63. Name the fifth chamber seen in the apical five-chamber view.
    The proximal ascending aorta (see question 62) (Fig. 14).

64. Which structures are visualized from the apical three-chamber view (also known as the apical long-axis view)?
    This view is the same imaging plane through the heart as that obtained from the parasternal long-axis view; the structures viewed are also the same (Fig. 15).
    Heart walls
        RV free wall
        IVS
        LV posterior wall
    Heart valves
        Mitral valve
        Aortic valve
    Vessels
        Aortic root
        Coronary sinus

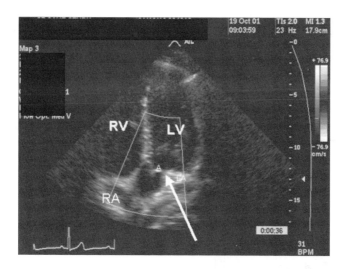

FIGURE 14. Apical five-chamber view. LV = left ventricle, RV = right ventricle, LA = left atrium, RA = right atrium, A = aorta. (See also Color Plates, Figure 5.)

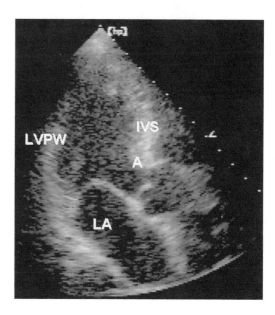

FIGURE 15. Apical three-chamber view. LVPW = LV posterior wall, LA = left atrium, A = aorta, IVS = interventricular septum.

65. List the sructures visualized from the apical two-chamber view.
   Heart walls (Fig. 16)
      LV inferior wall
      LV anterior wall
   Valves
      Mitral valve

66. What structures are visualized from the subcostal view?
   In the subcostal view, the ultrasound waves cross the liver to reach the heart. Although virtually any section plane through the heart can be obtained, the most commonly used planes are

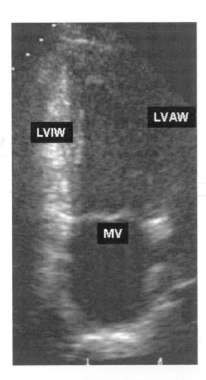

FIGURE 16. Apical two-chamber view. LVIW = inferior wall of the LV; LVAW = anterior wall of the LV; MV = mitral valve.

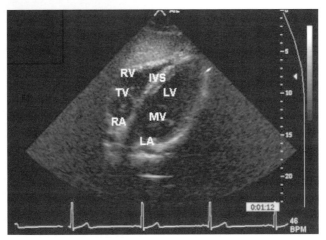

FIGURE 17. Subcostal view. LV = left ventricle, MV = mitral valve, LA = left atrium, RV = right ventricle, TV = tricuspid valve, RA = right atrium, IVS = interventricular septum.

identical to the apical four-chamber view (Fig. 17) or parasternal short-axis view. The subcostal view is particularly helpful when imaging from the chest (e.g., immediately after cardiac surgery) is not possible.

67. Describe the different LV segments, as seen from the standard echocardiographic views.

According to the new guidelines of the American Heart Association, in conjunction with the American Society of Echocardiography, American Society of Nuclear Cardiology, and several other cardiac imaging societies, the LV is divided into 17 segments. Basically the LV is considered to have six walls: anterior, anterolateral, inferolateral, inferior, inferoseptal, and anteroseptal. Each of these walls is subdivided further into a basal segment, a midventricular segment, and an apical segment (which has only four segments) and an apical "cap" devoid of LV cavity (Fig. 18).

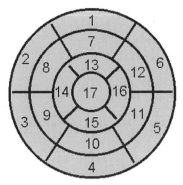

1. basal anterior	7. mid anterior	13. apical anterior
2. basal anteroseptal	8. mid anteroseptal	14. apical septal
3. basal inferoseptal	9. mid inferoseptal	15. apical inferior
4. basal inferior	10. mid inferior	16. apical lateral
5. basal inferolateral	11. mid inferolateral	17. apex
6. basal anterolateral	12. mid anterolateral	

FIGURE 18. Schematic of the left ventricle segmentation.

68. Compare the 3-D geometry of the two ventricles.
   The **LV** has an elliptical shape. This chamber appears circular in short-axis views and ovoidal in long-axis views.
   The **RV** is "wrapped around" the LV and is flattened anteroposteriorly. As a result of its complex structure, the RV appears foreshortened from most echocardiographic planes and must be assessed from as many imaging angles as possible. The RV is seen as a crude triangular structure from the apical four-chamber view and as a "sausage" or "half-moon" wrapping around the LV from the short-axis view. The true 3-D shape, volume, and function of the RV would be appreciated better from 3-D imaging rather than current 2-D echocardiography.

69. Explain the anatomic relationship between the two papillary muscles and the two leaflets of the mitral valve.
   Each of the two papillary muscles is connected to both mitral valve leaflets. Chordae from the anterolateral papillary muscle connect to the lateral aspects of the leaflets, whereas chordae from the posteromedial papillary muscle connect to the medial aspects of the leaflets.

70. What are the characteristics of the normal mitral valve?
   - Wide separation of the leaflets in diastole, with the anterior leaflet coming in close proximity to the septum
   - A high degree of leaflet coaptation in systole (6–12 mm of the tip part of the leaflets superimpose)
   - Leaflet thickness < 5 mm
   - Absence of valve calcification in the leaflet or annulus
   The subvalvular apparatus, an integral part of mitral valve evaluation and function, includes the chordae tendinae (thin and mobile structures tether the valves to the papillary muscles) and the papillary muscles. The integrity and lack of calcification of these strictures are assessed carefully as part of the mitral valve assessment.

71. What is the echocardiographic appearance of the normal mitral valve annulus?

The mitral annulus is the junction between the LA, the LV, and the mitral valve leaflets. It is a frequent site for calcification, especially along the posterior part of its circumference.

72. Describe the three-dimensional anatomy of the mitral valve annulus.

The mitral valve annulus is saddle-shaped, with the anterior and posterior borders farthest from the apex and the medial and lateral borders closest to the apex. From an echocardiographic perspective, the higher parts of the annulus (furthest from the apex) are seen in their correct location in the parasternal *long*-axis view but represent the lowest aspects of the annulus in the apical four-chamber view. As a result, the mitral valve may appear above the annulus in the apical four-chamber view and falsely suggest mitral valve prolapse but appear normally positioned in the long-axis view. *Only the long-axis view is used to diagnose mitral valve prolapse.* In the early days of echocardiography, before the complex shape of the mitral valve was realized, a false diagnosis of mitral valve prolapse was made in 30% of otherwise healthy subjects (Fig. 19).

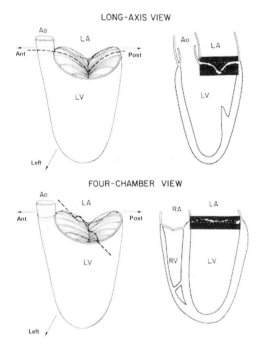

FIGURE 19. The saddle-shape of the MV. (From Levine RA, Triulzi MO, Harrigan P, Weyman AE: The relationship of mitral annular shape to the diagnosis of mitral valve prolapse. Circulation 75:756–767, 1987, with permission.)

73. Describe the M-mode anatomy of the mitral valve.

An M-mode study of the mitral valve from the parasternal long-axis view shows the two valve leaflets moving in mirror-image fashion, with systolic coaptation and diastolic separation. The diastolic valve motion reflects the period during which there is transvalvular blood flow, with two peaks noted in sinus rhythm: an early systolic peak (E point) and a late systolic peak (A point) (Fig. 20).

74. Describe the normal transmitral blood flow on Doppler.

In normal subjects, the LV fills in diastole. LV filling is not uniform but is accomplished during four successive phases, characterized by different LA/LV pressure gradients. The different phases of diastole are:

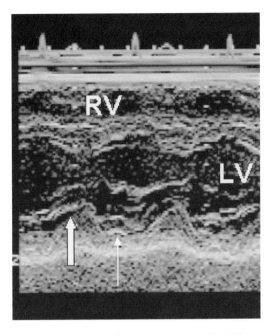

FIGURE 20. M-mode anatomy of the mitral valve. The M-mode study intercepts both mitral valve leaflets, moving in a mirror-image fashion. The leaflets coapt during systole (*thick arrows*) and separate during diastole (*thin arrows*). LV = left ventricle; RV = right ventricle.

    Isovolumic relaxation—when the mitral valve is closed, and there is no ventricular filling
    Early (rapid) diastolic filling—the passive LV filling stage designated by the transmitral Doppler E wave
    Diastasis—LV/LA pressure equalization with near-absent flow through the mitral valve
    Late diastolic (atrial) filling—atrial systole designated by the transmitral Doppler A wave

75. List the important parameters of the mitral E and A waves.
- The peak E wave velocity (mean of 0.6–0.7 m/sec at < 70 years old and 0.4 m/sec afterward)
- Peak A velocity (mean of 0.4 m/sec at < 50 years old and 0.6 m/sec afterward)
- E/A peak velocity ratio (mean of 2 m/sec at < 50 years old, 1 m/sec in patients 50–70 years old, and < 1 m/sec afterward)
- E wave deceleration time, which represents the time interval between the moment of peak velocity and the end of flow (> 140 m/sec at < 70 years old and > 90 m/sec afterward) (Fig. 21)

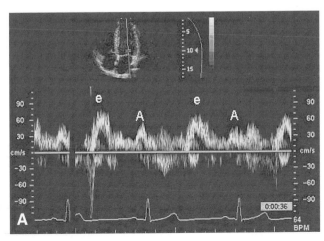

FIGURE 21. *A,* Pulsed wave Doppler of the MV, from the apical four-chamber view. e = e wave, A = A wave. (*continued*)

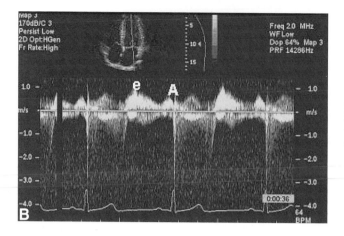

FIGURE 21. (*continued*) *B*, Continuous wave Doppler of the MV from the apical four-chamber view.

76. What is the importance of the E and A waves?

These parameters help characterize the LV diastolic function because they represent the filling of the heart during diastole. Also, the E wave velocity offers indirect information concerning the severity of mitral regurgitation.

77. The M-mode echo of the mitral valve has two peaks (the E and A points), the Doppler recording from mitral inflow has an E wave and an A wave, and the LV wall motion on tissue Doppler has two components (e and a). Why is the same nomenclature used for M-mode, Doppler, and tissue Doppler?

The E (e) and A (a) waves and peaks represent a measure of the same diastolic events:

- The Doppler E and A waves represent the two velocity peaks of transmitral blood flow in diastole.
- The M-mode E and A points reflect the corresponding points of maximum mitral leaflet excursion.
- The e and a waves reflect the corresponding myocardial excursion in diastole.

78. Under what circumstances will the A (a) peak/wave be absent?

When there is no mechanical activity (contraction) of the LA, most frequently in patients with atrial fibrillation.

79. What auscultatory finding corresponds to the Doppler A wave?

The fourth heart sound.

80. The normal aortic valve has three leaflets. How can the number of leaflets of the aortic valve be determined?

The number of leaflets can be assessed from the parasternal short-axis view at the level of the aortic valve. This *en face* view allows visualization of all three leaflets. The final assessment of the number of leaflets should be ascertained in early systole, when the leaflets separate along three lines (resembling the letter *Y*). The presence of a raphe (in the case of a bicuspid aortic valve) can mimic a valvular coaptation line in diastole and can be missed if the valve is evaluated only in diastole.

81. What is a nodule of Arantius?

The normal aortic valve leaflets are thin and mobile but display an area of focal thickening at the middle of their free edge, at the point of coaptation of the three leaflets. These normal structures enlarge with age and have a nodular aspect that first was described by the anatomist Arantius.

82. Are the mitral and the aortic valve annuli anatomically similar?

No. Although the *mitral annulus* is a well-defined fibrous structure at the confluence of the mitral leaflets, LA, and LV, the *aortic annulus* is not a discrete anatomic structure. The aortic annulus represents the circumference of the aortic valve, where the valve leaflets are attached to the aortic root. In the absence of calcification, neither the mitral annulus nor the aortic annulus is normally visualized by echocardiography.

83. Describe the M-mode anatomy of the aortic valve (parasternal long-axis view).

Typically the aortic valve has a rectangular box appearance, with a distance of approximately 2 cm between the two horizontal edges. In diastole, the aortic leaflets coapt and form a thin line. To understand this configuration, remember that M-mode depicts the motion of a set of points in time. The box shape does not describe the shape of the aortic valve, but rather the systolic motion (separation, open position, and finally reconvergence) of the two aortic leaflets (right and noncoronary) that are intersected by the ultrasound beam. The opening pattern of the aortic valve can be affected whenever the blood flow through the valve is diminished, as in patients with LV dysfunction or when there is an anatomic obstacle to valve opening (valvular, subvalvular or supravalvular stenosis) (Fig. 22).

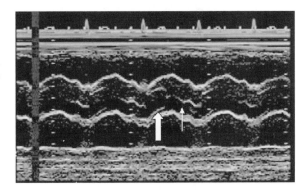

FIGURE 22. M-mode anatomy of the aortic valve. The typical aspect of the aortic valve on an M-mode study from the parasternal long axis view is roughly that of a rectangular "box." *Large arrows* = diastole; *small arrows* = systole.

84. Describe the normal Doppler blood flow pattern across the aortic valve.

The normal Doppler aortic tracing includes a steep acceleration slope and a less steep deceleration slope. The onset of flow occurs just after the onset of the Q wave of the electrocardiogram (ECG), at the end of isovolumic contraction. The aortic valve flow velocity is usually 1.0–1.8 m/sec (Fig. 23).

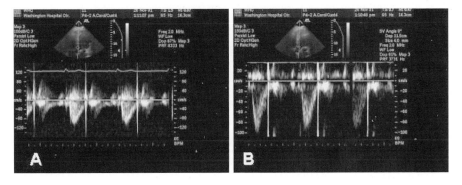

FIGURE 23. Normal aortic blood flow by CW (A) and PW (B) Doppler. The normal aortic blood flow is represented by a systolic Doppler tracing with a steep acceleration slope and a less steep deceleration slope. The velocity of blood flow through the aortic valve is of 1–1.8 m/sec.

85. What is the significance of the area under the aortic blood flow velocity curve?

This area (called the *time-velocity integral*) is proportional to the stroke volume.

86. How do the Doppler patterns (and blood flow) through the tricuspid and the pulmonary valve compare with the flow through mitral and aortic valves?

The blood flow through the tricuspid and pulmonic valves closely resembles flow through the mitral and aortic valves, but the flow velocities on the right side of the heart are lower than on the left side (Fig. 24).

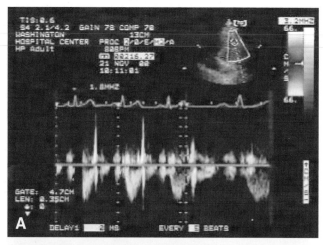

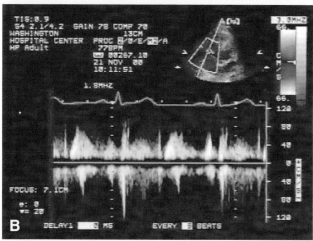

FIGURE 24. *A,* Normal pulmonic valve flow by Doppler. *B,* Normal tricuspid valve flow by Doppler. (See also Color Plates, Figures 6 and 7.)

87. How might the IVS in elderly patients differ from the septum in younger patients?

A common anatomic variant in elderly subjects is the so-called **sigmoid septum,** which represents a disproportionate upper septal hypertrophy at the base of the IVS. In contrast to the asymmetric hypertrophy of hypertrophic cardiomyopathy, the sigmoid septum usually does not cause increased subaortic obstruction or mitral regurgitation. Many believe that a sigmoid septum is due to long-standing hypertension (Fig. 25).

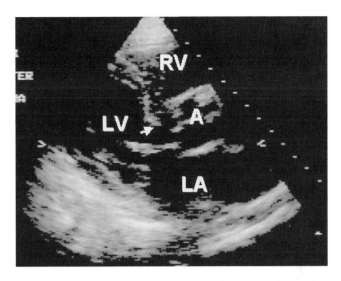

FIGURE 25. The sigmoid septum. A common anatomical variant in elderly subjects is the so-called sigmoid septum, a disproportionate hypertrophy of the base of the interventricular septum (*arrow*). LV = left ventricle, LA = left atrium.

88. What is the crista terminalis?

A muscular ridge coursing between the ostia of the SVC and the inferior vena cava (IVC). It separates the trabeculated anterior portion of the RA from the posterior, smooth-walled RA segment (Fig. 26). This structure can be appreciated best from the RV inflow view, which represents a modification of the parasternal long-axis view. It is believed to be a remnant of the sinus venosus.

FIGURE 26. Crista terminalis. The crista terminalis (*arrow*) is a muscular ridge coursing between the ostia of the superior and the inferior vena cava, and separates the trabeculated anterior portion of the right atrium from the posterior, smooth-walled right atrial segment.

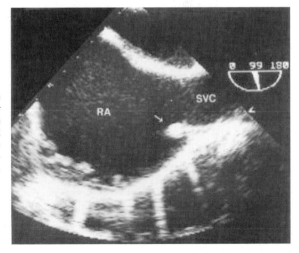

89. What is the moderator band?

A muscular trabeculation that traverses the RV apex and follows an oblique course. The moderator band can be seen easily by echocardiography and contains the right bundle branch.

90. A dilated coronary sinus can be due to several cardiac diseases. There is one anatomic variant, however, that also can result in a dilated coronary sinus without being indicative of a pathologic state. Discuss that variant.

In 0.3–0.5% of subjects, a persistent left SVC is present (versus the usual single SVC) draining into the coronary sinus. This causes dilation of the coronary sinus. A persistent left SVC is 10 times more frequent in patients with congenital heart disease. When a dilated coronary sinus is detected in the absence of other known causes (e.g., high RA pressure), agitated saline should be injected into a left arm peripheral vein; this agitated saline (contrast effect) opacifies the coronary sinus before it opacifies the RA.

Pitfalls

91. What are Lambl's excrescences?

These are thin (≤ 2 mm), linear, mobile structures attached to the atrial side of mitral and tricuspid valves or the ventricular side of aortic valves, near the leaflet closure lines (Fig. 27). Although the cause is uncertain, they are presumably "wear-and-tear" lesions. Lambl's excrescences are diagnosed by TEE and rarely by TTE because they are small. Lambl's excrescences often are identified mistakenly as vegetations.

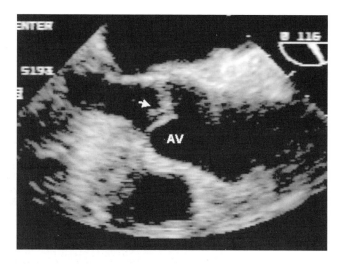

FIGURE 27. Lambl's excrescences. Lambl's excrescences (*arrow*) are small filiform processes attached to the ventricular surfaces of the aortic valve.

92. What is the eustachian valve?

The eustachian valve, also known as the *valve of the IVC*, is a normal ridge or membrane at the junction of the RA and IVC (Fig. 28). In utero, this valve directs blood from the IVC across the patent foramen ovale into the LA. This congenital remnant can be mistaken for a pathologic mass, such as a tumor, thrombus, or vegetation. Rarely, vegetations or blood clots can grow on the eustachian valve.

93. Define the Chiari network.

The Chiari network first was described by the anatomist Chiari in 1897. It is a highly mobile, fenestrated membrane that appears as an undulating linear density on the echocardiogram (Fig. 29). It extends obliquely across the RA from a site near the entrance of the IVC to a site near the opening of the coronary sinus. Chiari's network is found in approximately 1–5% of patients un-

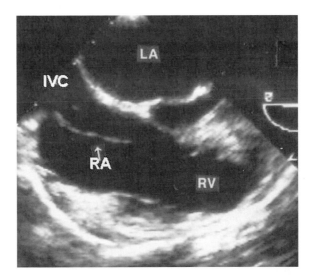

FIGURE 28. The eustachian valve. The eustachian valve (*arrow*), also known as the valve of the IVC, is a normal ridge or membrane at the junction of the right atrium and IVC. RV = right ventricle.

dergoing TTE and is more common in younger patients (believed to be a remnant of the sinus venosus valve). The importance of recognizing this congenital remnant lies mainly in its differentiation from pathologic RA masses, such as thrombus, vegetation, tumor, or catheter tips.

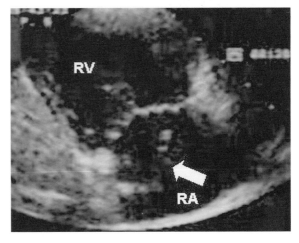

FIGURE 29. Chiari's network. Chiari's network (*arrow*) is a fenestrated membrane that is highly mobile and appears like an undulating linear density on the echocardiogram.

94. How can pectinate muscles in the LA appendage be distinguished from thrombi?

Pectinate muscles are muscular trabeculations in the walls of both atrial appendages and can be mistaken for masses or thrombi (on TEE). These muscular ridges are usually small and multiple and move in concert with the atrial wall. In contrast, thrombi typically have a different echodensity or texture than the atrial wall and may be pedunculated or mobile. Thrombi occur in conjunction with certain conditions, including atrial fibrillation, mitral stenosis, prosthetic mitral valve, dilated cardiomyopathy, or low-output states. Nevertheless, pectinate muscles cannot always be distinguished confidently from thrombi.

95. What is the transverse sinus?

A pericardial reflection between the LA and the great vessels, surrounded anteriorly by the ascending aorta, superiorly by the right pulmonary artery, and posteriorly by the LA. When it contains pericardial fluid, it may appear as a periaortic cavity.

96. Can certain TEE views of a normal aortic valve mimic a vegetation?

Yes. A commonly observed "mass" effect occurs when a cusp (usually the left coronary cusp) is cut tangentially. The appearance of the aortic cusp imaged *en face* may be mistaken for a vegetation or tumor. This pitfall is resolved easily with multiplane views of the aortic valve and emphasizes the importance of confirming true masses by viewing them in more than one imaging plane.

97. What is the structure indicated by the arrow in Figure 30?

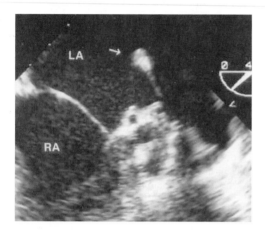

FIGURE 30. The Coumadin ridge (*arrow*) vs. LAA thrombus. LA = left atrium, RA = right atrium.

This echodensity, a ridge separating the LA appendage from the left upper pulmonary vein, is a normal variant. Its proximal portion is usually thin, and its distal portion is bulbous; its shape may resemble a cotton-tipped swab or a matchstick. It may be prominent in some patients and mimic a pathologic intracardiac mass, such as tumor or thrombus. It has been termed the *Coumadin ridge* because it is often misinterpreted as thrombus and mistakenly treated with warfarin (Coumadin).

98. What is the structure indicated by the arrow in Figure 31?

FIGURE 31. Lipomatous hypertrophy of the atrial septum (*arrowheads*). RV = right ventricle; RA = right atrium; LV = left ventricle.

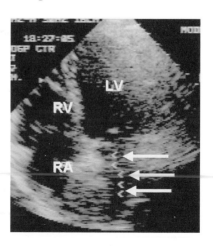

Lipomatous hypertrophy is the deposition of fat in the superior and inferior regions of the atrial septum. It is likely due to a proliferation of adipocytes rather than to true hypertrophy of individual cells. The pathognomonic bilobed or dumb bell shape of the atrial septum is due to sparing of the membrane of the fossa ovalis. The amount of fatty infiltration varies but can be impressive and can be mistaken for tumors such as myxoma, lipoma, and liposarcoma. Lipomatous hypertrophy is considered a benign finding but has been associated with several atrial arrhythmias.

99. What is the structure indicated by the arrow in Figure 32?

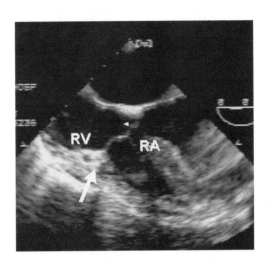

FIGURE 32. Adipose tissue in the tricuspid annulus. The tricuspid annulus at the atrioventricular (AV) groove normally contains variable amounts of adipose tissue (*arrow*). When excessive, it can be mistaken for a mass on echocardiography.

The tricuspid annulus at the AV groove normally contains variable amounts of adipose tissue. It also can be mistaken for a mass when visualized by echocardiography. Because of the motion of the AV groove toward the apex in systole, this echodense wedge, especially when excessive, can be misinterpreted as a tumor, thrombus, or abscess. Awareness of this pseudomass is important to avoid unnecessary and potentially dangerous surgery. MRI should be performed when the diagnosis remains in doubt.

NUCLEAR MEDICINE

Manuel D. Cerqueira, M.D. and Gabriel Adelmann, M.D.

100. What are the characteristics of a normal nuclear perfusion scan?

A normal nuclear perfusion scan shows equal uptake of radiotracer in all the myocardial segments, at rest and under conditions of stress. Care should be exercised not to misinterpret attenuation artifact caused by breast tissue or diaphragm for perfusion defects. A normal perfusion scan is shown in Figure 33.

101. How are the red blood cells labeled for an equilibrium radionuclide angiogram?

Equilibrium radionuclide angiogram commonly called *MUGA* (**mu**ltigated **a**cquisition), uses red blood cells radiolabeled by pretreatment with a stannous chloride solution that creates a favorable oxidation/reduction environment inside the cells. As a result, when the RBCs are exposed to technetium-99m pertechnetate, the radioactive compound is bound irreversibly to the hemoglobin in the red blood cells. The labeling can be done *in vitro* or *in vivo* or using a combination method. The cells circulate in the patient's intravascular space, and the ECG signal is used to acquire 16–32 individual time images or frames for each individual heartbeat. Each of the three planar views consists of 300–500 individual beats, which are summed (see Chapter 1).

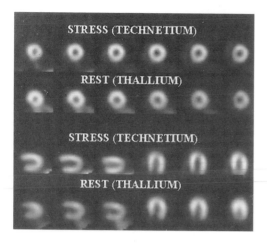

STRESS (TECHNETIUM)

REST (THALLIUM)

STRESS (TECHNETIUM)

REST (THALLIUM)

FIGURE 33. Normal myocardial perfusion, demonstrated by a dual isotope (stress with a techetium-99m tracer and at rest with thallium-201) SPECT perfusion scan. All the segments of the myocardium have equal radiotracer uptake. The dual isotope technique is discussed later in this chapter.

102. What are the characteristics of a normal study?

A normal MUGA scan shows a global ejection fraction > 50% and equal regional contribution (equal inward systolic endocardial motion of all the myocardial segments) to this global systolic function. A normal MUGA scan is shown in Figure 34.

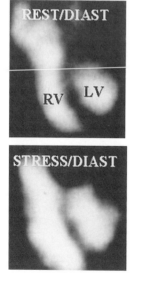
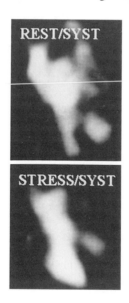

REST/DIAST

REST/SYST

RV   LV

STRESS/DIAST

STRESS/SYST

FIGURE 34. Normal left 45° anterior oblique MUGA scan at rest (*top*) and stress (*bottom*) for end diastole (DIAST) and end systole (SYST). At rest, the ejection fraction is 57%, and it increases to 70% with exercise stress. This is a normal response. A drop in ejection fraction by 5 ejection fraction units is abnormal and consistent with exercise-induced ischemia or some other form of cardiac disease.

103. What are the characteristics of a normal first-pass study?

A first-pass study is performed by injecting a radiotracer into a vein and taking individual images at 25–50 msec of the radioactivity, as it travels through the heart chambers. RV and LV ejection fraction can be calculated. The RV ejection fraction is > 35%, and the LV ejection fraction is > 50%. In addition, normal values have been described for:

- LV filling parameters (diastolic function)
- Pulmonary circulation time (contrast transit through the lungs, defined as the time interval between the first appearance of the radiotracer in the RV and its first appearance in the LV)
- Recirculation time (the time interval between the first opacification of the RV after intravenous administration of the radiotracers and the reappearance of the diagnostic agent in the RV, through physiologic venous return)

- The time of radiotracer persistence in the LV and RV, defined as the interval between the first appearance of diagnostic agent in the ventricular cavity and the moment when activity is no longer detected

The most important parameter is the LV ejection fraction. The other measurements are rarely used in clinical practice. A normal first-pass study is shown in Figure 35.

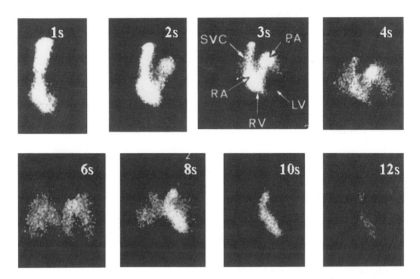

FIGURE 35. Normal first pass study. The radionuclide tracer is followed as it flows through the different heart chambers. SVC = superior vena cava, PA = pulmonary artery, LV = LV, RV = right ventricle, RA = right atrium. The *s* indicates the number of seconds between the intravenous injection of the radiotracer and the acquisition of the respective image. Individual images are acquired every 25–50 msec.

CHEST X-RAY

Gabriel Adelmann, M.D., Matthew R. Brewer, M.D., Rina Sternlieb, M.D., and Curtis E. Green, M.D.

104. List the main organs inspected on a chest x-ray.
Heart
Mediastinum
Lungs
Pleura
Skeleton of the thorax
Figure 36 illustrates normal chest x-rays from the posteroanterior (PA) and lateral views.

105. How is the heart visualized radiographically?
The *cardiac shadow* encompasses the myocardium and the intracardiac blood and the adjacent pericardium. In the normal subject, the heart valves and the pericardium are not visualized independently. This is because:
1. The heart valves are of the same radiographic density as the surrounding blood and myocardium.
2. The normal pericardium is thin and in close proximity to the cardiac border.
Generally, visualization of either the heart valves or the pericardium indicates the presence of disease (e.g., calcification).

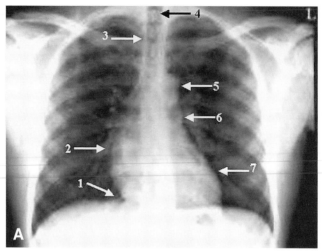

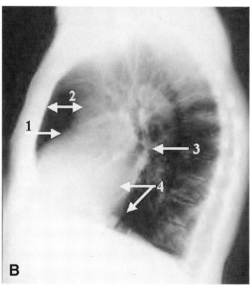

FIGURE 36. *A,* Normal chest x-ray, PA view. 1, cardiophrenic angle; 2, right atrium; 3, superior vena cava; 4, trachea; 5, aortic knob (superior arch of the left cardiac border); 6, pulmonary artery and left atrium (middle arch of the left aortic border); 7, left ventricle. *B,* Normal chest x-ray, lateral view. 1, right ventricle; 2, retrosternal border; 3, left atrium; 4, right atrium.

106. How is the mediastinum visualized radiographically?

The mediastinum is the area between the medial borders of the two lungs. On a frontal chest x-ray, the lower two thirds of the mediastinum are occupied by the heart and related vessels, and its borders coincide with the cardiac borders (see later). The upper third of the mediastinum (the superior mediastinum) is seen as a relatively high-density (white) area bordered:

- Inferiorly, by the superior border of the aortic arch
- Laterally, by the medial borders of the apical lobes of both lungs
- Superiorly, by the neck shadow

107. What is the normal width of the mediastinum?

Because the apparent width of the mediastinum varies widely with body habitus, degree of inspiration, projection (PA versus AP), rotation, hypertension, and age, there is no fixed measurement to distinguish normal from abnormal.

108. List the organs that are projected in the superior mediastinum.
- Esophagus
- Trachea
- Thyroid
- Thymus
- Lymph nodes

109. How are the lungs visualized radiographically?
1. The air-filled bronchi and pulmonary alveoli present almost no resistance to the progress of x-rays (minimal attenuation) and are depicted in black on the radiographic image.
2. The blood-filled pulmonary vessels and the cartilaginous airway walls, so-called water density structures, cause a greater x-ray attenuation than the pulmonary alveoli and are depicted in shades of gray.

110. What are the characteristics of normal pulmonary vasculature?
Normal pulmonary vessels are generally well-defined structures, gradually branching toward the periphery. In the standing position, the vasculature of the inferior half of the lungs is significantly more abundant than that of the apical halves, because of the effect of gravity.

111. How is the skeleton of the thorax visualized radiographically?
The chest x-ray depicts the different components of the thoracic skeleton (ribs, vertebrae, clavicles, scapulae, sternum) as white areas, representing the significant x-ray attenuation produced by the bones. The specific bones that are seen depend on the radiographic view that is being used. The skeletal structures themselves are shown poorly on a chest x-ray aimed primarily to show cardiac and pulmonary detail; if skeletal structures are of primary interest, spine or rib studies should be ordered.

112. Name the main radiographic views of the chest used in clinical practice.
The frontal view (PA or AP) and the lateral view.

113. List the cardiac borders on a frontal film.
Lateral borders (left and right)—coincide with the inferior two thirds of the mediastinal borders
Inferior border—usually not visible because of the adjacent diaphragm
Superior border—not visible, continuous with the aortic arch and hilar vessels

114. What are the structures composing the left border of the heart on a frontal film?
The left border of the heart is composed of three arches. In relationship to the left wall of the thorax, the superior and inferior arches are convex, and the middle arch is *depicted* as concave, although, in reality, the pulmonary artery trunk and the LA appendage are convex. In craniocaudal sequence, the arches are composed of the following structures:
Superior arch—the left subclavian artery and the aortic arch
Middle arch—the pulmonary trunk and the LA appendage
Inferior arch—the LV (see Figure 36A)

115. What are the structures composing the right border of the heart on a frontal film?
The right border of the heart includes two arches only, both convex in regard to the right wall of the thorax:
1. The **superior arch** comprises the SVC and the azygos vein.
2. The **inferior arch** comprises the RA border (see Figure 36A).

116. Which heart chambers do *not* form a border on a PA view?

The RV and the LA (with the exception of the LA appendage) do not form borders on a frontal (i.e., AP or PA) view. A lateral film is needed for radiographic evaluation of these structures.

117. What are the normal dimensions of the heart on a frontal chest x-ray?

The dimensions of the heart are described best as the ratio between the maximum transverse diameter of the heart and the maximum transverse diameter of the thorax on a nonrotated, end-inspiratory frontal film. This ratio is called the *cardiothoracic ratio* (CTR), and its normal value in adults is ≤ 0.5. A CTR > 0.5 indicates cardiac enlargement.

118. Does the CTR vary with age?

In the newborn, the normal CTR is approximately 0.66, owing to the relatively underdeveloped lungs in newborns.

119. What is the normal appearance of the pulmonary trunk on a frontal chest x-ray?

The pulmonary trunk is normally concave or mildly convex in adults and convex in children. A mildly convex pulmonary trunk in an adult should be interpreted in light of other radiographic findings (see Figure 36A).

120. What is the normal appearance of the LA appendage on a frontal chest x-ray film?

The LA appendage is the only portion of the LA visible on the frontal chest x-ray and represents the lower half of the middle arch of the left cardiac border. This arch is normally concave or mildly convex in adults.

121. Describe the normal appearance of the LV on a frontal chest x-ray.

- It has a rounded apex.
- The long axis of the LV (i.e., the imaginary line connecting the mid RA with the LV apex) is pointing downward.
- The apex of the LV does not come into contact with the lateral wall of the thorax (see Figure 36A).

122. What is the normal appearance of the azygos vein?

The azygos vein is a convex structure visible just above the proximal right main bronchus on a frontal chest x-ray and has a transverse diameter < 7 mm. This vascular structure is important to identify because its enlargement may indicate the presence of right-sided congestion.

123. What is the normal appearance of the RA on a frontal chest x-ray?

The normal RA border is ≤ 5.5 cm to the right of the midline and is in contact with the right hemidiaphragm at the costophrenic angle.

124. List the cardiac borders on a left lateral chest x-ray.

Anteriorly: the RV
Posteriorly: the LA (superiorly) and the RA (the caudal portion of the posterior border) (see Figure 36B)

125. Describe the normal cardiac dimensions on a left lateral chest x-ray.

Lateral films allow assessment of the dimensions of the RV. As in the case of LV assessment on a frontal chest x-ray, assessment of the cardiac dimensions on a lateral film is not performed in an absolute quantitative way (diameter in centimeters) but is based on the relationship with the surrounding thoracic structures.

1. The normal RV comes into contact with the sternum along a distance that does not exceed the lower one third of the distance between the sternal angle and the diaphragm.

2. The posterior border of the normal LA generally is represented by a straight line (this border is neither concave nor convex).

**126. Does the presence of a normal heart shadow and of normal pulmonary vascularity in-
dicate the absence of cardiac disease?**

No. Although these findings may correspond to a normal heart, myocardial disease can be radiographically inapparent. The negative predictive value of a normal chest x-ray for heart disease
is relatively low. Typical examples include LV hypertrophy or ischemia that does not cause cardiac dilation or dysfunction.

3. SYSTOLIC AND DIASTOLIC FUNCTION OF THE VENTRICLES

CARDIAC CATHETERIZATION

Gabriel Adelmann, M.D., Benjamin Kleiber, M.D., and Luis Gruberg, M.D.

1. List abnormalities of left ventricle (LV) structure that can be detected by contrast ventriculography.
- LV dilation
- LV hypertrophy
- Rupture of the LV, right ventricle (RV), or interventricular septum (IVS)
- Filling defects caused by tumor or thrombus

2. List abnormalities of LV function that can be detected by contrast ventriculography.
- **Decreased contraction** (hypokinesis)
- **Absent contraction** (akinesis)
- **Segmental dyssynergy,** seen when a myocardial segment is bulging out in systole rather than moving toward the central axis of the ventricle (dyskinesis)
- **Hyperdynamic contraction** of the LV (e.g., cavity obliteration, as seen in hypertrophic cardiomyopathy)

3. What are the angiographic characteristics of dilated cardiomyopathy (DCM)?
The main angiographic characteristic is LV enlargement with increased end-systolic and end-diastolic volumes and a globally or segmentally reduced LV ejection fraction. Occasionally a thrombus can be seen in the LV.

4. Name the typical findings of *ischemic* DCM on contrast ventriculography.
Typically, DCM of ischemic origin is characterized by segmental (rather than global) hypokinesis of the LV, with relative sparing of the RV.

5. What are the sensitivity and specificity of ventriculography for distinguishing ischemic from idiopathic DCM?
Although the characteristics outlined in question 3 may suggest the cause of DCM in a patient, they lack specificity. Occasional patients with idiopathic DCM show segmental ventricular involvement, whereas patients with ischemic DCM may show global LV dysfunction.

6. List the forms of hypertrophic cardiomyopathy that can be distinguished by means of contrast ventriculography.
- Mild concentric hypertrophy, frequently seen in patients with hypertension or aortic stenosis
- True hypertrophic obstructive cardiomyopathy (HOCM)
- Apical hypertrophy

7. What are the typical findings of mild concentric hypertrophy on contrast ventriculography?
- Increased thickness of the LV walls, equally involving all the myocardial segments
- A variable LV ejection fraction, which can be normal or increased in the initial stages and decreased (occasionally, significantly so) in the late stages of the disease

8. Describe the angiographic findings in asymmetric apical hypertrophy.

Patients with asymmetric apical hypertrophy have a marked thickening of the anteroapical wall of the LV. In the right anterior oblique view, the LV free wall often shows a marked increase in end-diastolic thickness (resembling a spade) and an extremely vigorous contraction with almost total obliteration of the ventricular cavity at end-systole (Fig. 1).

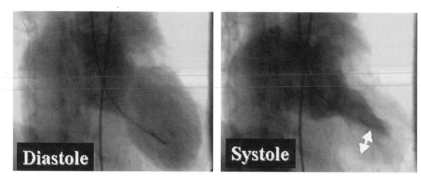

FIGURE 1. Apical hypertrophy. Marked increase in left ventricular end-diastolic thickness (*double arrow*), with near-total obliteration of the ventricular cavity at end-systole.

9. Describe the angiographic findings in patients with HOCM.

The typical angiographic finding is that of a thickened IVS bulging into the LV outflow tract (LVOT) in systole and diastole. It also is possible to see the systolic anterior movement (SAM) of the mitral valve's anterior leaflet and the associated mitral regurgitation (Fig. 2).

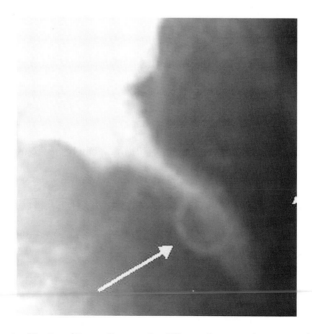

FIGURE 2. Hypertrophic obstructive cardiomyopathy. LV gram demonstrating near-total systolic obliteration of the left ventricular cavity. Note the pigtail catheter in the LV cavity (*arrow*).

10. What is postextrasystolic potentiation?

According to the Frank-Starling law, within certain limits, the LV stroke volume is directly proportional to the end-diastolic volume (myocardial stretch). At the end of a prolonged diastole, such as that seen in beats immediately succeeding a premature beat ("compensatory pause"), the LV has a higher volume (is more filled with blood) than after a normal diastole. This leads to increased stroke volume.

11. How can postextrasystolic potentiation be shown in the catheterization laboratory?

Ventricular premature beats can be induced in the catheterization laboratory, and postextrasystolic pressure gradients can be measured. This maneuver commonly is used in patients with HOCM (Fig. 3).

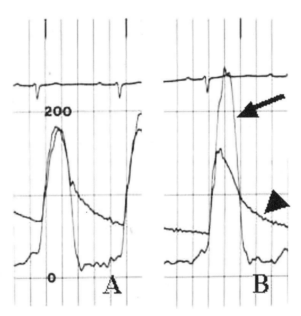

FIGURE 3. Hypertrophic obstructive cardiomyopathy. Increased gradient after PVC simultaneous left ventricular (*arrow*) and aortic (*arrowhead*) pressure tracings. A = normal beat; B = postextrasystolic beat.

12. What are the angiographic findings in restrictive cardiomyopathy?

The most frequent angiographic **structural finding** is LV hypertrophy. This finding lacks sensitivity and specificity, however. The **functional** hallmark of restrictive cardiomyopathy is diastolic ventricular dysfunction, which can be assessed in the catheterization laboratory by measuring the variation in intraventricular pressure as a function of time (dp/dt). This laborious measurement would not have a clear influence on patient management, however, because there is no specific treatment for diastolic dysfunction. Quantitative measurements of diastolic function rarely are performed clinically, and the main functional parameter assessed by ventriculography is LV systolic function.

ECHOCARDIOGRAPHY

Gabriel Adelmann, M.D., Steven A. Goldstein, M.D., and Neil J. Weissman, M.D.

13. What are the main phases of systole, and how can they be determined?

Isovolumic contraction period (pre-ejection period)—defined as the part of ventricular systole between mitral valve closure and aortic valve opening. It can be determined as the interval between the end of the A wave on the Doppler pattern of mitral inflow and the onset of blood flow through the LVOT.

Ejection period—defined as the part of systole during which there is flow through the aortic valve. It can be assessed as the duration of transvalvular aortic flow on a Doppler tracing or, on an M-mode study, as the time interval during which the aortic valve leaflets are open.

14. What is LV systolic dysfunction?

A decrease in myocardial contractility, resulting in decreased LV ejection fraction. The ejection fraction (EF) is calculated as:

$$EF (\%) = [(LVEDd - LVESs) / LVEDd]$$

where LVEDd is the end-diastolic LV volume and LVESs is the end-systolic LV volume.

The greater the degree of systolic dysfunction, the lower the ejection fraction. Most clinicians believe that an ejection fraction $< 50\%$ is considered abnormally decreased.

15. What is the difference between LV ejection fraction, stroke volume, and cardiac output?

LV ejection fraction is the percent decrease of LV volume in end-systole compared with end-diastole.

Stroke volume is the volume of blood expelled with each systole contraction into the aorta.

Cardiac output is the volume of blood expelled into the aorta during 1 minute.

A cardiac output compatible with life can be maintained even in face of severe decreases in LV ejection fraction by two main compensatory mechanisms: (1) cardiac dilation, which results in an increased stroke volume for the same ejection fraction, and (2) tachycardia, which increases the total volume of blood expelled into the aorta per minute (cardiac output) based on a higher number of cardiac contractions per unit of time.

16. How are the two phases of ventricular systole affected by systolic dysfunction?

Systolic dysfunction results in a prolongation of the isovolumic contraction time and a shortening of the ejection time.

17. Name the causes of ventricular systolic dysfunction.

Systolic dysfunction can be idiopathic (as in primary DCM) or secondary to diseases, such as ischemic heart disease and valvular disease (e.g., late stages of mitral insufficiency, aortic insufficiency, or aortic stenosis), or exposure to toxic (e.g., ethanol, cocaine, doxorubicin [Adriamycin]) or infectious (e.g., viral) agents.

18. What are the two basic echocardiographic characteristics of systolic ventricular dysfunction?

Systolic dysfunction is noted by a decreased endocardial motion and a decreased myocardial thickening in systole. These abnormalities sometimes are appreciated visually and usually reported in a semiquantitative fashion. The LV function accordingly is classified as normal, mildly reduced (hypokinetic), moderately reduced, or severely reduced (severely hypokinetic or akinetic = no movement from systole to diastole). These assessments can be reasonably accurate in a patient with good endocardial border definition, provided that the observer is experienced and integrates data from several tomographic planes.

19. How can LV systolic dysfunction be diagnosed by M-mode echocardiography?

The LV systolic function can be assessed by measuring the change in LV dimensions from diastole to systole on the M-mode. M-mode in the setting of LV dysfunction shows an "increased E point–septal separation," which represents the distance between the anterior mitral leaflet at the point of its maximum diastolic excursion and the IVS. A poor LV systolic function is associated with an E point–septal separation > 1 cm.

20. What is systolic endocardial motion, and what is its role in the evaluation of LV function?

LV systolic endocardial motion represents the motion (excursion) of the endocardial segments toward the center of the ventricle. Normal LV systolic function is expressed echocardiographically by a normal endocardial excursion in addition to endocardial thickening. It is impossible to assess LV contractility accurately in patients in whom the endocardial border is not well visualized. In these cases, the use of second harmonic imaging or of echocardiographic contrast agents typically increases the quality of endocardial delineation.

21. Define the classification of different degrees of myocardial segmental motion abnormalities.

1. **Hypokinesis** is diminished contraction of a myocardial segment. Hypokinesis can be mild, moderate, or severe.

2. **Akinesis** is absence of myocardial contraction (Fig. 4).

3. **Dyskinesis** is the motion of a given segment in systole in an opposite direction from the normal segments (i.e., the normal segments have an inward motion in systole, toward the center of the ventricle, whereas a dyskinetic segment bulges out in systole).

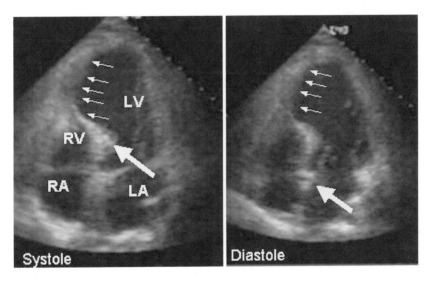

FIGURE 4. Akinetic myocardial segment. Note the absence of systolic endocardial excursion in the upper two parts of the interventricular septum (*thin arrows*), as opposed to the normal excursion of the basal segment (*thick arrows*).

22. Why is it important to distinguish between hypokinesis and the more severe degrees of systolic LV dysfunction?

- The different degrees have a different influence on overall cardiac function (a hypokinetic myocardial segment causes a less severe reduction in LV ejection fraction than an akinetic segment).
- The different degrees have an impact on establishing the probability of functional recovery after revascularization. The recovery chances of an akinetic or a dyskinetic segment are substantially lower than those of a hypokinetic segment. Myocardial viability is more probable for lower degrees of dysfunction.

23. Discuss the role of echocardiography in establishing the cause of systolic dysfunction.

Echocardiography is the method of choice for noninvasive diagnosis and grading of systolic dysfunction. It provides information that may suggest the cause of the ventricular dysfunction. A segmental pattern that spares the RV suggests an ischemic process, whereas a global, biventricular decrease in contractility is more likely a cardiomyopathy. The specificity of these findings is only modest, however, and echocardiography cannot determine definitively the cause of LV dysfunction.

24. How can LV function be assessed quantitatively with echocardiography?

Two-dimensional echocardiography can be used for quantitative assessment of LV systolic function by means of Simpson's rule (Fig. 5). The LV volume is assessed in systole and diastole by dividing the ventricle into several slices (≤ 20) and electronically summing up the resulting volumes of each disk of the LV cavity at that level. This allows the calculation of the LV volume at end-diastole and end-systole and subsequent calculation of ejection fraction. This is usually performed in two orthogonal views (four-chamber and two-chamber views).

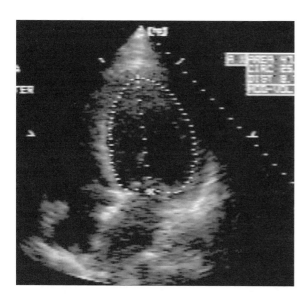

FIGURE 5. Left ventricular tracing used for Simpson's rule to calculate LV volume and ejection fraction.

25. What are the limitations of quantitative assessment of LV function with echocardiography?

The endocardial border tracing requires good delineation of the entire endocardial border. In the absence of good endocardial border delineation, there can be a high degree of variability.

26. What is normal diastolic function?

The ability of the LV to easily accommodate an adequate filling volume to maintain normal cardiac output while operating at a low pressure. Essentially, this means the capacity of the ventricular walls to move outward to accommodate diastolic filling, without substantial increases in intracavitary pressure. In normal subjects, this movement occurs even during exercise at rapid heart rates, when the duration of diastole is significantly shortened.

Abnormalities of this process are termed *diastolic dysfunction*.

27. List the most important causes of LV diastolic dysfunction.
- LV hypertrophy
- Myocardial scar

- LV wall infiltration (e.g., amyloid)
- Pericardial disease

The first two causes are the most frequent.

28. List the four phases of diastole.

1. Isovolumic relaxation time (IVRT)
2. Early rapid diastolic filling (E wave), which is the passive filling from the pressure gradient between the left atrium (LA) and the LV.
3. Diastasis (the interval between the end of the E wave and the beginning of the A wave)
4. Late filling resulting from atrial contraction (A wave, absent in subjects who are not in sinus rhythm), which also is called active filling because it occurs as a consequence of LA systole

29. Which phases of diastole are assessed by echocardiography?

The echocardiographic assessment of LV diastolic function usually is based on measurement of the E and A waves from Doppler.

30. What is IVRT?

The time between closure of the aortic valve (end of ejection) and the opening of the mitral valve (beginning of filling). During this brief period (normally 60–100 msec), the ventricular volume remains constant (isovolumic) (Fig. 6).

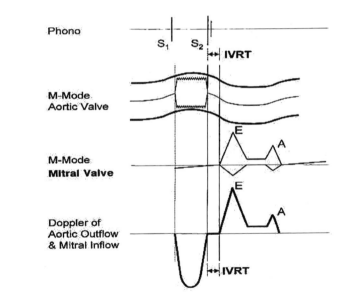

FIGURE 6. IVRT.

31. How can IVRT be measured noninvasively?

IVRT can be measured using several noninvasive methods, singly or in combination, for timing the physiologic events that define this time interval. The phonocardiogram shows aortic valve closure as the onset of the aortic component of the second heart sound, whereas M-mode and Doppler echocardiography can determine aortic valve closure and mitral valve opening (see Figure 6).

32. What are the three abnormal patterns of LV diastolic filling as determined by the mitral inflow velocity pattern?

1. Impaired passive filling/relaxation, a relatively early sign of diastolic dysfunction, is noted with a small E and a larger A (with an E/A ratio < 1).

2. A restrictive pattern, a later manifestation of diastolic dysfunction, is manifest by a high LA pressure and rapid but brief filling of the LV with the onset of diastole. In this situation, the E/A ratio is much greater than 1.

3. *Pseudonormalization* is a situation between 1 and 2, whereby diastolic dysfunction has progressed pass just impaired passive filling but not yet a true restrictive pattern. In this scenario, the E/A ratio could appear "normal" with the E wave slightly larger than the A wave (Fig. 7).

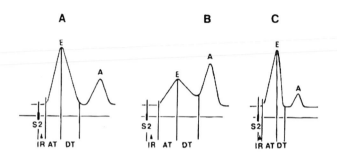

FIGURE 7. Impaired relaxation, "restrictive" pattern, and "pseudonormal" pattern. (Modified from Feigenbaum H: Echocardiography, 5th ed. Philadelphia, Lippincott Williams & Wilkins, 1994, p 525, with permission.)

33. How can impaired relaxation (early diastolic dysfunction, such as in the elderly) be distinguished from a restrictive pattern of LV filling (severe diastolic dysfunction, such as with an infiltrative cardiomyopathy)?

Impaired relaxation results in impaired early diastolic filling and in increased atrial contribution to total LV filling. It is characterized by:
- Reduced mitral E wave velocity
- Increased mitral A wave velocity
- Prolonged mitral deceleration time
- Lengthened IVRT

The **restrictive pattern** results from abnormal ventricular compliance, causing a rapid rise in LV diastolic pressure and a relatively small atrial contribution to filling, because the LA/LV pressure gradient already is elevated at the time of atrial contraction. The echocardiographic characteristics of this pattern include:
- Increased mitral E wave velocity (> 2.0 msec)
- Decreased mitral A wave velocity
- A shortened IVRT (<160 msec)

34. How can the normal and pseudonormal LV filling pattern be distinguished?

The **similarities** between the two patterns include:
- An E/A ratio between 1 and 2
- An E wave deceleration time of 160–240 msec

The pseudonormal pattern is **different** from normal in that it is associated with:
- A shortened IVRT
- An abnormal E/A ratio with the Valsalva maneuver (ratio becomes > 1)
- Specific changes in the pulmonary vein flow
- Characteristic findings using special techniques, such as tissue Doppler imaging or Doppler color propagation studies

The use of pulmonary venous flow patterns is the most helpful method to distinguish normal from pseudonormal patterns.

35. Discuss the influence of the patient's age on the E and A waves of the transmitral flow.

There is a gradual decrease in myocardial relaxation with age, resulting in a slower filling of the LV with a decrease in E wave velocity. Consequently, more of the LV filling occurs at the end of diastole (greater contribution of the atrial systole to ventricular filling, resulting in a taller A wave). In patients 60–70 years old, the two waves are approximately equal, with the A wave often being taller than the E wave after age 70.

36. What is cardiomyopathy?

Cardiomyopathy refers to a heterogeneous group of diseases characterized by alterations in the myocardial structure (hypertrophy, dilation, or myocardial infiltration) resulting in systolic or diastolic myocardial dysfunction. The term *cardiomyopathy* has been used to designate either idiopathic myocardial dysfunction or dysfunction secondary to other conditions (e.g., ischemia, exposure to toxic agents).

37. Name the three basic physiologic categories of cardiomyopathy.

(1) Dilated, (2) hypertrophic, and (3) restrictive. Most of these can be primary (idiopathic, genetic) or secondary to another condition (e.g., valvular disease, exposure to toxic agents).

38. List the main echocardiographic findings in patients with HOCM.
- Severe LV hypertrophy with a septal thickness usually > 1.7 mm
- SAM of the mitral valve
- Subaortic pressure gradient resulting from the SAM
- Mitral regurgitation, also caused by SAM

39. Which of the diagnostic features of HOCM mentioned in question 38 are specific to HOCM?

Technically speaking, none. LV hypertrophy can occur with hypertension, but isolated septal thickening from hypertension is unusual. SAM of the mitral valve is rare in the absence of HOCM but could occur with LV hypertrophy and a small, hyperdynamic LV cavity leading to an outflow gradient. SAM of the mitral chordae also is a common finding that is a normal variant and not diagnostic of HOCM.

40. What are the characteristics of the ventricular hypertrophy associated with HOCM?

Although the classic finding is a septal thickening out of proportion to the other walls, there are variants of HOCM with thickening at:
- The basal portion of the IVS
- The apex
- All the LV segments

41. What is SAM of the anterior leaflet of the mitral valve?

SAM is a two-dimensional echocardiography and M-mode echocardiography finding in patients with HOCM. The anterior mitral leaflet moves anteriorly (toward the ventricular septum) after the onset of systole and returns to its normal position just before the onset of ventricular diastole. This motion is believed to be due to the Venturi effect of the rapidly exiting blood in the narrowed LVOT, which "lifts" the anterior mitral leaflet and apposes it to the IVS. This is similar to the lifting of the wing of an airplane when exposed to high-velocity air currents (Fig. 8).

42. Does the degree of SAM correlate with the degree of obstruction?

Some investigators have indicated that the pattern or degree of SAM can predict the degree of obstruction. The closer the leaflet comes to the septum and the longer the duration of leaflet apposition to the septum (septal contact), the greater the severity of obstruction. Although this finding is only semiquantitative, when SAM touches the septum and becomes "flat" throughout most of systole, one can be reasonably sure that a high degree of obstruction is present. Conversely, if

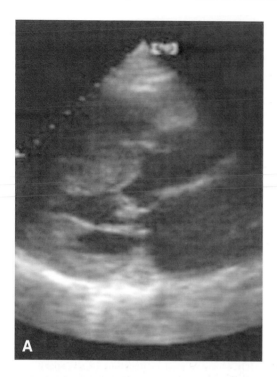

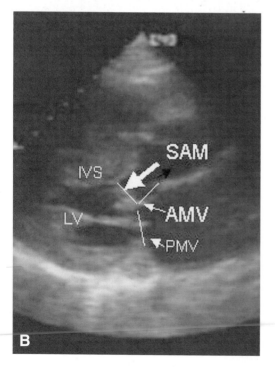

FIGURE 8. *A,* Hypertrophic obstructive cardiomyopathy (HOCM) and systolic anterior movement (SAM). *B,* In this HOCM patient, the tip of the anterior mitral valve leaflet (AMV) deviates toward the interventricular septum (IVS) in systole. Thus, the shape of the leaflet approximates an angled line. Contrast this with the straight line representing the posterior leaflet.

the leaflet merely moves anteriorly, then drops backward without touching the septum, a lesser degree of obstruction is likely to be present. Nonetheless, Doppler-determined gradients are used to assess the degree of obstruction and to follow the effectiveness of therapy, such as β-blockers, myotomy/myectomy, dual-chamber pacing, and alcohol ablation of the IVS.

43. What is the subaortic obstruction in patients with HOCM?

The subaortic obstruction is a pressure gradient between the apical and the basal portions of the LV resulting from the dynamic obstruction of the outflow tract caused by the anterior mitral valve leaflet. The dynamic nature of this gradient (worse later in systole) results from the relatively unimpeded blood flow through the outflow tract initially, which "lifts" the mitral leaflet toward the septum, worsening the gradient as the mitral leaflet contacts the septum. Also, several clinical interventions (see question 44) typically increase this gradient.

44. Which interventions increase (or decrease) the peak Doppler velocity of the intracavitary jet in patients with HOCM?

The peak velocity is increased by interventions that:
- Increase cardiac contractility (e.g., the first normal beat after an extrasystole)
- Decrease the ventricular cavity size (e.g., during Valsalva maneuver strain phase) (Fig. 9)
- Cause peripheral vasodilation (e.g., amyl nitrite inhalation)

Conversely, β-blockers (which decrease contractility) and squatting (which increases LV cavity size) typically cause a decrease in peak velocity and gradient at the level of the subaortic obstruction.

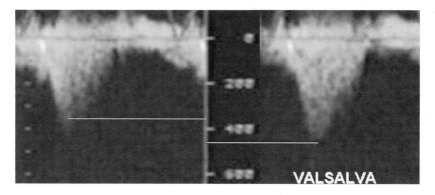

FIGURE 9. Increased HOCM gradient with Valsalva. The Valsalva maneuver often results in an increased LVOT gradient in patients with HOCM.

45. How can echocardiography assist the management of HOCM?
- Assessment of LVOT pressure gradient
- Assessment of LVOT pressure gradient response to therapeutic interventions (e.g., medication)
- Guidance of *alcohol ablation,* which is a controlled necrosis of the hypertrophic portion of the IVS produced in the catheterization laboratory by intracoronary injection of ethanol

Echocardiography is used to assess the extent of myocardium supplied by the septal artery supplying the portion of the septum to be ablated. This is achieved by intracoronary administration of an echocardiographic contrast agent (Optison) before the instillation of ethanol.

46. List some of the typical two-dimensional echocardiographic and Doppler features of a DCM.
- Four-chamber enlargement (Fig. 10)
- Impaired LV and RV systolic function

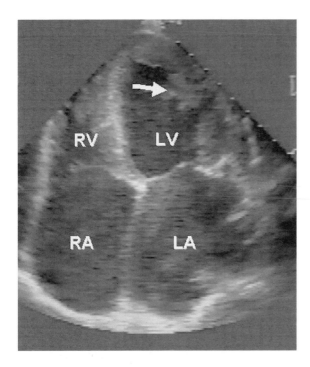

FIGURE 10. Four-chamber enlargement in a patient with dilated cardiomyopathy. Note the significant enlargement of the two atria. Due to the foreshortened cut through the left ventricle, the LV cavity does not appear exceedingly large, but the mural thrombus (*arrow*) is extremely suggestive for severe LV dysfunction, which was confirmed from other echocardiographic views.

- Diastolic dysfunction
- Increased LV heart mass (usually caused by LV dilation with normal wall thickness)
- Pulmonary hypertension (dilated pulmonary artery, RV, and right atrium (RA) with elevated tricuspid regurgitation velocity)
- Complications associated with DCM:
  Mitral regurgitation frequently present secondary to LV dilation and altered geometry and to mitral annular dilation
  Apical LV thrombus

47. What is the frequency of LV thrombus in DCM, and where is it usually located?

The most common location for a thrombus in DCM is the LV apex. An apical clot is present in 10–30% of patients with DCM who are not given anticoagulation.

48. What are the most important echocardiographic prognostic factors in DCM?

The following echocardiographic findings are associated with a poor prognosis:
- Severely impaired LV ejection fraction
- Short E wave deceleration time
- An abnormal E/A ratio (restrictive pattern) persistence after therapy (associated with high mortality)
- Increased pulmonary artery pressure

49. In patients with DCM, an important finding is the reduced rate of rise in LV pressure (*dp/dt*) in systole. Can this parameter be determined by echocardiography?

Most patients with DCM have coexisting mitral regurgitation. Because the velocity of mitral regurgitation is proportional to the gradient between the LV and the LA during systole, the rate of rise in the velocity of the mitral regurgitation jet correlates with the *dp/dt*.

50. What are the causes of restrictive cardiomyopathy?

Idiopathic and secondary to other conditions, such as hypertension or myocardial infiltration

51. Name the most important echocardiographic characteristics of restrictive cardiomyopathy.
- Abnormal diastolic function, in the presence of a normal systolic function
- LA and RA dilation
- Increased pulmonary artery pressure
- Increased LV end-diastolic pressure manifest as a decreased contribution of atrial systole to ventricular filling (low A wave) and an E/A ratio > 1
- Structural changes of the LV (most commonly LV hypertrophy) frequently associated with RV hypertrophy

52. List the echocardiographic findings used for distinguishing restrictive cardiomyopathy from constrictive pericarditis.

The elements **common** to the two conditions include:

Atrial enlargement

Dilated inferior vena cava and hepatic veins

E/A ratio > 1

Constrictive pericarditis is **different** from restrictive cardiomyopathy in the following respects:

1. It may be associated with a thick pericardium (better delineated by magnetic resonance imaging [MRI] or computed tomography [CT] scan than by transthoracic echocardiography)

2. LV size and systolic function are usually normal.

3. Constrictive pericarditis is not uniformly associated with LV hypertrophy or RV hypertrophy.

4. There may be an abrupt posterior motion of the ventricular septum in early diastole ("septal bounce") and a flattened diastolic motion of the posterior wall of the LV. These two features (best assessed with M-mode echocardiography) reflect one of the basic hemodynamic characteristics of constrictive pericarditis: Most of LV filling occurs in early diastole, causing a rapid increase in intracavitary pressure and a characteristic IVS motion.

5. There is an increase in the LV IVRT (> 20%) on the first beat after inspiration.

53. Discuss the most useful finding for distinguishing restrictive cardiomyopathy from constrictive pericarditis.

The most useful finding present with constrictive pericarditis is an exaggerated variation of the amplitude of the mitral and tricuspid early diastolic filling wave (E wave) between inspiration and expiration. During inspiration, the RV has an increased venous return. The increased RV volume causes the IVS to bow toward the LV with a subsequent decrease in LV volume. On echocardiography, the increased RV volume during inspiration corresponds with an increase in the tricuspid E velocity and a decrease in the mitral E wave. Opposite changes are noted during expiration. This finding is termed *respiratory variation* of the Doppler inflow patterns and typically is not present in restrictive cardiomyopathy.

54. What is the clinical significance of a restrictive pattern of LV filling?

The term *restrictive*, although generally accepted, is not an accurate term because most patients with this pattern do *not* have a restrictive cardiomyopathy. It usually implies a late stage of diastolic dysfunction and is associated with a severe decrease in LV compliance. Patients with this pattern usually have elevation of mean LA pressure at rest. It is seen most often in patients with coronary artery disease, ischemic cardiomyopathy, and DCM. It is also typical of restrictive cardiomyopathy, but restrictive cardiomyopathy is far less common than the aforementioned conditions.

55. What is arrhythmogenic RV dysplasia?

A primary cardiomyopathy of unknown cause characterized by progressive loss of RV myocardium with replacement by fatty or fibrofatty tissue and associated with ventricular arrhythmias and sudden death in adolescents and young adults.

56. What are the two-dimensional echocardiography findings suggestive of arrhythmogenic RV dysplasia?

RV dysplasia can manifest in many different forms; RV dysplasia may have a dilated RV, aneurysms or outpouchings of the RV, focal or global RV wall thinning, or abnormal global or regional RV systolic wall motion. MRI, not echocardiography, is the imaging procedure of choice for the diagnosis of this condition.

57. Describe the types of cardiac involvement that may occur with sarcoidosis.

Sarcoidosis may affect the myocardium, pericardium, valves, and blood vessels (including coronary arteries) (Fig. 11). Clinical manifestations of sarcoid are due to the typical granulomas, which may occur in any location and cause:

- Cor pulmonale, owing to irreversible pulmonary fibrosis
- Rhythm and conduction abnormalities, including sudden death
- DCM
- Pericardial disease
- Valve disease

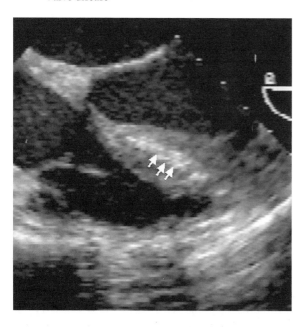

FIGURE 11. Cardiac sarcoidosis. Note abnormal myocardial texture and motion due to sarcoid granulomas in the interventricular septum (*arrows*). This is the second most frequent location of sarcoid granulomas (the left ventricular free wall is most frequent).

58. Name the most frequent serious cardiac manifestation of sarcoidosis.

Cor pulmonale.

59. What are the most frequent locations of cardiac sarcoid granulomas?

In decreasing order of frequency, these granulomas appear in the LV free wall, ventricular septum, RV, papillary muscle, RA, and LA. Often granulomas involve only a small portion of the heart and are clinically silent. The most common manifestation of granulomas in the myocardium is regional wall motion abnormalities.

60. What are some of the echocardiographic findings in sarcoidosis?

The most common echocardiography-detected manifestation in sarcoidosis is *cor pulmonale*. The echocardiographic features of cor pulmonale include dilated RA and RV, RV hypertrophy, and a series of echocardiographic and Doppler findings consistent with pulmonary hypertension. The second most common finding is a *DCM* (dilated LV with global hypokinesis). Small focal aneurysms, especially of the ventricular septum, may be seen.

61. What are the characteristics of cardiac carcinoid?

The predominant lesion of cardiac carcinoid is fibrosis of the tricuspid and pulmonary valves, producing characteristic thickening and retraction associated with restricted motion of the valves with incomplete coaptation. These changes result in severe tricuspid regurgitation, tricuspid stenosis (usually mild), and varying degrees of pulmonic stenosis. An excess production of serotonin and other biologically active agents is the pathogenic mechanism in this condition.

62. State the main cause of death in patients with carcinoid.

Approximately half the deaths in carcinoid patients are due to heart failure resulting from severe tricuspid regurgitation.

63. Which patients with carcinoid tumors develop carcinoid heart disease?

Cardiac involvement occurs in approximately 30% of patients with carcinoid tumors. It is seen almost exclusively in patients with hepatic metastases and includes plaque like deposits on the endocardium and right-sided heart valves. Left-sided heart valve lesions are much less frequent and occur in patients with a patent foramen ovale or pulmonary carcinoid.

64. What are the typical features of amyloid heart disease?

Amyloid, a fibrillary protein with a B-pleated sheet structure, may deposit in the heart. Clinical features of cardiac amyloidosis include heart failure (usually with restrictive physiology) and arrhythmias (especially atrial fibrillation and heart block). Pericardial effusion and cardiac tamponade have been described.

65. List the typical two-dimensional echocardiography features of amyloid heart disease.

- Small or normal LV cavity size
- Concentric LV hypertrophy, sometimes mimicking hypertrophic cardiomyopathy
- Decreased LV contractility
- Increased atrial septal thickness and biatrial dilation
- Nonspecific valvular thickening
- Increased myocardial echogenicity, which may have a "sparkling" quality (Fig. 12)

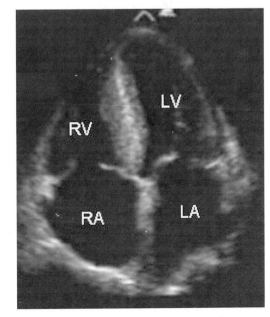

FIGURE 12. Hypertrophied, "sparkling" myocardium, biatrial enlargement with a small left ventricle and leaflet thickening in a patient with amyloid cardiomyopathy.

- Small pericardial effusion
- A typical restrictive Doppler velocity pattern (late in the disease); Doppler pattern may be normal in the early stages of disease

66. Are there echocardiographic or Doppler parameters that help assess prognosis in cardiac amyloidosis?

Yes. Predictors of poor outcome in cardiac amyloidosis include LV hypertrophy and decreased LV contractility (systolic dysfunction). The combination of a decreased fractional shortening ($<20\%$) and a mean LV wall thickness of ≥ 15 mm is associated with an actuarial medium survival of only 4 months. The parameters of LV diastolic dysfunction also are independent predictors of cardiac mortality. Patients with early cardiac amyloidosis often have an impaired relaxation pattern of LV filling. These patients have a significantly better prognosis (almost double 1-year survival rate) than patients with advanced cardiac amyloidosis and a restrictive filling pattern.

67. What are the cardiac effects of anthracyclines?

The anthracyclines, including daunorubicin (Cerubidine) and doxorubicin (Adriamycin, Rubex), are the major drugs that cause chemotherapy-induced cardiomyopathy. The frequency of serious cardiomyopathy is 1–10% at total doses < 450 mg/m^2. The risk increases markedly ($>$ 20%) at total doses > 550 mg/m^2. Preexisting cardiac disease, concomitant use of cyclophosphamide, and previous chest irradiation all increase the risk of cardiomyopathy.

68. Is there a role for serial echocardiographic evaluation of patients undergoing cancer chemotherapy with doxorubicin?

All patients requiring anthracycline chemotherapy should have a baseline evaluation of ventricular function. This is often done by echocardiography. Alternatives include nuclear ventriculography (multigated acquisition [MUGA]), MRI, and gated single-photon emission computed tomography (SPECT) with thallium. If the initial ejection fraction is $\geq 50\%$, the risk of cardiomyopathy is small, but the ejection fraction should be determined again after dose levels of 300 mg/m^2 and 400 mg/m^2 and after each subsequent dose of doxorubicin.

Chemotherapy should be stopped:
- If the ejection fraction decreases by $\geq 10\%$ compared with baseline
- If the ejection fraction decreases to $< 50\%$

69. In which patients is doxorubicin contraindicated?

In patients with baseline ejection fraction $\leq 30\%$. In patients with an ejection fraction of 30–50%, chemotherapy can be considered provided that the ejection fraction remains $> 30\%$ and does not decrease by $> 10\%$.

70. List the most frequently encountered cocaine-induced cardiovascular conditions.

- Myocardial ischemia, manifested as angina pectoris or acute myocardial infarction
- Cardiac arrhythmias
- Sudden cardiac death
- Myocarditis
- DCM
- Aortic dissection

Myocardial ischemia is the most frequent cardiovascular complication of cocaine use.

71. Describe the cardiac manifestations of acquired immunodeficiency syndrome (AIDS).

1. **Pericardial effusion** is one of the most common forms of cardiac involvement in human immunodeficiency virus (HIV) infection. The varied clinical presentation includes asymptomatic pericardial effusion, pericarditis, cardiac tamponade, and constrictive pericarditis. Approximately 20% of AIDS patients have pericardial effusions detectable by echocardiography. Pericardial ef-

fusion may be a marker of end-stage HIV infection because it is associated with a low CD4 cell count and could be due to opportunistic infections, malignant neoplasms, or direct viral pericarditis. Echocardiography is an ideal technique for detecting pericardial effusions.

2. **Myocarditis** may cause global or regional LV dysfunction. The autopsy incidence of this finding may approach 30% of asymptomatic patients.

3. **DCM** has a prevalence of 10–30% by echocardiographic and autopsy studies. DCM occurs late in the course of HIV infection and usually is associated with a significantly reduced CD4 count. The pathogenesis of cardiomyopathy is unclear.

4. **Infective endocarditis** in patients with AIDS usually occurs in intravenous drug users.

5. **Pulmonary hypertension** has a prevalence of 1 in 200 patients (compared with 1 in 200,000 in the general population). The pathogenesis may be due to concomitant pulmonary disease or direct HIV-associated pulmonary hypertension, which is a diagnosis of exclusion.

6. **Malignant neoplasms** in AIDS patients include cardiac Kaposi's sarcoma and lymphoma and have a grave prognosis.

7. **Drug-related cardiomyopathy** occurs in AIDS patients.

Early recognition, usually using echocardiography, and prompt treatment are important to prevent significant morbidity from these manifestations of AIDS.

72. Should HIV-positive patients undergo periodic screening by electrocardiogram (ECG) and echocardiogram?

Although there is no consensus or general recommendation for periodic screening of HIV-positive patients with ECG and two-dimensional echocardiography, this approach has been advocated for two reasons:

1. Cardiac abnormalities are common (found at autopsy in two thirds of patients with AIDS) and varied (e.g., pericardial effusion, myocarditis, DCM, or endocardial involvement at any stage of the disease). The cardiac complications are detected easily by echocardiography.

2. Cardiac complications often are clinically silent or subtle in the initial stages and often are overshadowed by manifestations in other organs, primarily lungs and brain.

73. What is the hypereosinophilic syndrome, and what are its cardiac manifestations?

The idiopathic hypereosinophilic syndrome (Löffler's endocarditis) is a relatively rare disorder, characterized by overproduction of eosinophils and endocardial fibrosis. Cardiac involvement is the major source of morbidity and mortality. Typical cardiac findings include endocardial fibrosis and mural thrombus.

74. Summarize the typical echocardiographic findings in the hypereosinophilic syndrome.

- Increased wall thickness with "layering" of the endocardial echoes, most evident at the apex of the LV or RV (or both); the endocardial deposits can obliterate the ventricular apex
- Thickening and fibrosis of the posterior mitral and anterior tricuspid leaflets, causing valvular regurgitation, occasionally severe
- Normal or small ventricles, with normal ventricular function; the "covered" LV apex also may have preserved function
- Dilated atria

MAGNETIC RESONANCE IMAGING

Gabriel Adelmann, M.D., and Anthon R. Fuisz, M.D.

75. What are the main elements of information provided by MRI regarding the cardiac chambers?

Ventricular structure—thickness, volume, and mass
Ventricular function—global and regional systolic function; diastolic function

76. Does MRI have a role in clinical practice for the assessment of ventricular structure and function?

Despite the high degree of accuracy, MRI measurements seldom are carried out for clinical purposes; today these measures are mainly of research interest because:

- MRI is a complex, costly, sometimes uncomfortable, and not widely available imaging modality.
- The relevant diagnostic and prognostic information in patients with structural or functional problems of the ventricles usually is provided by echocardiography. (For a comparison between the advantages and disadvantages of MRI and echocardiography, see Chapter 1.)

In patients with inadequate transthoracic echocardiography windows, however, MRI is a reasonable alternative to transesophageal echocardiography.

77. How can the ventricular volume be measured by MRI?

Similar to echocardiography and cardiac catheterization, LV volume is measured based on the intracardiac blood pool. The delineation of the LV endocardial border is based on the different electromagnetic properties of the blood compared with the myocardium.

78. How can the LV mass be measured by MRI?

The areas of multiple short-axis slices through the LV are measured and multiplied by the number of slices. This yields the myocardial volume (not to be confused with the LV *chamber* volume). By multiplying this volume by the specific density of the myocardium (1.05 g/cm^2), an accurate estimate of the LV mass is obtained.

79. How does the assessment of LV volume and mass by MRI compare with that based on echocardiography and cardiac catheterization?

The **similarity** consists in the methodology: All the noninvasive techniques calculate the LV volume as the sum of the volumes of several LV slices, measured in systole and diastole. The **difference** resides in the fact that in calculating the LV volume and mass:

1. **Echocardiography and cardiac catheterization** usually are based on geometric assumptions (it is postulated that the LV cavity has no gross irregularities, such as aneurysms, and consequently the measured slices are representative of the LV as a whole).

2. **MRI** effectively images the LV in its three-dimensional complexity, owing to its intrinsic ability to distinguish electromagnetic signals emitted from tissues situated at different locations within the patient's body. No geometric assumption is needed, and the resulting calculations are precise.

80. How does MRI compare with echocardiography and cardiac catheterization for assessment of LV mass and volume?

Because of the high accuracy of the images and measurements it provides, MRI is considered the gold standard for assessment of LV mass and volume.

81. What are the clinical correlates of LV mass increase?

LV mass has been shown to be a prognostic factor in diseases associated with LV hypertrophy (systemic hypertension, aortic stenosis). More importantly, the regression of LV mass after successful treatment of the underlying condition (antihypertensive therapy, aortic valve replacement) has been shown to have prognostic value in these patients.

82. If all the relevant information necessary for patient management generally is provided by echocardiography, why bother with tedious LV mass and volume measurements by MRI?

These calculations are important for research purposes. It has been shown that for the same degree of reduction in blood pressure, there could be a substantial difference between the degree of regression in LV hypertrophy induced by different antihypertensive agents. Similarly the total LV mass regression after aortic valve replacement is of prognostic value.

83. What are the clinical correlates and the practical importance of LV volume increase?

Measurements of the LV volume are of prognostic importance in patients with LV dilation (volume overload conditions and late stages of pressure overload conditions). Although MRI-derived volume calculations are more accurate and reproducible, the prognostic information supplied by echocardiographic measurement of the LV diameter usually is considered sufficient. The American Heart Association guidelines for patient management in congestive heart failure or valvular heart disease are based primarily on LV end-systolic and end-diastolic diameter and not on the corresponding LV volumes.

84. How can MRI assess the global LV systolic function?

LV ejection fraction can be measured precisely by MRI, based on end-systolic and end-diastolic LV volume measurements. LV ejection fraction can be measured at rest and under pharmacologic stimulation (dobutamine stress test).

85. Where does MRI assessment of global LV systolic function fit into clinical practice?

MRI assessment has a modest role in clinical practice, mainly owing to the high costs, reduced availability, and intrinsic complexity of a cardiac MRI study. (Despite its semiquantitative nature, LV functional assessment by echocardiography is sufficiently accurate for practical management in most patients.) In patients who cannot be studied adequately with transthoracic echocardiography, MRI becomes a more reasonable choice. MRI is used sometimes when there is significant disparity between echocardiographic and radionuclide assessments of LV function.

86. How can the regional function of the LV be assessed by MRI?

Similar to assessment by echocardiography, cardiac catheterization, or gated nuclear imaging, assessment is based on the presence and extent of myocardial thickening and the degree and direction of endocardial border motion in systole (normal, hypokinetic, akinetic, or dyskinetic)

87. Discuss myocardial tagging.

The greatest challenge in assessing the systolic function of a myocardial segment is following the motion of the segment accurately throughout the cardiac cycle (from end-diastole to end-systole). This assessment can be problematic when using non-MRI techniques:

- **With echocardiography,** the motion of the heart as a whole during the cardiac cycle (the "twist" of the heart with each contraction) may lead to comparison of different (albeit adjacent) segments at end-systole versus end-diastole.
- **Cardiac catheterization and gated nuclear imaging** are "summation" imaging modalities, in which clear distinction of different myocardial segments is not possible.

Ideally, to assess the systolic function of a given segment accurately, one should be able to (1) "label" that segment and (2) follow its motion throughout the cardiac cycle. These two goals can be achieved by MRI myocardial tagging; tagging is superimposing an electronically generated grid on the image of the heart (Fig. 13). This grid deforms with cardiac motion, following (tagging) the different myocardial segments throughout the cardiac cycle and allowing precise definition of the function of an individual myocardial segment.

88. What are the practical applications of myocardial tagging?

Despite its great intuitive appeal, the tagging method still is used primarily as an investigative tool. In addition to the problems of cost and availability, the postprocessing of myocardial tagging also is laborious and time-consuming.

89. Define the myocardial strain rate.

Myocardial strain rate is a parameter referring to the magnitude and direction of deformation of a myocardial region of interest throughout the cardiac cycle. Myocardial strain rate is assessed by MRI tagging and is altered in pathologic conditions. The motion of an infarcted area

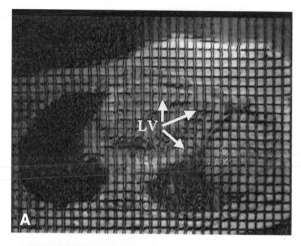

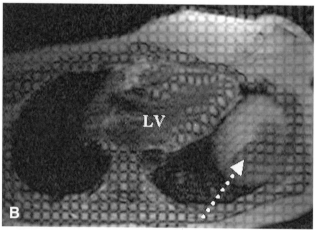

FIGURE 13. Myocardial tagging. *A,* Diastolic frame. Note that all the cells of the grid have a square shape. *B,* Systolic frame. The cells of the grid are deformed, demonstrating normal myocardial excursion in systole (normal contraction). Note that the grid over the dome of the diaphragm (*dotted arrow*) is not deformed at all, because this muscle does not have cardiac cycle-dependent motion. An akinetic myocardial segment would demonstrate a similar image.

consists more of "stretching" (owing to the action of normal neighboring segments pulling on the infarcted segment) than intrinsic contraction. Currently, this method is primarily of research interest.

90. Discuss the role of MRI in the assessment of diastolic function of the ventricles.

Diastolic function refers to the capacity of the ventricles to accommodate blood from the atria during diastole; the diastolic function is the filling function of the ventricles. The ventricular filling can be assessed by measuring the diastolic volume changes of the ventricles against time, which allows derivation of the early-to-peak filling rate and the percentage of LV filling occurring during early diastole. Additional parameters that can be assessed by MRI include mitral inflow velocities and pulmonary vein flow velocities (see Chapter 6).

91. Summarize the role of MRI in the diagnosis of cardiomyopathy.

- Assessment of the LV and RV function and identification of small decreases in myocardial function
- Accurate visualization of the pericardium, helping to distinguish between constrictive pericarditis and restrictive cardiomyopathy
- Identification of specific MRI findings (i.e., tissue characteristics) associated with specific types of cardiomyopathies

92. What are the MRI features of arrhythmogenic RV dysplasia?

- Marked dilation of the RV, in the absence of other discernible causes
- Fatty replacement of the RV wall
- Presence of focal wall motion abnormalities

Arrhythmogenic RV dysplasia is one of the more challenging diagnoses to make by MRI (or any other imaging modality), and patients thought to have this rare condition should be referred to experienced tertiary care centers for definitive diagnosis.

93. List some of the pitfalls of diagnosis of arrhythmogenic RV dysplasia.

1. Mistaking the normal epicardial fat for fatty infiltration of the ventricular wall
2. Mistaking mild abnormal segmental LV or RV hypokinesis (often after attempts at ventricular tachycardia ablation) as a sign of arrhythmogenic RV dysplasia
3. Problems with ECG gating and image quality resulting from ventricular premature beats, which are common in these patients

94. What is the role of MRI in the management of DCM?

MRI can be used to provide accurate assessment of:

- LV and RV size and function
- Myocardial viability (i.e., the reversibility of contraction abnormalities, produced by chronic ischemia, after blood flow is reestablished by revascularization)

In clinical practice, ventricular function routinely is assessed by echocardiography, and myocardial viability is determined by nuclear or echocardiographic methods. MRI techniques to show viability are becoming more available and are easy and rapid to perform (Fig. 14).

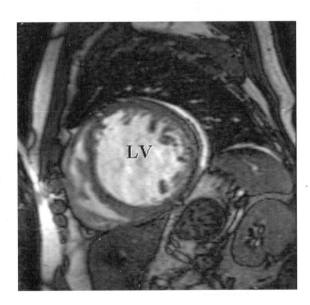

FIGURE 14. Dilated cardiomyopathy. Note the severely dilated left ventricle. Three-dimensional reconstruction in the same patient demonstrated a spherical shape of the LV, characteristic of advanced stages of left ventricular dysfunction.

95. Describe the role of MRI in the management of HOCM.

MRI can detect the thickened septum and dynamic LVOT obstruction typically associated with HOCM and a substantially thickened LV apex in patients with apical hypertrophy (Fig. 15). MRI also can be used for assessment of LV mass and of the LV mass changes in response to therapy. Echocardiography still remains the procedure of choice to diagnose HOCM.

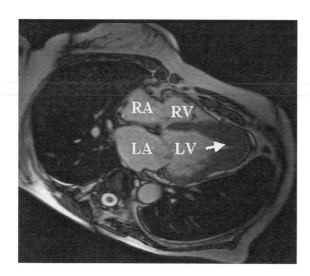

FIGURE 15. LV apical hypertrophy (*arrow*).

96. Describe the role of MRI in the management of restrictive cardiomyopathy.

The clinical role of MRI is mainly to distinguish restrictive cardiomyopathy from constrictive pericarditis. This distinction is notoriously difficult by echocardiography, and even direct pressure measurements in the catheterization laboratory may be inconclusive, owing to the significant impact of loading conditions on the hemodynamics of these patients. MRI demonstration of thickened pericardium is significant circumstantial evidence in favor of the diagnosis of constrictive pericarditis.

97. What are the MRI features of hemochromatosis?

Hemochromatosis is one of the easiest MRI diagnoses, based on the typical image of an "absent liver" (MRI "image void" owing to hepatic iron deposits). Myocardial involvement also is diagnosed as areas of absent signal, owing to the same mechanism.

98. What are the MRI features of sarcoidosis?

Cardiac MRI in patients with sarcoidosis occasionally may show myocardial infiltrative patterns, but the diagnostic value of these findings has yet to be proved.

NUCLEAR MEDICINE

Manuel D. Cerqueira, M.D., Gabriel Adelmann, M.D., and Dorothea McAreavey, M.D.

99. What is the role of nuclear cardiology in the diagnosis of LV dysfunction?

MUGA, first-pass studies, or ECG-gated SPECT perfusion imaging can be used to measure global and regional LV function and determine the possible causes in patients in whom function is abnormal.

100. What is the role of nuclear cardiology in the diagnosis of myocarditis and can it be used to monitor cardiotoxicity resulting from chemotherapeutic drugs such as doxorubicin?

Although the diagnosis of myocarditis or cardiotoxicity generally is based on a combination of clinical, ECG, and radiologic factors, nuclear cardiology is a valuable tool for:

- Assessment of patient prognosis, based on measurement and changes in LV volume
- Assessment of the presence and severity of myocardial inflammation (this is an evolving indication; at present, it cannot be recommended uniformly because of problems with the sensitivity and specificity of available radiotracers)

MUGA provides an objective and reproducible measurement of LV function and an accurate method for serial monitoring of patients receiving cardiotoxic drugs such as doxorubicin.

101. What are the findings on thallium-201 imaging in a patient with myocarditis?

The most frequent finding is a homogeneous distribution of the perfusion tracer. In occasional patients, fixed focal defects may be shown.

102. Discuss the role of nuclear cardiology in the diagnosis of DCM.

Although echocardiography remains the main diagnostic modality for DCM, the assessment of LV ejection fraction by means of nuclear studies also is widely used. In this setting, nuclear studies have the significant advantage of not only showing the end result of ischemia (i.e., ventricular dysfunction), but also its initial cause, most frequently ischemic heart disease.

103. Can nuclear perfusion imaging help in differentiating idiopathic from ischemic DCM?

Yes. The presence of perfusion defects including $> 40\%$ of the myocardium strongly argues in favor of an ischemic cardiomyopathy. Occasional patients with normal coronary arteries and a DCM have been shown, however, to display large, fixed defects, especially at the apex. A definitive diagnosis cannot be established based on gamma camera imaging alone. Positron emission tomography (PET) assessment of myocardial glucose metabolism can be used to assess perfusion defects characterized as fixed, based on gamma camera imaging. Some of these defects are revealed by PET to show a metabolism/perfusion mismatch (diminished perfusion and enhanced glucose use) and consequently to represent areas of severe chronic ischemia, so-called viable or hibernating myocardium, rather than scar.

104. What is the prognostic value of LV function assessment by nuclear cardiology?

Nuclear measurement of LV function are valuable in the follow-up and management of patients with ischemic and nonischemic DCM because it offers important information regarding:

- Prognosis (the lower the ejection fraction, the higher the morbidity and mortality)
- Guidelines for daily physical activity
- Monitoring of aggressive medical therapy

105. Discuss doxorubicin cardiotoxicity.

Doxorubicin, a chemotherapy agent used to treat various tumor types, causes cardiotoxicity in a dose-dependent fashion. Many patients have cardiotoxicity in the absence of clinical symptoms. When clinical symptoms finally develop, it is too late to prevent progression of LV dysfunction, and many of these patients die from cardiac causes rather than the tumor for which they were being treated. Patients with prior cardiac disease or radiation treatment are at increased risk for toxicity. If evidence of cardiotoxicity can be diagnosed before the development of overt clinical symptoms, stopping treatment prevents further deterioration of LV dysfunction, and many patients improve overall function.

106. Summarize the role of nuclear cardiology in guiding the proper clinical use of doxorubicin.

It is recommended that all patients have a baseline measurement of LV ejection fraction prior to clinical use of doxorubicin.

1. If the ejection fraction is $\leq 30\%$, treatment with doxorubicin should not be given, and alternative agents should be considered.

2. For patients with an ejection fraction of 30–50%, there is an increased risk for cardiotoxicity; it is advised ejection fraction be measured before each dose.

3. For ejection fraction $> 50\%$, treatment can be given until the patient reaches a total dose of 450 mg/m^2 body surface area, when a repeat measurement should be done. A decrease in ejection fraction of 10 units (e.g., from 60% to 50%) is a sign of mild toxicity, and the use of other agents should be considered. If the ejection fraction decreases by > 15 units and the absolute ejection fraction value is $< 45\%$, this represents clear toxicity and further treatment should not be given.

107. What are the radionuclide findings in a patient with HOCM?

LV function is usually hyperdynamic but may be decreased in the late stages of the disease. This information is valuable in establishing the optimal treatment (β-blockers and calcium blockers are appropriate in patients with normal or increased LV systolic function) and in assessing prognosis (a decreased LV function implies a poor prognosis).

Asymmetric septal hypertrophy is detected as a disproportionately increased septal thickness compared with that of the posterior LV free wall on a myocardial perfusion scan.

Echocardiography is the imaging modality of choice for HOCM.

108. What is the role of nuclear perfusion imaging in the assessment of HOCM patients for possible coexistent coronary artery disease?

In these patients, coronary artery disease cannot always be detected by perfusion imaging. It has been reported, however, that some patients have reversible, exercise-induced perfusion defects in the absence of epicardial coronary artery stenosis. These defects tend to be small and diffuse, indicating the presence of small vessel disease and the increased oxygen demands imposed by hypertrophied and hypercontractile myocardium.

109. If nuclear perfusion imaging is unreliable for detection of coronary artery disease in HOCM patients, does this mean these studies are useless in this population?

It has been suggested that the presence of reversible perfusion defects in young patients with HOCM may be a marker of a poor prognosis. Consequently, perfusion scans may be considered in this population because patients with positive studies may be candidates for early defibrillator implantation.

110. What is the role of nuclear perfusion imaging in the management of HOCM patients?

With the possible exception of detection of reversible perfusion defects in young patients (see question 109), nuclear studies generally are not indicated. Echocardiography represents the diagnostic modality of choice.

111. List the findings of nuclear functional imaging in patients with a restrictive cardiomyopathy.
- Normal or decreased LV end-diastolic volume
- Normal or mildly decreased LV ejection fraction
- Dilated atria

112. State the significance of a fixed perfusion defect in patients with restrictive cardiomyopathy.

In addition to the "usual" significance (myocardial scar), this finding may be present in patients with amyloidosis, sarcoidosis, systemic sclerosis, and cardiac tumors.

113. What is the role of nuclear cardiology in the diagnosis of a restrictive cardiomyopathy?

As in the case of HOCM, nuclear imaging has a secondary role in diagnosis and management.

114. Summarize the findings on nuclear studies in patients with hypertensive heart disease.

Function and perfusion imaging studies are helpful for the assessment of:
- LV systolic function and its response to therapy
- LV diastolic function (peak diastolic filling rates)
- Coexistent coronary artery disease

115. What are the limitations of nuclear studies in the diagnosis of ischemic heart disease in patients with systemic hypertension?

Patients with LV hypertrophy often show an abnormal ejection fraction response to exercise, even in the absence of epicardial coronary artery stenosis. In these patients, nuclear perfusion studies are preferable to radionuclide angiography and accurately diagnose the presence or absence of coronary artery disease.

116. Can nuclear studies be used to monitor patients after cardiac transplantation?

Nuclear cardiology studies provide important information regarding some of the main concerns after cardiac transplant, including:
- LV and RV performance in the early postoperative period and on follow-up
- Graft rejection
- Coronary arteriopathy

117. Summarize the specific technical challenges of nuclear studies in post-transplant patients.

Several anatomic peculiarities of the donor heart must be taken into account in the context of radionuclide angiography and perfusion imaging. These characteristics include:
- Increased cardiac mobility, owing to the absence of the containing pericardium
- Paradoxic septal motion
- Leftward rotation and posterior displacement of the apex, which may make the LV cavity appear small or nonexistent with planar studies; SPECT overcomes this difficulty
- The presence of redundant RA and LA tissue retained from the native heart

118. What is the significance of ventricular dysfunction after cardiac transplantation?

The significance of this finding depends on the time when it becomes apparent:
- Ventricular dysfunction ≤ 1 week after transplantation is most likely not due to rejection, but rather to preexisting damage to the donor heart.
- Ventricular dysfunction occurring 1 week after transplantation, in the absence of another explanation, is most likely secondary to rejection.
- Ventricular dysfunction occurring years after transplantation may be due to chronic rejection or the development of obstructive coronary disease.

119. Does the presence of normal LV function, as shown by radionuclide techniques, rule out rejection of the cardiac graft?

No. Most patients with mild rejection and some patients with moderate or severe rejection shows normal LV function. Nuclear studies cannot be used instead of periodic biopsy. The **negative predictive value of a normal study for the absence of graft rejection** is low. **The positive predictive value of an abnormal study for the presence of rejection** is high, however. Even subtle decreases in the LV ejection fraction (by 4%) have been shown to correlate with "conversion" of biopsy results from negative to positive. Conversely, stabilization or improvement in ejection fraction correlates with histologic resolution of graft rejection. Meticulous technique and exact reproduction of the same imaging angles from study to study are essential for accurate diagnosis of these subtle changes in ejection fraction.

120. What is the utility of radionuclide/antibody imaging in patients after cardiac transplant?

Antimyosin antibodies may be coupled to radioactive tracers (most often, technetium), and used for detection of cardiac transplant rejection. At present an adjunct to biopsy, this method is envisioned by some as a *future* noninvasive alternative to serial myocardial biopsies.

121. Discuss allograft vasculopathy.

Allograft vasculopathy is a form of graft rejection, manifesting as diffuse occlusive disease of the mid and distal coronary arteries. The typical angiographic finding is that of coronary "pruning" and occlusion. The usual "alarm mechanism" represented by angina pectoris is absent in these patients because of denervation of the transplanted heart. An aggressive, proactive approach is necessary for timely identification of this occult, but potentially life-threatening disease. At present, there is still insufficient information regarding the value of perfusion studies for this purpose. The American Heart Association guidelines for the practice of nuclear cardiology consider nuclear profusion studies in this setting as a class IIb indication.

122. What is the only class I indication for nuclear studies in patients after cardiac transplant?

Assessment of LV performance by radionuclide angiography.

123. What is the information provided by first-pass studies regarding LV diastolic function?

Similar to gated or MUGA studies, first-pass studies allow assessment of such LV diastolic parameters as peak diastolic filling rate, time-to-peak filling rate, and filling fractions. A typical radioactivity curve of the intraventricular blood pool is shown in Figure 16. These curves and the derived parameters are not used routinely in clinical practice.

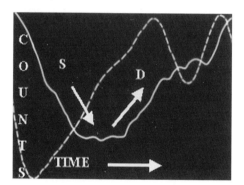

FIGURE 16. Time-activity (counts or volume) curve (*solid lines*) of the intraventricular blood pool and the first derivative curve (*dashed line*). The derivative curve helps to identify the peak rates and the time at which they are achieved. The number of radioactive counts is expressed on the vertical axis, against time on the horizontal axis. During systole (S), there is a decrease in the intraventricular blood pool radioactivity because of ejection of blood into the systemic circulation. Conversely, in diastole (D) the LV fills with blood, and the counts (volume) increase correspondingly. The temporal course of this filling is one of the parameters that characterize the diastolic function of the LV.

124. What is the nuclear procedure of choice for assessment of RV function?

First-pass studies for assessment of RV ejection fraction. For this purpose, the radiotracers should be administered slowly, rather than using a rapid bolus, as is necessary for LV ejection fraction determinations.

CHEST X-RAY

Matthew R. Brewer, M.D., Rina Sternlieb, M.D., Gabriel Adelmann, M.D., and Curtis E. Green, M.D.

125. List the chest x-ray findings in a patient with chronic congestive heart failure (CHF).
- Cardiac dilation (cardiomegaly)
- Pulmonary venous congestion
- The presence of Kerley B lines (interstitial edema)
- An enlarged pulmonary artery trunk

For radiographic findings in acute heart failure (pulmonary edema), see question 140.

126. Does a normal chest x-ray rule out the diagnosis of CHF?

No. CHF is a clinical diagnosis. The various imaging modalities, including radiography, can show the underlying structural changes of the heart (cardiomegaly) and the repercussion of LV dysfunction on the pulmonary vasculature (congestion). Early stages of CHF or heart failure that has responded to therapy may not have either of these findings and be missed on chest x-ray.

127. When is the heart considered to be enlarged on a chest x-ray study?
The radiologic criteria for the diagnosis of **cardiomegaly** include:
- On a frontal posteroanterior film, a cardiothoracic index > 0.5 (Fig. 17)
- On a lateral film, the contact between the RV and the sternum extends cranially beyond the lower third of the distance between the sternal angle and the diaphragm (see Figure 40 in Chapter 6)

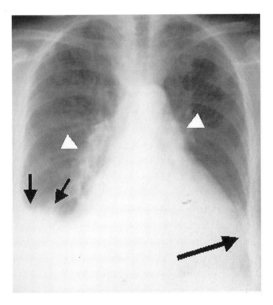

FIGURE 17. Cardiomegaly in a 56-year-old patient with recurrent myocardial infarction and congestive heart failure. Note the dilated left ventricle (*long arrow*), right pleural effusion (*short arrows*), and dilated pulmonary trunk and right main pulmonary artery (*arrowheads*).

128. What are the pitfalls of the radiographic diagnosis of cardiomegaly?
In a **false-positive diagnosis:**
1. On an anteroposterior frontal film, the cardiac shadow may appear larger than it truly is because of the phenomenon of magnification (see Chapter 1).
2. On a study that is not performed at end inspiration, the dimensions of the thorax are not maximized, a fact that may lead to a false "increase" in the cardiothoracic index.
3. In obese patients, there may be apparent cardiomegaly on posteroanterior and lateral films.
A **false-negative diagnosis** may result from lung overinflation in patients with pulmonary emphysema.

129. Cardiomegaly on chest x-ray can be due to one of two major causes (or both). Name these conditions.
1. Dilation of the ventricles (LV, RV, or both) or atria (or both)
2. Pericardial effusion

130. Name the most frequent cause of cardiomegaly.
LV dilation. This condition is noticeable on a frontal film (cardiothoracic index increase) and, possibly, on a lateral film (which visualizes the RV, most frequently enlarged secondary to LV dysfunction).

131. Does LV hypertrophy cause cardiomegaly?
No. In general, LV hypertrophy is not associated with dilation or heart failure (increased pulmonary venous pressure) and does not cause cardiomegaly.

132. What are the radiographic signs of LV dilation besides the increased cardiothoracic ratio?
- Indentation of the gastric bubble by the inferiorly displaced apex (the gastric bubble is seen as a radiotransparent [i.e., black] area in the left upper quadrant; in patients with LV dilation, there is an impression [indentation] on the upper border of the gastric bubble)
- A bulge of the posterior contour on a lateral chest x-ray film, below the level of the LA (Fig. 18)

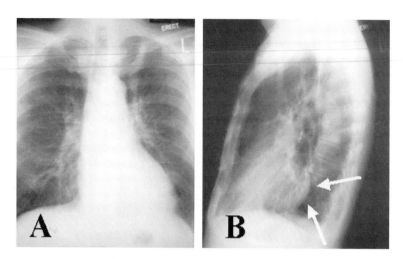

FIGURE 18. In this patient with a history of recurrent myocardial infarction, the LV dilatation was missed on the PA film (A) and was diagnosed on a lateral film (B), which showed a posterior bulge of the cardiac shadow (*arrows*).

133. How sensitive is chest radiography for LV dilation?
The LV must be almost twice its normal size before it can be detected reliably on the chest radiograph.

134. State the diagnostic importance of the position of the LV apex on a frontal chest x-ray.
In normal subjects, the apex is directed inferiorly. Several patterns of deviation from this normal position have been described, but the sensitivity and specificity of these patterns for the diagnosis of LV and RV dilation are low.

135. What are the radiologic signs of RV dilation?
In patients with **early** RV dilation, the contact between the RV and the sternum, as shown on a lateral film, extends cranially above the lower one third of the distance between the sternal angle and the diaphragm (see Figure 40 in Chapter 6).

In **later stages** of RV dilation, there is posterior displacement of the LV and leftward rotation of the heart, which cause the RV to become apparent on the posteroanterior film as the left heart border (the RV is normally not a border-forming structure on the frontal chest x-ray). Cardiac rotation causes the apex to assume a horizontal orientation.

136. What are the pitfalls of the radiographic diagnosis of RV dilation?
A **false-positive** diagnosis of RV dilation is possible in a distorted relationship between the RV and the sternum. The most frequent underlying conditions are:
- Pectus excavatum
- Distorted anatomy of the sternum, as a result of sternotomy

- The presence of abnormal tissue in the mediastinum (e.g., fat, tumor)

A **false-negative** diagnosis of RV dilation can be made in patients with pulmonary hyperinflation resulting from emphysema. This is important to keep in mind because severe pulmonary emphysema also can be associated with RV dilation and failure.

137. What are Kerley B lines?

Small horizontal lines seen in the peripheral zone of the lungs in patients with chronic heart failure. They are believed to represent a disturbance in lymphatic drainage as a result of the increased pulmonary venous pressure.

138. State the significance of an enlarged pulmonary artery trunk in patients with heart failure.

An enlarged pulmonary artery trunk is indicative of an increased pulmonary artery pressure, generally secondary to LV failure (see Figure 17). For a discussion of pulmonary artery trunk dilation, see Figure 40 in Chapter 6.

139. Describe the pulmonary findings on the chest x-ray in patients with heart failure.

In patients with CHF, there is an elevated LA pressure causing increased pulmonary venous pressure (pulmonary venous hypertension). There are different stages of pulmonary venous hypertension, corresponding to the different degrees of LA (pulmonary capillary wedge) pressure elevation.

With **moderately** increased wedge pressure, there is dilation of the pulmonary vessels of the upper lobe and contraction of the lower lobe vessels. This results in vascular markings that are more pronounced in the upper than in the lower lobes (in normal subjects, owing to gravity, the lower lobe pulmonary vessels are approximately twice the size of the upper lobe vessels). This finding is termed *redistribution* or *cephalization* of the pulmonary circulation.

With **moderately to severely** increased capillary wedge pressure, there is interstitial pulmonary edema, as evidenced by (1) a "reticular" pattern in the lower pulmonary lobes, representing the accumulation of fluid in the interstitium between the pulmonary alveoli (Fig. 19), and (2) blurring of the pulmonary vasculature in the upper lobes.

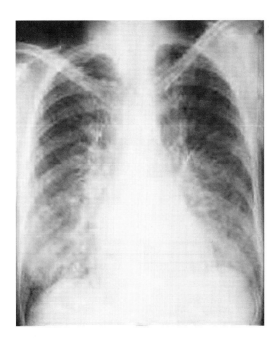

FIGURE 19. Interstitial pulmonary edema. The heart is enlarged, and there is redistribution of pulmonary blood flow to the upper lobes. Note the blurring of the pulmonary vessels and the increased interstitial markings (seen as indistinct white areas, especially prominent in the vicinity of the hili).

With **severely** increased capillary wedge pressure, there is alveolar pulmonary edema with blurring of the entire surface of the lung fields.

There is not always a good correspondence between the pulmonary capillary wedge pressure and the degree of congestion seen on chest x-ray. Some patients may manifest full-blown pulmonary edema with only moderately increased capillary wedge pressure, whereas others may not show the complete x-ray findings even with higher increases in wedge pressure.

140. Is it possible to distinguish between patients with acute pulmonary edema superimposed on chronic CHF and patients with acute pulmonary edema without prior heart failure by chest radiography?

In patients with acute pulmonary edema that is not superimposed on chronic CHF, the chest x-ray shows:

- A typical "butterfly" distribution of the pulmonary edema fluid (i.e., predominantly in the pulmonary hili)
- A nondilated LV and LA

A typical clinical setting for these findings is the pulmonary edema associated with myocardial infarction.

141. Is LV systolic failure the only cause of increased pulmonary venous pressure?

No. There are numerous additional causes of pulmonary venous hypertension:

Inability of the LV to maintain a normal stroke volume. This can be secondary to:

Decreased diastolic relaxation of the LV (diastolic LV dysfunction)
Obstructed LV filling in diastole, owing to mitral stenosis
Obstructed LV emptying in systole, owing to aortic stenosis
Systolic reflux of blood into the LA, owing to mitral regurgitation
Diastolic reflux of blood into the LV, owing to aortic insuffiency

Increased blood volume that exceeds the capacity of the pulmonary venous system (volume overload) and leads to accumulation of fluid in the pulmonary interstitial space, this can occur with atrial septal defect.

142. How can the pulmonary vascular changes seen on chest x-ray help establish the cause of cardiomegaly?

Numerous conditions can lead to dilation of the heart chambers or fluid accumulation in the pericardial space. Cardiomegaly can be associated with normal, increased, or decreased pulmonary vascular markings. By assessing the pulmonary vasculature, the cause of cardiomegaly can be narrowed.

Normal pulmonary vasculature
CHF after diuretic therapy
Pericardial effusion
Pericardial cyst

Increased pulmonary vasculature
Primary DCM
Secondary DCM (ischemic, valvular, or toxic)

Decreased pulmonary vasculature
Pulmonary atresia without ventriculoseptal defect
Ebstein's anomaly

143. In a patient with pulmonary congestion, does the absence of LV dilation on a chest x-ray mean there is no LV dysfunction?

No. The presence of LV dilation is *not* an essential component of this diagnosis. A normal LV size on chest x-ray does not rule out:

- Diastolic dysfunction in a hypertrophic, nondilated LV
- Acute LV dysfunction, as can be seen in patients with acute myocardial infarction or rup-

tured papillary muscle (acute mitral regurgitation) or in patients with mitral or aortic valve destruction resulting from infective endocarditis

144. What are the radiographic characteristics of DCM?

DCM is characterized by different degrees of cardiomegaly and pulmonary venous hypertension (congestion) (Fig. 20).

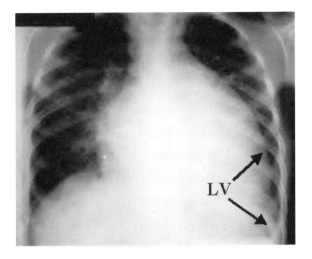

FIGURE 20. Dilated cardiomyopathy. Note the severely dilated left ventricle (*arrows*), as well as the *absence* of pulmonary congestion in this well-diuresed patient.

145. What are the radiographic characteristics of hypertrophic cardiomyopathy?

Isolated LV hypertrophy is not noticeable on the chest x-ray. Associated pulmonary venous hypertension or LV dilations are the only signs that can be detected on chest x-ray.

146. What are the radiographic characteristics of restrictive cardiomyopathy?

Restrictive cardiomyopathy does not have distinctive radiographic findings.

147. When should the diagnosis of compensated LV failure be suggested by a chest x-ray?

Whenever there is evidence of a condition potentially resulting in LV failure (e.g., cardiomegaly, coronary or valvular calcification), in the absence of pulmonary venous congestion, the possibility of compensated cardiac failure should come to mind.

148. What lesions present with normal pulmonary vascularity and cardiac enlargement?

Cardiomegaly may be due to true cardiac dilation or to pericardial effusion. The normal lung vasculature indicates the presence of compensatory mechanisms, either intrinsic or secondary to diuretic therapy. The differential diagnosis includes *p*ericardial effusion and increased *p*reload/afterload treated by *p*rescription, occasionally in the presence of *m*yocardiopathy. The mnemonic to remember this is: *3 PM.*

4. ISCHEMIC HEART DISEASE AND MYOCARDIAL ISCHEMIA

CARDIAC CATHETERIZATION

Gabriel Adelmann, M.D., Benjamin Kleiber, M.D., and Andrew E. Ajani, MBBS, FRACP

1. What elements of information can be obtained in the catheterization laboratory (cath lab) regarding the impact of coronary artery disease (CAD) on the myocardium?

Information about myocardial structure, function, and microcirculation.

2. List the main structural changes of the myocardium that occur as a consequence of CAD.

Abnormal regional systolic function.

3. What is the role of cardiac catheterization in the identification of LV structural changes?

In addition to the above, CAD can result in the following left ventricle (LV) structural changes:
- Dilation
- Aneurysm
- Calcification
- Rupture (pseudoaneurysm)

4. Summarize the angiographic hallmarks of LV rupture.

LV rupture may involve:
- The **LV free wall,** in which case it rapidly leads to tamponade and death, unless there is pseudoaneurysm formation (see question 5)
- A **papillary muscle,** resulting in acute, severe mitral regurgitation
- The **interventricular septum (IVS),** resulting in ventricular septal defect, expressed as opacification of the right ventricle (RV) at the time of contrast material injection into the LV (Fig. 1)

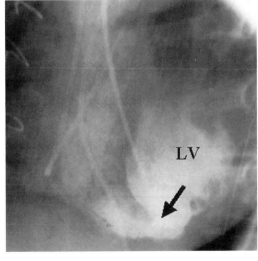

FIGURE 1. Interventricular septal rupture (*arrow*), 5 days after an acute anteroseptal myocardial infarction. LV = left ventricle.

5. What is the hallmark of LV pseudoaneurysm as visualized by cardiac catheterization?

LV pseudoaneurysm is a form of myocardial rupture, in which the transmural hemorrhage is contained ("sealed off") by an intrapericardial clot. Angiographically a pseudoaneurysm appears as an area of localized, contained contrast material extravasation from the LV cavity into the pericardium (Fig. 2).

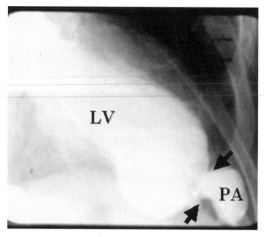

FIGURE 2. LV pseudoaneurysm (PA). Note the "narrow neck" of the contrast collection.

6. What are the similarities and differences between the angiographic appearance of an LV aneurysm and that of a pseudoaneurysm?

The **similarity** between these two conditions is a distorted LV shape, with an area of contrast extension beyond that seen in normal subjects. The **differences** are:

1. An **aneurysm** has a broad base and represents a "gradual bulge" in the LV contour.

2. A **pseudoaneurysm** has a narrow base, corresponding to an abrupt discontinuity at the site of myocardial rupture.

7. What is the significance of myocardial calcification?

Myocardial calcification, easily observed by fluoroscopy (generally carried out before the catheterization), suggests an old, calcified myocardial infarction (MI). Myocardial calcification generally can be considered as a sign of chronic ischemic heart disease.

8. Describe the changes in LV function caused by ischemic heart disease and identified by left ventriculography.

Myocardial ischemia causes diastolic and systolic LV dysfunction. The first to occur in the *ischemic cascade* is **diastolic dysfunction,** but this typically is not shown by left ventriculography. The impact of coronary ischemia on LV function, as identified in the catheterization laboratory, consists of different degrees of **systolic wall motion abnormalities,** ranging from hypokinesis to akinesis to dyskinesis. For a discussion of these contraction abnormalities, see Chapter 3.

9. How can myocardial perfusion be assessed in the cath lab?

Coronary catheterization classically has been used for visualization of the epicardial coronary arteries. The final consequence of epicardial coronary stenosis is a decrease in coronary capillary blood flow, however. Coronary catheterization uses *direct* assessment of the coronary arteries as *indirect* evidence of myocardial ischemia. It has been suggested that coronary catheterization also can give important information regarding the microcirculation, based on demonstration of:

- Myocardial "blush" (i.e., the presence of a ground-glass appearance of the heart muscle on injection of contrast material into the coronaries; the presence of this blush indicates integrity of the microcirculation) (Fig. 3)
- The speed (number of heart beats) with which the myocardial blush clears (indicating the runoff of blood from the myocardial capillaries)

Based on these parameters, a myocardial blush score has been established and has been found to be predictive of cardiac mortality in MI patients after thrombolysis. Briefly stated, patients who have either absent myocardial blush or blush that does not clear from the microvasculature over a relatively long period have a substantially higher mortality than patients in whom myocardial blush is present and clears within three heartbeats. The absence of myocardial blush has been postulated to represent the absence of actual microcirculation in the involved segment, whereas a persistent myocardial blush has been attributed to extravasation of contrast material from damaged myocardial capillaries.

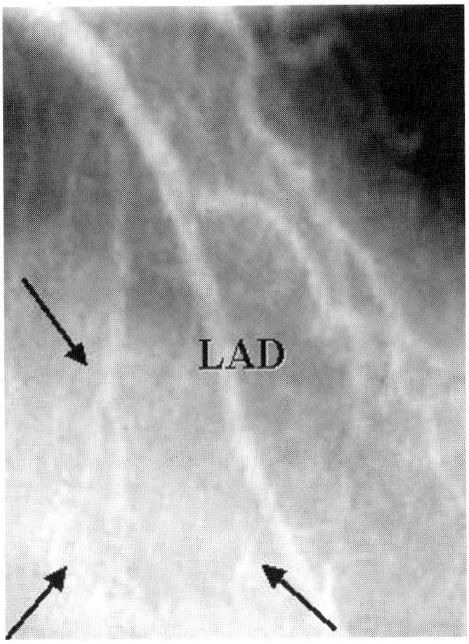

FIGURE 3. Myocardial blush. Note the ground glass appearance (*arrows*) of the myocardium supplied by a normal LAD.

10. Is it possible to identify myocardial viability in the cath lab?

Although myocardial viability is an issue generally addressed in the echocardiography or nuclear medicine laboratory, the following angiographic characteristics have been suggested to indicate viability:

- Transient myocardial **blush**
- **Post-extrasystolic potentiation** (see Chapter 3)

11. What is myocardial staining?

Myocardial staining is a complication of percutaneous transluminal coronary angioplasty (PTCA) and consists of extravasation of contrast material into the myocardium, resulting in a "stain" that does not correspond to the LV cavity and is persistent over a relatively long period (Fig. 4).

ECHOCARDIOGRAPHY

Gabriel Adelmann, M.D., and Neil J. Weissman, M.D.

12. What information can echocardiography provide regarding the impact of coronary ischemia on the myocardium?

- **Structural LV or RV changes** (dilation, scar, aneurysm, myocardial rupture after infarction)
- **Functional LV or RV changes** (hypokinesis, akinesis, dyskinesis)

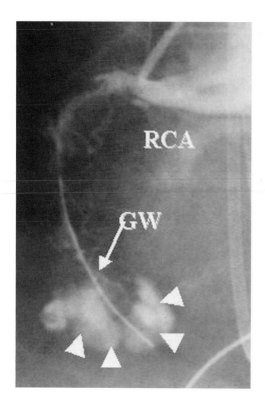

FIGURE 4. Myocardial staining (*arrowheads*) as a complication of PTCA. Although this image bears a superficial resemblance to an LV gram, it was obtained after intracoronary injection of contrast into the RCA, with extravasation into the myocardium through perforation of the vessel wall. GW = guidewire

13. Can echocardiography help distinguish acute from chronic ischemia?

No. Regional hypokinesis, akinesis, or dyskinesis can be seen as a result of chronic, long-standing ischemic heart disease or in the setting of acute myocardial ischemia.

14. Describe the echocardiographic features of a myocardial scar.

There is no pathognomonic echocardiographic sign for myocardial scar, but visualization of a thin, bright, noncontractile segment is highly suggestive. Identification of a scar suggests that the probability of functional recovery after revascularization is low.

15. Describe the echocardiographic features of a LV aneurysm.

LV aneurysm is defined as a localized area of LV dilation that moves outward during systole ("bulging") (Fig. 5). An aneurysm results from replacement of the myocardium with scar tissue that does not have the same mechanical properties as normal heart muscle and does not contract. LV aneurysms most frequently involve the apex and frequently harbor clots. The formation of aneurysm is an expression of adverse LV remodeling after MI.

16. What degree of myocardial bulging defines an LV aneurysm?

There is no precise definition of the severity of myocardial bulging that constitutes an aneurysm.

17. Explain the difference between an LV aneurysm and an LV pseudoaneurysm.

An LV **aneurysm** involves all of the normal cardiac layers (endocardium, myocardium, epicardium) and has a wide base; it is a "bulge" of the LV.

An LV **pseudoaneurysm** does not involve all of the normal cardiac layers because it is caused by an area of muscle rupture. A pseudoaneurysm has a narrow base, which is the communication of the LV chamber with the pericardial space (Fig. 6).

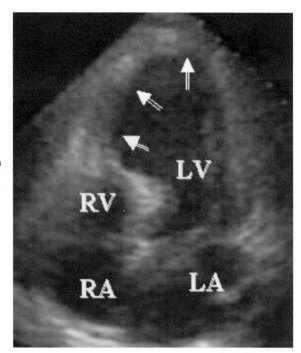

FIGURE 5. Left ventricular aneurysm (*arrows*), four-chamber view. LV = left ventricle, LA = left atrium, RV = right ventricle, RA = right atrium.

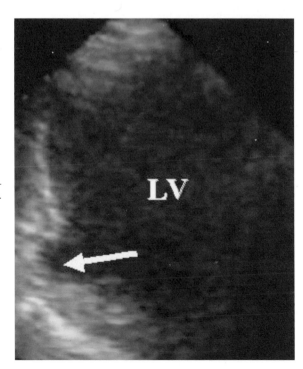

FIGURE 6. Left ventricular pseudoaneurysm (*arrow*). LV = left ventricle.

18. Which acute or subacute complications of MI can be shown by echocardiography?
- **LV pseudoaneurysm** (rupture of the LV free wall, with a sealing pericardial clot)
- **Rupture of the papillary muscle with acute mitral regurgitation**
- Ischemic rupture of the IVS, with creation of ventriculoseptal defect (Fig. 7.)

Unsealed LV rupture rarely is seen because these patients die before there is time to perform an echocardiographic study.

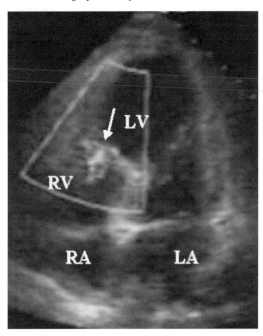

FIGURE 7. Ventricular septal defect (*arrow*) in a patient after myocardial infarction. LV = left ventricle, LA = left atrium, RV = right ventricle, RA = right atrium. (See also Color Plates, Figure 8.)

19. What is the role of echocardiography in the diagnosis of myocardial ischemia?
Echocardiography may show the presence of ischemic heart disease based on:
- Findings consistent with chronic ischemia (see questions 12 and 13)
- Identification of LV dysfunction at rest, consistent with either acute or chronic ischemia
- Identification of new-onset LV dysfunction with concurrent physical exercise or dobutamine stimulation (exercise/dobutamine echocardiography), diagnostic of inducible ischemia. In these patients, there is underlying CAD (stenosis in the subepicardial portion of the coronaries), with the potential to cause ischemia (reduced blood flow in the capillary microcirculation)

20. How can ischemic heart disease be diagnosed by exercise or dobutamine echocardiography?
Normal LV function at rest does not signify the absence of significant coronary stenosis. In these patients, increasing the oxygen demands of the myocardium by physical exercise or dobutamine-induced tachycardia and inotropic stimulation causes dysfunction in the segments supplied by a stenotic coronary artery. In these segments, the *contractile reserve* is diminished. The blood supply through the stenotic artery is sufficient for the resting state of the myocardium but insufficient for the stimulated myocardium:

1. Previously normal segments may become hypokinetic or akinetic.
2. Hypokinetic segments may become akinetic (this change is much more difficult to assess than development of LV dysfunction in previously normal segments).
3. The LV cavity may increase, owing to stress-induced global ischemia leading to LV dilation.

21. How is the assessment of resting LV function and exercise-induced changes performed?

LV function at rest and stress is assessed on a semiquantitative basis. The different myocardial segments are assessed qualitatively as normal, hypokinetic, akinetic, or dyskinetic.

22. Present the practical steps of an exercise echocardiographic stress test.

1. The LV is imaged from the parasternal long-axis, short-axis, two-chamber, and four-chamber views at baseline while resting. Selected beats displaying each of the views are digitized and played in an "endless loop" format. This process is repeated for each of the echocardiographic views. A representative heartbeat must have each of the following:
   - Optimal visualization of all the myocardial segments normally seen from that view
   - A true longitudinal or transverse cut without foreshortening
   - Not an extrasystolic or postextrasystolic beat, which may show global and segmental LV contractility different from those of "normal" heartbeats

2. The four representative heartbeats (one for each echocardiographic view) are displayed side by side, in a "quad screen" format.

3. The patient exercises on a treadmill with electrocardiogram (ECG), heart rate, and blood pressure monitoring. The stress test is stopped:
   - When 85% of the target heart rate is reached (if the patient is able to exercise further, this is highly desirable because the exercise tolerance has diagnostic and prognostic value beyond the ECG and echocardiographic findings)
   - If there is a decrease in blood pressure, severe arrhythmia, or ECG signs or clinical symptoms suggestive of ischemia (most commonly, chest pain)
   - If the patient feels he or she cannot continue any further (generally, because of fatigue, shortness of breath, or lower limb pain)

4. Immediately after stopping the treadmill, the patient is guided as rapidly as possible back to the examination bed and the echocardiographic views described in the first step are obtained within 90 seconds (preferably within 60 seconds) of terminating the exercise.

5. The representative images at rest and stress are rearranged so the rest and stress beats are side by side.

6. The images are compared in regard to their technical standards (it is essential to ascertain that, for each view, the LV is imaged from the same angle).

7. The images are compared in regard to the changes in LV contractility and chamber size. The normal response to exercise is global hyperkinesis and decrease of the LV chamber dimensions. Abnormal responses include:
   - The lack of a hyperkinetic response
   - The development of hypokinesis or akinesis in a previously normal segments
   - Exercise-induced LV dilation

8. The echocardiographic, ECG, and clinical findings are integrated into a final conclusion referring to the probability and localization of significant coronary stenosis.

23. Discuss the particular technical challenges posed by exercise echocardiography.

Exercise echocardiography combines the most difficult task of cardiac ultrasound (i.e., the assessment of segmental and global LV function) with the most challenging situation (stress-induced tachycardia with respiratory interference). Immediately after exercise, patients are:
   - Tachypneic, a fact that accentuates the intrathoracic cardiac motion and the interposition of air-filled, poorly echogenic lung tissue between the heart and the transducer
   - Tachycardic, which also increases the cardiac motion in the chest cavity

In addition, it is essential to perform the postexercise echocardiographic study as rapidly as possible, while the patient is still tachycardic. It has been shown that exercise-induced contraction abnormalities may subside rapidly with decreasing heart rates (within 90 seconds). Stress echocardiography requires substantial experience on the part of the sonographer and on the part of the physician who interprets the study.

24. What are the steps of a dobutamine stress echocardiographic study?

Dobutamine stress echocardiography is similar to exercise echocardiography, but the tachycardic and inotropic responses are elicited by an infusion of dobutamine. Dobutamine is infused gradually at increasing doses until 85% of the target heart rate is reached. Generally the dobutamine protocol involves three or four steps of increases of 5–10 µg of dobutamine every 3 minutes. If, at the end of the dobutamine protocol, that heart rate is not achieved, low doses of atropine are administered (typically, ≤ 1.0 mg). The LV is imaged from the same views as those used for exercise echocardiography. At the end of this study, there are four successive quad screens to interpret, each showing the LV under resting conditions and under successively increasing doses of dobutamine. The interpretation of the dobutamine stress test is similar to that of the exercise stress test.

25. When should echocardiographic contrast material be used in the setting of stress echocardiography?

One of the main challenges of stress echocardiography is to visualize the LV adequately from the different imaging windows. In patients in whom all views cannot be obtained, intravenous administration of echocardiographic contrast material produces an intense opacification of the LV chamber, allowing clear delineation of the endocardial border. This may salvage an otherwise uninterpretable study. Although the use of contrast agents is necessary in only 3–5% of regular echocardiography studies, they are used more frequently in the setting of stress echocardiography.

Echocardiographic contrast material also is used for myocardial contrast echocardiography (MCE) assessment of perfusion at rest and under stress conditions (see later).

26. When should I order an exercise stress test and when should I order a dobutamine stress test for the diagnosis of ischemic heart disease?

Whenever feasible, an exercise stress test is preferable because of the additional information provided by the patient's exercise tolerance and symptomatic status under physical exertion. A dobutamine stress test is indicated in the following settings:

1. The patient is unable or unwilling to exercise.
2. It is estimated that the patient will not be able to exercise long enough to reach 85% of the target heart rate.
3. The clinical question to be answered pertains not to the *presence* of ischemia, but to the *reversibility* of ischemic myocardial dysfunction (i.e., myocardial viability). For assessment of the probability that hypokinetic or akinetic myocardial segments will return to normal function after revascularization (myocardial viability; see later), a dobutamine stress test is necessary.

27. What are the different patterns of myocardial contractility response to dobutamine stimulation, and what is their clinical significance?

PATTERN	BEFORE	AFTER	SIGNIFICANCE
1	Normal	Hyperkinetic	Normal response
2	Normal	Hypokinetic	Inducible ischemia
3	Hypokinetic	Hyperkinetic	Normal response
4	Hypokinetic	Improves, then worsens (biphasic response)	Viable myocardium
5	Hypokinetic/akinetic	Hypokinetic/akinetic	Myocardial scar

28. Distinguish the significance of pattern 3 in question 27 from that of pattern 2.

Pattern 2 shows **normal myocardial function at rest,** with myocardial dysfunction observed only under conditions of stress; this phenomenon is termed *inducible ischemia.*

Pattern 3 shows **decreased function even at rest,** which indicates a more severe and long-standing degree of myocardial ischemia or a previous subendocardial infarction.

29. What is the explanation for the biphasic response to dobutamine stimulation with viable myocardium?

Although the complete explanation is still unclear, it is postulated that viable segments are able to respond to catecholamine stimulation by an *increase* in contractility *at low doses,* whereas the use of *higher doses* produces a *decrease* in contractility owing to worsening ischemia.

30. Why is it not possible to show myocardial viability by exercise stress test?

As practiced at most centers in the United States, exercise echocardiography uses a treadmill (as opposed to the exercise bicycle used in many European countries), so it is impossible to image the effects of low-level exercise without interfering with the patient's ability to exercise to peak exercise.

31. How do dobutamine echocardiography, exercise echocardiography, and nuclear perfusion tests compare in regard to detection of myocardial ischemia?

These three modalities have similar sensitivity and specificity, of approximately 85–90%.

32. How does stress echocardiography compare with nonimaging stress ECG in regard to the detection of myocardial ischemia?

Stress echocardiography (by either exercise or dobutamine stimulation) has a higher sensitivity and specificity for ischemic heart disease (around 90%) than nonimaging stress ECG (generally around 80%).

33. How does dobutamine echocardiography compare with nuclear perfusion scans for the detection of myocardial viability?

Dobutamine echocardiography has a lower sensitivity than nuclear perfusion scans for the detection of myocardial viability. Dobutamine has a higher specificity, however, for detection of viable segments that respond to revascularization with an improvement in contractility.

For clarification, it was stated earlier that myocardial viability is synonymous with functional recovery after revascularization. This statement is an oversimplification. A myocardial segment affected by chronic ischemia is often a mix a viable myocytes and of myocardial scar. Viability is not an "all-or-none" phenomenon, but rather represents a histologic and functional spectrum. Sometimes a patient in whom revascularization (with the attending morbidity and mortality) has been undertaken based on a viability study does not show functional improvement after the intervention.

Dobutamine echocardiography is less apt than nuclear perfusion studies to pick up all the viable segments but is more apt to show selectively segments that probably would improve their systolic function after revascularization.

34. If dobutamine echocardiography is more apt than nuclear perfusion studies to show viable myocardial segments that would benefit from myocardial revascularization, what is the role of nuclear cardiology in this setting?

1. In some patients, it is technically impossible to obtain echocardiographic images of diagnostic quality.

2. Although improvement in systolic function after revascularization remains the main goal of interventional cardiology, there are additional benefits that may be derived from the presence of an "open artery," including greater electrical stability (decreased incidence of ventricular arrhythmia) and a lower likelihood of adverse myocardial remodeling (LV dilation or aneurysm formation). Good clinical judgment and individualization of treatment are necessary before a patient is sent for a revascularization procedure for these indications alone.

35. Does every patient with coronary lesions technically amenable to revascularization need a viability study?

No. Patients with normal or mildly impaired function do not need a viability study. For patients with moderately or severely impaired LV function, viability testing is the subject of intense debate. Despite the intuitive appeal of this approach, the absolute necessity of a viability study has never been proved conclusively. A multicenter, large-scale study currently is addressing this question.

36. What are the indications for echocardiographic stress testing?
- In patients with suspected ischemic heart disease based on the risk factor profile or the presence of clinical symptoms (or both)
- After MI, for prognostic assessment (what is the likelihood of a recurrent ischemic event?), activity prescription (what is the "safe" amount of physical exercise that the patient can undertake after he or she returns home?), and evaluation of medical therapy (is the patient "sufficiently protected" against exercise-induced ischemia by the medications he or she is taking?)
- When myocardial revascularization is contemplated (viability studies)
- In patients scheduled for noncardiac surgery; in this population, stress echocardiography or nuclear studies are indicated based on the probability of ischemic heart disease (risk factors, clinical symptoms) and on the type of surgery (certain surgical procedures, such as vascular surgery, imply a higher risk for perioperative ischemic events, whereas others, such as cataract surgery, imply a minimal risk)

37. List some additional echocardiographic techniques (besides classic echocardiography and echocardiographic stress test) for detecting the impact of coronary ischemia on the myocardium.
- Myocardial contrast echocardiography (MCE)
- Tissue Doppler imaging
- Myocardial tissue characterization

38. What is MCE?
A technique based on intravenous administration of echocardiographic contrast material, consisting of minuscule microbubbles with a protein, lipid, or synthetic shell enclosing a small volume of gas. These microbubbles are echogenic, and when they perfuse into the myocardial microcirculation, they cause *myocardial opacification*. MCE can be applied under either rest or stress conditions.

39. Discuss the role of MCE in the diagnosis of ischemic heart disease.
Although the concept of MCE was introduced many years ago, only recently has this method started emerging as a viable diagnostic technique. MCE has not yet been proven to work in the routine clinical setting, however. MCE is the subject of intense ongoing research, and the future will show its place in the diagnostic algorithm of patients with ischemic heart disease. If MCE does gain widespread acceptance, it will be possible to obtain a complete assessment of ischemic heart disease (myocardial microcirculation, LV function) in a single echocardiographic study. This would represent an ideal (complete, harmless, cheap, widely available, fast, portable) "one-stop shop" in the diagnosis of myocardial ischemia, while also providing information regarding the cardiac valves and pericardium.

40. What is tissue Doppler?
As its name indicates, tissue Doppler is an extension of the Doppler technique applied to the moving cardiac tissues, rather than flowing blood (see Chapter 11). The motion of ischemic myocardium differs from that of normal myocardium in regard to:
- Velocity
- Timing
- Characteristics in the subendocardial versus the subepicardial area
- The parameters of diastolic function (diastolic function is the first to be affected by myocardial ischemia)

41. What is the role of tissue Doppler in the diagnosis of ischemic heart disease?

These characteristics can be used for the diagnosis of myocardial ischemia.

At present, tissue Doppler can be viewed as an adjunct, rather than a replacement, of classic echocardiography for the diagnosis of myocardial ischemia (and for almost any other of its indications).

42. Discuss echocardiographic myocardial tissue characterization and its role in the diagnosis of ischemic heart disease.

Diagnostic ultrasound is based on a rigorous filtering and electronic processing of the echoes bouncing back from the tissues to the transducer. In this process of filtering, a certain component of the echo is discarded. This is the so-called backscattered echo (i.e., echoes that have multiple directions of propagation and cannot serve for the creation of the final diagnostic image). It has been shown, however, that the characteristics of these backscattered echoes depend on the histologic properties of the tissue that the echo bounces off of. Analysis of the backscatter pattern has been suggested as a method for diagnosing myocardial ischemia. Although described many years ago, this method has not found widespread acceptance and remains of research interest only.

MAGNETIC RESONANCE IMAGING

Gabriel Adelmann, M.D., and Anthon R. Fuisz, M.D.

43. Summarize the main issues regarding ischemic heart disease that can be clarified by magnetic resonance imaging (MRI).

- The **presence** of CAD in a given patient (does the patient have ischemic heart disease or not?)
- Its **extent** (how large is the area involved?)
- Its **reversibility** (can it be "fixed " by revascularization procedures, or has the affected myocardial territory been replaced by fibrotic tissue [scar]?)

44. What is myocardial viability?

The reversible nature of the ischemic systolic dysfunction of a myocardial segment when the blood flow is re-established. Reversible ischemic systolic dysfunction may be caused by:

- A **previous** episode of acute ischemia with residual myocardial dysfunction (*myocardial stunning*); the therapy in these patients may be conservative or interventional (revascularization)
- Severe, **chronic** ischemia (*myocardial hibernation*); the therapy is coronary revascularization.

45. What is the practical importance of showing myocardial hibernation?

This is an area of intense debate. Although some authorities advocate revascularization (i.e., PTCA or coronary artery bypass graft [CABG] surgery) of any significant coronary arteries stenosis that is technically amenable to such procedures, others suggest that, before subjecting the patient to an invasive procedure (with the attending complications), definite proof for the reversible nature of myocardial dysfunction should be obtained. Large-scale studies are needed to compare the outcome of patients in whom revascularization was based on technical considerations alone (feasibility of the revascularization procedure) with that of patients in whom the decision to perform a revascularization procedure was based on demonstration of myocardial hibernation.

46. State the main MRI methods to address the presence, extent, and reversibility of ischemic heart disease.

Direct coronary artery visualization (for a discussion of these methods, see Chapter 5)

Assessment of the consequences of stenosis in the epicardial coronary artery on the capillary blood flow to the corresponding myocardium (microcirculation) by:

Myocardial perfusion
Myocardial function
Viability with delayed hyperenhancement techniques

47. Define myocardial perfusion and the factors that influence it.

Myocardial perfusion is the blood flow delivered to a certain volume of myocardium per unit of time. Myocardial perfusion depends on:

The degree of development of the microcirculation (genetically determined number of capillaries per unit of myocardium)

The blood flow through the microcirculation, in turn dependent on:

The presence or absence of narrowing of the epicardial segment of the coronary artery (i.e., coronary artery stenosis)

The degree of collateral flow

48. How can myocardial perfusion be identified by MRI?
- Directly measuring and quantifying the blood flow through a coronary segment
- Assessment of the blood flow through the entire heart, based on determination of the degree of oxygenation in the hemoglobin in the coronary sinus
- Quantitative and semiquantitative methods of myocardial perfusion assessment, based on the patterns of contrast enhancement. Contrast enhancement seems to be the best method of myocardial perfusion assessment.

49. What is myocardial contrast enhancement?

Myocardial perfusion can be identified based on the degree of "brightening" of the different segments when a contrast agent (gadolinium) is administered. The degree of myocardial brightening is termed *enhancement* and represents myocardial perfusion.

50. How is the use of gadolinium different in the setting of myocardial perfusion studies from the use in direct coronary artery visualization?

Gadolinium is not a blood-pool contrast agent (i.e., it is not confined to the intravascular space but diffuses into the myocardium). This property makes it ideal for assessment of myocardial perfusion but prevents it from allowing adequate distinction between the coronary arteries and the surrounding myocardium. Gadolinium is an **essential part** of perfusion studies but is **not used** for direct visualization of coronary arteries.

As new blood-pool contrast agents are being developed, this distinction may disappear in the future.

51. Practically, how can gadolinium be visualized in the myocardium?

Intravenously injected gadolinium can be followed as it progresses through the RV, through the LV, and into the myocardium (from the epicardium to the endocardium). Myocardial perfusion studies are first-pass studies, because they are based on following the progress of the contrast substance on its first pass through the central circulation, before it has time to return to the right heart by the systemic veins (i.e., before its recirculation).

52. What are the different patterns of contrast enhancement and their significance for the diagnosis of ischemic heart disease?

Early transient enhancement—present at approximately 30 seconds after contrast material injection and absent 10 minutes afterward; this pattern is characteristic of normal myocardium

Delayed transient enhancement—onset slower than in normal segments, but contrast is absent 10 minutes later; this is characteristic of ischemic but viable myocardium (Fig. 8A)

Delayed hyperenhancement—slow onset of enhancement that reaches a higher intensity than normal segments; this is characteristic of nonviable myocardium (scar) (Fig. 8B)

These patterns correspond to the semiquantitative method of enhancement assessment. Quantitative assessments also are possible but are used rarely for clinical purposes.

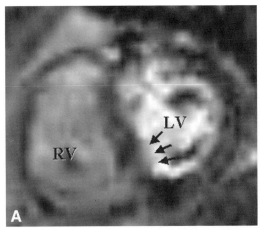

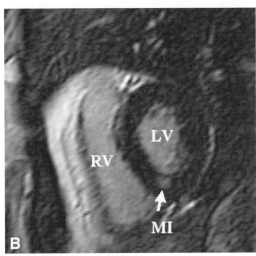

FIGURE 8. *A,* In this patient, the myocardial uptake of MR contrast agent had a slower than normal onset and was absent 10 minutes after injection. This pattern is termed *delayed transient enhancement* and is characteristic of viable myocardium. The logical next step is to refer this patient for cardiac catheterization and possible revascularization. *B,* Delayed hyperenhancement sequence showing small infarction in the inferior wall (*arrow*) in a patient with an unstable lesion in the right coronary artery.

53. Why is breath holding important in the performance of an MRI perfusion study?

One of the main challenges of MRI perfusion studies is motion artifact, which can be minimized by breath holding. The relevant information in an MRI perfusion test can be acquired over five or six heartbeats, which is easily achievable by cooperative patients. Practically, patients are asked to hold their breath for as long as they can comfortably do so, which almost always covers this crucial period.

54. Can a myocardial perfusion study be performed in patients unable to hold their breath?

Yes, but quantitative or semiquantitative analysis is more difficult because cardiac images must be registered in a special, time-consuming process.

55. What is the average duration of an MRI myocardial perfusion study?

20–30 minutes. This duration also covers the time necessary for assessment of cardiac size and function.

56. Under what physiologic conditions should myocardial perfusion be assessed?

1. At rest
2. After administration of a pharmacologic stress agent, such as adenosine or dipyridamole

The second condition is called *vasodilatory stress* and is based on the principle that the capillary bed (microcirculation) of a stenotic coronary artery is unable to dilate further under pharmacologic stimulation. Although normal myocardium becomes "brighter" (more enhanced) after simultaneous intravenous administration of gadolinium and vasodilatory agents, ischemic microcirculation does not show an increased enhancement under these conditions.

57. My patient has an anterior myocardial wall akinesis (shown by echocardiography) after MI. Perfusion MRI showed the presence of delayed hyperenhancement in the anterior wall. Should this finding encourage me to refer the patient for coronary revascularization?

No (see question 56). The presence of delayed hyperenhancement signifies the absence of myocardial viability. This is opposite to the significance of delayed redistribution seen with thallium imaging.

> **Delayed** gadolinium **hyperenhancement** signifies the **absence** of viability.
> **Delayed** thallium **redistribution** signifies the **presence** of viability.

58. How can ischemic heart disease be diagnosed based on myocardial function?

Myocardial segments supplied with blood from a stenotic coronary artery have a *decreased* systolic function. The assessment of functional decrease may be used for establishing the presence, the extent, and the reversibility of the underlying coronary ischemia. As in the case of perfusion assessment, assessment of LV contractility may be performed **at rest** or **under pharmacologic stimulation with the inotropic sympathomimetic agent dobutamine.** Normal myocardial segments have a sustained increase in contractility under dobutamine stimulation, whereas ischemic segments may show one of the following two response patterns:

1. Hypokinesia or akinesia of previously normal segments. In these patients, systolic function under resting conditions is normal but decreases under dobutamine stimulation; this pattern is termed **inducible ischemia.**

2. Initial improvement in function of a hypokinetic segment, followed by hypokinesia or akinesia (biphasic response). In these patients, the transient improvement in function under dobutamine stimulation shows the viability of this myocardial segment (hibernating myocardium), but the coronary stenosis is so significant that systolic function cannot be maintained under increasing stress.

59. Is the degree of endocardial motion (e.g., normokinesis, hypokinesis) the only criterion for ischemic heart disease based on LV systolic function?

No. The degree of myocardial thickening also can be appreciated (the normal myocardium increases its thickness during systole; ischemic myocardium has reduced or absent systolic thickening; infarcted myocardium is replaced by scar tissue and appears "thinned out" and akinetic). Because of its higher image resolution, MRI generally is better than echocardiography for assessment of this parameter (Fig. 9).

60. What is the next practical step after demonstration of coronary ischemia (under resting or stress conditions) by either perfusion or dobutamine studies?

Cardiac catheterization and revascularization, as needed.

61. Does an MRI myocardial perfusion or dobutamine study allow continuous ECG monitoring of the patient?

The patient's ECG always is continuously monitored. ST and T wave changes cannot be assessed reliably, however, while the patient is in the bore of the magnet. Pre-MRI and post-MRI 12-lead ECG should be performed to detect the unusual patient with lasting ST or T wave changes after pharmacologic stress.

62. What are the sensitivity and the specificity of MRI perfusion and dobutamine studies (ischemia/viability)?

Definitive large-scale studies using this technique in "real-world" patients have yet to be done. Smaller studies have shown accuracy similar to that of radionuclide techniques (85–95% accurate). Newer hardware and software for MRI machines should improve the accuracy further.

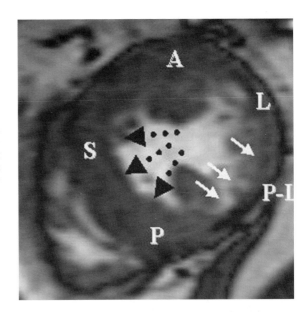

FIGURE 9. Inferolateral left ventricular wall thinning (*white arrows*) compared with normal myocardium (*black arrows*). This finding is consistent with a history of previous posterolateral myocardial infarction.

63. Discuss the current role of MRI in diagnosing coronary ischemia by perfusion or dobutamine studies?

In current clinical practice, dobutamine studies are performed under echocardiographic visualization, and perfusion studies generally are carried out in the nuclear laboratory (in the future, contrast echocardiography may become an alternative to nuclear perfusion studies). In view of the wide availability, diagnostic accuracy, and cost-effectiveness of these procedures, MRI perfusion and dobutamine studies rarely are performed except in sites with the appropriate expertise. If the promise of a "one-stop shopping" assessment of ischemic heart disease (coronary anatomy, myocardial function, myocardial viability) is fulfilled in the future, MRI may assume a more prominent role in the future.

64. How can MRI be used for assessment of the myocardial energetic balance?

Although MRI has become a synonym of high-quality images, one of the most exciting developments of the MRI principle is a nonimaging modality. This is termed *MRI spectroscopy* and can show the presence and the amount of specific chemical elements in the heart, based on their electromagnetic characteristics. Phosphorus is the main element of interest for metabolic energetic assessment. The amount of phosphorus in the myocardium is proportional to the amount of high-energy compounds (e.g., adenosine triphosphate [ATP]) and can be detected by MRI spectroscopy. At the time of this writing, this application is still experimental.

NUCLEAR MEDICINE

Overview

*Manuel D. Cerqueira, M.D., Gabriel Adelmann, M.D., and
Ernest K. Amegashie, M.D.*

65. Discuss the physiology regarding myocardial ischemia that can be determined by nuclear cardiology studies.

Simply stated, myocardial ischemia consists of reduced blood flow through the myocardial capillaries. This reduction in blood flow may be associated with a preserved microvasculature and structural integrity of the myocytes or may be caused by replacement of the myocardium with scar tissue. Myocardial ischemia or MI causes different degrees of LV systolic dysfunction, consisting of decreased endocardial motion (hypokinesis, akinesis) and decreased myocardial thickening in systole. The decrease in blood flow and myocardial function may be evident under conditions of rest or stress and can be assessed by means of nuclear functional and perfusion studies.

66. List clinical data regarding myocardial ischemia that can be assessed by nuclear studies.
- The **presence** of ischemia
- The **extent** of ischemia
- The **reversibility** of ischemia
- The severity and distribution of regional **myocardial dysfunction** caused by ischemia

67. How can the presence and extent of ischemia or obstructive CAD be identified by nuclear cardiology procedures?
The presence and extent of ischemia can be shown as:
- A decreased radionuclide uptake in the affected myocardial segments
- A decreased regional systolic function of the LV, manifest as decreased endocardial motion (different degrees of hypokinesis or akinesis) and decreased myocardial thickening

68. Is it possible to assess the absolute quantity of radiotracer (and the blood flow) to a certain segment of the myocardium, based on how bright this segment appears?
This assessment is not yet possible with current gamma camera techniques (this is an area of intense research). With the current technology, the degree of brightness of a myocardial segment always should be compared with that of the neighboring segments **in the same patient.** The nuclear image is calibrated according to the brightest region included in the picture, which may be extracardiac. In a patient with substantial hepatic uptake of radiotracer, the myocardium may have a relatively low brightness, even in normal patients. Conversely, in a patient without substantial extracardiac uptake, a significantly decreased brightness in a myocardial segment may indicate ischemia.

Using the positron emission tomography (PET) camera, absolute regional blood flow can be assessed quantitatively. In common practice, however, a semiquantitative approach, similar to that used for gamma camera imaging, is applied most often.

69. Does the presence of radionuclide uptake by a myocardial segment signify preserved coronary microcirculation and myocyte integrity?
Generally, yes, if it is present at rest and under conditions of stress.

70. Does the absence of radionuclide uptake by a myocardial segment signify that the coronary microcirculation and myocyte integrity in that segment are compromised?
The absence of radionuclide uptake is seen in the following settings:
- Failure to deliver blood via large coronary arteries
- Lack of integrity of the microcirculation
- Lack of uptake or retention of radiotracer by myocardial cells **at the time and under the physiologic conditions when the imaging is performed**

When using thallium-201, imaging may be performed immediately after radiotracer injection (generally, under conditions of exercise or pharmacologic stress) and at a later time (generally, under resting conditions). In some patients in whom thallium initially was not taken up by the myocardial cells, the uptake pattern may change on late imaging. The significance of the different uptake patterns is discussed later in this chapter.

71. How can you predict the potential for ischemic or hibernating myocardium to regain contractility after revascularization using nuclear cardiology techniques?
- Using thallium-201 (stress/redistribution/reinjection protocols or late imaging, at 24 hours): Areas that fail to show thallium uptake at 4 hours may not be infarcted, but only hibernating (viable), as shown by present uptake if additional amounts of tracer are administered (reinjection) or if imaging is repeated at 24 hours after the stress injection. These areas are likely to improve contractility after revascularization.

- Using F-18 deoxyglucose (FDG) (PET imaging): PET documentation of FDG uptake is the most accurate method for identifying viable myocardium.

72. How can the severity and regional distribution of ischemia-induced LV dysfunction be assessed in the nuclear cardiology laboratory?

By imaging the wall motion at peak exercise, using first-pass or multigated acquisition (MUGA) assessment of wall motion, or through ECG gating of the perfusion studies. Gated perfusion studies are acquired at least 15 minutes after termination of stress, and only people with severe ischemia have abnormal wall motion so far out from termination of stress. This persistent hypocontractility is referred to as *stunned* myocardium.

73. List the clinical indications for a cardiac nuclear study in ischemic heart disease.

- Assessment of myocardial ischemia in symptomatic or select asymptomatic patients
- Assessment of prognosis in patients with known CAD
- Assessment of myocardial ischemia before noncardiac surgery

74. Which patients with known ischemic heart disease benefit from myocardial perfusion scans?

Patients with:
- Chronic stable ischemic heart disease
- Unstable angina
- Acute MI

75. What are the indications for perfusion imaging in patients with chronic stable ischemic heart disease?

According to the American Heart Association (AHA) guidelines, the following are class I (general consensus in favor of the procedure, the procedure is standard of practice) indications for nuclear perfusion scans in this setting:

1. Diagnosis of ischemia in symptomatic patients, for identification of the culprit coronary arteries; this is especially important in patients with multivessel disease in whom PTCA is planned. In this setting, a partial revascularization strategy consisting of intervention limited to the culprit arteries, rather than on all the existing stenoses (*total revascularization*) may be preferable.

2. Diagnosis of ischemia in asymptomatic patients at high risk for ischemic heart disease.

3. Assessment of myocardial viability in patients with LV dysfunction, for establishing candidacy for revascularization.

4. Assessment of patients after PTCA or CABG surgery, either symptomatic or asymptomatic but with abnormal ECG response to exercise, or patients in whom exercise is not possible.

76. List the indications for myocardial perfusion imaging in patients with unstable angina.

According to the AHA guidelines, in this setting there is a class I indication for nuclear scans aimed at demonstration of:
- The **presence** of ischemia
- The **site** of ischemia
- The **extent** of ischemia
- The **influence** of ischemia on the regional and global LV function
- The response of ischemia to therapy.

Figure 10 shows the resolution of anterior myocardial ischemia after PTCA.

77. Which patients are ideal candidates for screening for ischemic heart disease by nuclear perfusion imaging?

- Patients with intermediate pretest probability of CAD
- Patients with abnormal baseline ECG tracing
- Patients who are unable to exercise

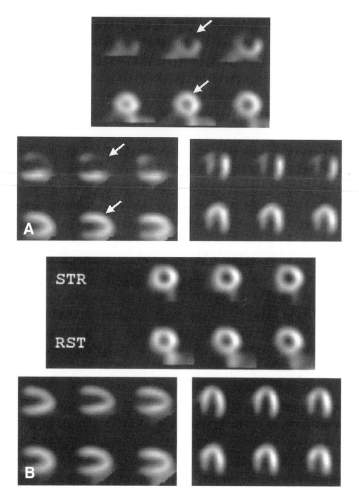

FIGURE 10. *A,* SPECT myocardial perfusion images with stress (*top rows*) and at rest (*bottom rows*) in a patient with anterior myocardial ischemia (*arrows*). *B,* The same patient studied after PTCA to LAD. Note that at the same level of exercise as before the procedure there is no inducible ischemia.

78. What are the indications for myocardial perfusion imaging in patients with MI?

According to the AHA guidelines, the main indications (class I) for nuclear scan in patients with MI refer to:

- Assessment of resting ventricular function
- Assessment of the presence and extent of stress-induced ischemia (post-MI assessment)

Perfusion imaging may be useful in other settings in the case of MI patients, but these are not class I indications. For a detailed discussion of these indications, see the AHA guidelines for radionuclide cardiac imaging and the guidelines for management of patients with MI.

79. What are the indications for myocardial perfusion imaging in patients before noncardiac surgery?

CAD is highly prevalent in patients undergoing vascular surgical procedures and in high-risk patients scheduled for other noncardiac surgery. In these patients, the bulk of the perioperative mortality and morbidity is due to ischemic heart disease (perioperative MI). Assessment for CAD, even in asymptomatic patients, if they belong to one of the two aforementioned categories, has become the standard of care.

80. Discuss the significance of the different patterns of thallium-201 uptake in patients being assessed for CAD in preparation for noncardiac surgery.

1. A normal perfusion scan has high negative predictive value for perioperative ischemic events. These patients are at a low risk for cardiac death or nonfatal MI during or immediately after the surgical procedure.

2. The presence of fixed perfusion defects is a less-than-ideal scenario, owing to the myocardial scarring that it represents. This uptake pattern does not imply a high risk for perioperative ischemic events, however. The patient's heart includes healthy myocardium and myocardial scar, but not ischemic myocardium that may become ischemic and possibly infarct around the time of the surgery.

3. The presence of reversible perfusion defects, which indicates myocardial ischemia, is the highest risk situation, however. There are myocardial segments that may become infarcted at the time of surgery or soon thereafter. The positive predictive value of a nuclear scan for perioperative ischemia is much lower than the negative predictive value (although one may be confident that the patient with a normal scan would not experience such events, only 15–30% of patients with a positive scan have perioperative events).

81. Do all patients scheduled for noncardiac surgery require a nuclear perfusion scan?

No. Patients in need of such assessment include:

- Patients scheduled for vascular surgery (the presence of atherosclerotic disease in extracardiac territories strongly suggests the possibility of occult coronary involvement)
- Patients with significant risk factors for CAD
- Asymptomatic or stable patients with known CAD, in whom it is necessary to identify the presence of inducible ischemia (i.e., such as may be precipitated by the major stress of surgery)

82. Are there any contraindications to performing nuclear cardiology studies?

Pregnant or potentially pregnant patients should not be studied using radionuclide techniques. Risks to the fetus are greatest in the first trimester and decrease over time. The most common contraindication for a nuclear study is the absence of a clear indication. According to Bayes' theorem, nuclear studies have low clinical value in patients with either a low probability of ischemic heart disease or with high pretest probability for such disease. In the former group, nuclear studies may lead to unnecessary invasive procedures (high probability of false-positives results), whereas in the latter group, they may lead to unnecessary time expense before coronary catheterization, which is generally necessary in these patients.

83. Does the presence of coronary artery stenosis on a *coronary angiogram* imply that the corresponding myocardial segment will show ischemia on a nuclear perfusion study?

No. Several other factors must be taken into account.

1. The **severity** of the stenosis: Generally, stenosis involving < 50% of the coronary lumen, in the absence of superimposed thrombus, is considered to have no hemodynamic significance (i.e., not to cause significant reduction of blood flow in the microcirculation either at rest or with stress). Stenosis in the 50–70% range may or may not limit coronary blood flow at peak stress.

2. The **type** of coronary stenosis (i.e., the composition of the atherosclerotic plaque): An organized, fibrotic plaque is much less likely to become thrombosed and occluded than a vulnerable, lipid-rich atherosclerotic lesion. Vulnerable plaques may cause abnormal coronary flow reserve that improves when the plaque becomes stable.

3. The **presence** of collateral blood supply to a myocardial segment, despite significant

stenosis in its "legitimate artery" (i.e., the corresponding coronary artery): These collateral vessels often measure 15–30 μ only and are not seen easily on coronary angiography.

84. Does the absence of significant (> 50%) coronary stenosis on a *coronary angiogram* rule out ischemia in the corresponding myocardial segment?

No. Several factors must be taken into account.

1. Coronary angiograms occasionally may not fully visualize significant coronary stenosis.

2. "Mild" coronary stenosis may become extremely significant, if there is superimposed thrombosis; native or pharmacologic thrombolysis may dissolve the clot before there is a chance to visualize it by angiography.

3. In occasional patients, the degree of endothelial dysfunction is disproportionately greater than the severity of the stenosis, as appreciated by angiography; in these patients, mild coronary stenosis may cause vasospasm, often absent at the time of coronary catheterization.

4. Occasionally the true culprit for ischemia is myocardial bridging (systolic "choking" of a coronary artery that has an intramyocardial, rather than epicardial, course); this may be missed if the person performing the study mistakenly equates the concept of *coronary ischemia* with that of *coronary stenosis*.

85. What do these considerations about coronary catheterization have to do with nuclear cardiology?

Nuclear perfusion studies and coronary catheterization are used for diagnosing myocardial ischemia. To understand better the difference between the information provided by these two types of studies, one needs to review the definition of ischemia. Briefly stated, coronary ischemia is a decrease in blood flow to the capillary **microcirculation,** affecting to different degrees the integrity and function of **myocytes,** and is caused in most cases by a stenosis in the **epicardial** portion of the artery. The different imaging modalities detect ischemia either

- **Directly,** by assessing the amount of radionuclide reaching the coronary microcirculation and subsequently taken up by myocytes; this is done by nuclear perfusion studies (contrast echocardiography and cardiac MRI have been proposed as alternatives to nuclear studies for this indication and are the subject of intense current research, but are not generally available in a clinical setting), *or*
- **Indirectly,** by demonstration of epicardial coronary artery stenosis; this classically is done by coronary angiography (cardiac MRI has made tremendous progress in this field and is envisioned by many as the angiographic procedure **of the future**).

86. Should the nuclear perfusion study be performed before or after coronary catheterization?

Generally, nuclear perfusion scans are performed before cardiac catheterization. One of the main roles of nuclear cardiology is to act as a "gatekeeper" for invasive procedures (i.e., to prevent unnecessary invasive procedures). In occasional patients, it may be reasonable, however, to perform a nuclear scan after coronary catheterization. Consider the following examples:

1. A patient with an intermediate probability for coronary ischemia (atypical chest pain, nonspecific ECG changes, the presence of multiple risk factors). The reasonable diagnostic algorithm in this patient consists of performing a nuclear study first and to proceed to cardiac catheterization only if this study shows significant (in terms of severity and extension) perfusion abnormalities.

2. A patient with known three-vessel disease and severe chronic angina, in the absence of localizing ECG changes, in whom the coronary angiography shows complex stenotic lesions, some of them (but not all) amenable to revascularization. In this patient, it is important to know whether the anginal syndrome is caused by vessels technically amenable to CABG surgery or PTCA. (One is able to revascularize only "fixable" arteries, but these may not be the ones responsible for myocardial ischemia). This information can be obtained by means of a nuclear perfusion study.

87. List the advantages of nuclear perfusion imaging compared with treadmill exercise testing alone in the diagnosis of ischemic heart disease.

- A substantially higher sensitivity (90% versus 50–60%) and specificity (90% versus 60–70%)
- Localization of the diseased arteries (on stress ECG, one looks for the *presence* of ST segment depression, but the specific localization of the ECG changes or the magnitude of depression does not establish the site or extent of coronary ischemia)
- Assessment of the extension of ischemia
- A higher prognostic value

88. If current nuclear technology allows assessment of LV perfusion and function in the same study, what role remains for echocardiography in the management of these patients?

Echocardiography is suited uniquely to offer information not only concerning LV function, but also the heart valves and pericardium, which are not assessed by nuclear studies. The coexistence of valvular disease, whether secondary to the coronary ischemia or independent of it, substantially alters the management of these patients. Additionally, echocardiography (especially transesophageal echocardiography) may show the presence, extent, and severity of aortic atherosclerosis, an important element of information in patients who are candidates for revascularization because manipulations of the aorta are an inherent component of CABG surgery and PCTA.

Echocardiography and nuclear studies complement each other for the assessment of ischemic heart disease.

Radionuclide Tracers

Manuel D. Cerqueira, M.D., and Gabriel Adelmann, M.D.

89. How are tracers used in nuclear cardiology?

Simply stated, nuclear cardiology measures blood flow in the heart chambers and muscle. This diagnostic modality uses tracers that track the blood flow. These tracers may be followed as they course through the heart chambers (providing an assessment of the ventricular function) and in the myocardium (providing an assessment of myocardial perfusion). The amount of tracer in the myocardium depends on the blood flow reaching the heart and the number and cellular integrity of the myocytes. Within certain limits, the cellular uptake of radionuclide tracers increases proportionately with blood flow (linear relationship).

90. What are the characteristics of an ideal perfusion tracer?

Beside obvious requirements related to safety, cost, and availability, a perfusion tracer must emit a type of radioactivity that can be accurately detected by the **gamma camera** and is proportional in intensity with the concentration of **radiotracer** in a given tissue (in turn, the concentration of tracer in a given tissue depends on the blood flow and on the cellular uptake); the agent must have predictable pharmacokinetics. In addition, the tracer should be taken up in direct proportion to myocardial blood flow over the entire physiologic range encountered in the heart.

91. List factors that affect the uptake of a perfusion tracer by myocardial cells.

- The magnitude of blood flow through the corresponding epicardial coronary arteries
- The integrity of the capillary microcirculation
- The integrity of the myocytes

92. Which characteristics of radiotracer uptake by the myocardial cells are important for the diagnosis of heart disease in the nuclear cardiology laboratory?

- **Presence** of uptake
- **Intensity** of uptake
- **Variation** in uptake pattern with time

93. Which radiopharmaceutical tracers are used for myocardial perfusion imaging?

- Thallium-201
- Technetium (Tc): This radioactive compound can be attached to several physiologically active molecules, such as Tc-99m-sestamibi (Cardiolite) and Tc-99m-tetrofosmin (Myoview). The additional moiety makes the radionuclide tracer concentrate in the heart.

94. Describe the pharmacodynamics of thallium-201.

Thallium is an unstable radionuclide produced by a cyclotron and emits photons that can be detected with a gamma camera. Thallium has a relatively long biologic half-life (72 hours) and is transported by blood to the myocardial cells, where it is taken up by in an active process using the Na^+, K^+-ATPase pump. The initial myocardial uptake is followed by a continuous exchange across the myocardial membrane, between the intracellular and the extracellular spaces. The ability to engage in this transmembrane exchange of thallium is characteristic of myocytes and is not present in areas of scar tissue (fibrosis).

95. What is thallium redistribution, and why is it important in nuclear cardiology?

Thallium redistribution is the transmembrane exchange of radionuclide between the myocytes and the extracellular space. After its initial intravenous injection, the radioactive tracer accumulates in the well-perfused areas of the myocardium and does not accumulate in areas of ischemia or fibrosis. This initial **distribution** is followed, however, by a slower process whereby the radiotracer leaves the cells in which it initially had accumulated, reaches the intercellular space, and from there is taken up by the segments of the myocardium that are ischemic but not replaced by scar. This process is termed **redistribution** and is the base of the viability assessment by radionuclide methods.

96. How can one distinguish normally perfused myocardial segments from ischemic segments and from myocardial scar, based on a thallium-201 perfusion scan?

Normal—high uptake and retention of thallium-201 with stress and rest
Ischemia—normal uptake at rest and diminished or absent uptake after stress
Scar or infarct—severely diminished or absent uptake at rest and stress

97. Can thallium-201 be used for assessment of LV function?

Yes, by performing ECG-gated planar or single-photon emission computed tomography (SPECT) studies. Because of the low energy and long half-life of thallium-201, attenuation is increased, however, and only 3–4 mCi of radiotracer can be administered, which results in low counts compared with technetium-99m perfusion tracers. These low count images are not as reliable for calculation of ejection fraction.

98. The pharmacodynamics of myocardial thallium-201 uptake closely resembles those of an ion ubiquitous in biologic systems. Name that ion.

Thallium-201 is a potassium analogue and equilibrates across the cellular membrane according to the same gradient as the potassium ion.

99. Why is it important to perform thallium-201 perfusion studies under fasting conditions?

Glucose intake-induced hyperinsulinemia causes a drop in thallium-201 levels (in parallel with a drop in potassium levels), slowing down the process of redistribution and potentially leading to underestimation of the extent of viable myocardium. It is important to perform thallium-201 studies under fasting conditions. When patients eat before stress or resting injections, there is greater blood flow to the stomach and mesenteric vessels, and this results in a high background activity. In nonfasting patients, the uptake of thallium-201 in the stomach may be higher than in the heart, resulting in scaling problems on the image display.

100. Describe the general pharmacodynamics of Tc-99m-based agents.

Tc-99m is a generator-produced radionuclide agent with a half-life of 6 hours, much shorter than the 72 hours of thallium-201, which results in a more rapid decay and higher counts. The shorter half-life results in a lower radiation dose to the patient and the possibility to administer 30 mCi, with a consequent improvement in image resolution. The attenuation also is much lower than with thallium. The Tc-based agents are taken up by the myocardial cells and subsequently bind irreversibly to the intracellular membranes. Because of their irreversible cellular binding, these tracers can be imaged later after the injection, allowing one to inject the radioisotope under acute conditions, such as MI or acute chest pain. Imaging can be deferred until a later time, when the patient is in stable condition. This provides a "snapshot" of the coronary perfusion in the acute setting. The absence of redistribution with technetium means that patients must be injected twice: once at rest and once after stress.

101. Name the most commonly used Tc-based radiotracers.

Tc-sestamibi, Tc-tetrofosmin, and Tc-teboroxime. The physiologic properties of these different compounds vary according to the specific ligand.

102. What are the characteristics of Tc-99m-sestamibi and Tc-99m-tetrofosmin?

The sestamibi moiety is an organic compound belonging to the class of the isonitriles. Tetrofosmin is a highly lipophilic molecule. Both of these compounds are taken up by myocytes from the blood and bound to the mitochondria, with little subsequent redistribution.

103. What is the place of Tc-99m radiotracers in clinical practice?

Sestamibi and tetrofosmin are the most frequently used Tc-based tracers in current clinical practice. They allow accurate detection of ischemia and are most appropriate for gated SPECT studies.

104. What are the characteristics and what is the role of Tc-99m-tetrofosmin in clinical practice?

The pharmacokinetics, clinical uses, and protocols are similar to those for Tc-sestamibi. Tetrofosmin has:

- A lesser degree of hepatic uptake on rest imaging (an advantage because the nuclear image is calibrated based on the highest intensity radioactive signal, whether cardiac or extracardiac; a high degree of hepatic uptake may result in "weaker" images of the heart)
- A slightly lower cellular extraction from blood (a potential disadvantage because it may result in a lower radioactive count and a lower quality image)

105. What is technetium-teboroxime, and what are its pharmacokinetic properties?

Tc-teboroxime is a Tc-based diagnostic agent, with properties notably different from those of Tc-sestamibi and Tc-tetrofosmin. These properties are due to the lipophilic nature of the teboroxime moiety and include:

- A lower influence of the roll-off effect on the dynamics of the tracer
- Possible reversibility and redistribution of myocardial uptake
- A fast washout from the myocardium

106. Explain the practical implications of the unique pharmacokinetics of Tc-teboroxime.

1. **Lower influence of the roll-off effect:** Within certain limits, radiotracer uptake is proportional to blood flow; however, this linear relationship no longer is preserved at higher flow rates (roll-off effect). It is relatively simple to distinguish a myocardial segment that gets no perfusion at all from one that gets normal perfusion (i.e., to distinguish a severe coronary stenosis from normal), but it is much harder to distinguish between normals and areas of mild coronary stenosis because in both of these settings the local blood flow is relatively high and influenced by the roll-off effect. Teboroxime is less subject to the roll-off effect, which makes it able to detect

milder degrees of coronary stenosis, which would be "lumped together" with normals if other technetium-based tracers were used.

2. **Possible reversibility and redistribution:** there is potential detection of myocardial viability.

3. **Fast washout from the myocardium:** Imaging immediately after administration of the radiotracer is necessary.

Despite these unique characteristics, teboroxime has an extremely short half-life within the myocardium (on the order of minutes), which makes it less practical for clinical use.

107. Discuss the respective advantages and disadvantages of thallium-201 and technetium-99m radiotracer imaging.

Technetium-99m, the most widely used isotope for demonstration of myocardial ischemia, has the **advantage** of producing a better quality image than thallium; additionally, because technetium-99m-sestamibi and technetium-99m-tetrofosmin do not redistribute, they can be injected at the time of acute ischemia and be imaged later, while preserving a "frozen snapshot" of the myocardial flow at the time of its injection.

Thallium-201, the standard for myocardial perfusion imaging before the advent of Tc, has the **advantage** of redistributing, being able to show myocardial viability. Its **disadvantage** is that it produces relatively lower image quality than Tc. Thallium cannot be injected when immediate imaging is impossible (e.g., unstable patients) because its myocardial uptake changes over time. Myocardial viability assessment necessitates the presence of the patient for at least 4 hours after the initial injection or their return to the medical facility 18–24 hours later.

108. Summarize the advantages and disadvantages of thallium-201 and Tc-99m protocols and of a special protocol involving the use of both isotopes (dual isotope protocol).

	THALLIUM	TECHNETIUM	DUAL ISOTOPE
Ischemia	Yes	Yes	Yes
Comments about ischemia assessment	Images of lower quality than with technetium	Current gold standard for nuclear detection of ischemia	Based on the exercise/ technetium component of the test
Viability	Yes	Yes, but not optimal	Yes
Comments about viability assessment	The great advantage of this isotope; not possible with classic technetium tracers	Yes, but not optimal	Based on the thallium-201 resting component of the test
LV function (gated SPECT)	Yes	Yes	Yes
Comments about gated SPECT	Lower quality than with technetium	High quality, owing to the high number of counts; gold standard for gated SPECT	Based on the technetium component of the test

Methods: Planar and Positron Emission Tomography

Manuel D. Cerqueira, M.D., and Gabriel Adelmann, M.D.

109. Name the two basic nuclear cardiology imaging methods used for performing perfusion studies.

Gamma camera imaging and PET.

110. What is the underlying principle of gamma camera imaging?

Gamma camera imaging is based on detection of the gamma radiation emitted by intravenously administered thallium or Tc-based agents. This provides an assessment of myocardial perfusion and LV systolic function.

111. Describe the degree of three-dimensional detail provided by gamma camera imaging, in regard to the presence, localization, and extension of myocardial perfusion defects and of LV dysfunction.

Planar imaging is essentially a summation technique, whereby photons emitted from all the regions of the myocardium are superimposed to form a single image.

SPECT imaging displays a series of myocardial slices (section planes) in three different axes: *short, vertical,* and *horizontal.* This approach is similar to computed tomography (CT) scanning and is made possible by computer-guided acquisition, reconstruction, and reorientation of the nuclear images.

112. Which imaging angles (views) are used on planar studies?

Planar imaging (regardless of whether it is aimed at demonstration of myocardial perfusion or at assessment of LV function) uses three standard views: *anterior, left anterior oblique,* and *left lateral.* Optimal imaging requires sufficient radioactivity emission from within the heart, correct patient positioning, appropriate image magnification, and adequate display of images. Figure 11 shows a planar perfusion thallium study and a planar MUGA study and indicates the myocardial segments shown from each view.

113. What parameters can be assessed by planar studies?

LV perfusion (by visualization of the myocardium) and LV function (by visualization of the intracardiac blood pool, MUGA) (see Figure 11).

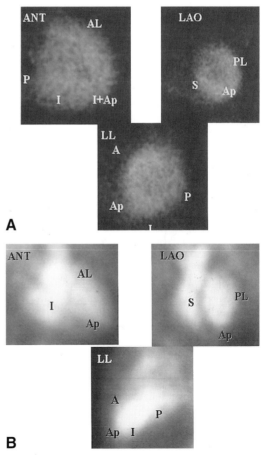

FIGURE 11. *A,* Planar perfusion thallium-201 study demonstrating the myocardium in white. The central darker area in all these images represents the cavity of the left ventricle. ANT = anterior, LAO = left anterior oblique, LL = left lateral, AL = anterolateral, I = inferior, Ap = apex, P = posterior, PL = posterolateral, AS = anteroseptal, A = anterior, S = septum. *B,* Planar MUGA, demonstrating the blood pool in white, and the myocardium in black. A = anterior, P = posterior, I = inferior, Ap = apex, A-L = anterolateral, P-L = posterolateral, S = septum.

114. What is the role of planar imaging in current practice?

Planar imaging largely has been supplanted by SPECT imaging (see question 115). Planar imaging still is used for the occasional patients who cannot fit within the SPECT camera (owing to weight restrictions) or are not willing to hold their left arm over their heads for 15–20 minutes and lay underneath a rotating gamma camera.

115. What does the term *SPECT* mean?

The acronym stands for **s**ingle-**p**hoton **e**mission **c**omputed **t**omography:

1. The energy particles (photons) emitted by the heart are detected "one by one" (as **single photons**) by the gamma camera; this is in opposition to the "coincidence counting" (see question 135), characteristic of PET.

2. It is a **tomographic** method (i.e., provides slices at different depths through the heart rather then superimposing or collapsing all the walls on top of each other as is done with planar imaging).

3. The **tomographic** display of the heart is based on computerized processing of radioactive data acquired by a gamma camera.

116. What is *image reorientation,* as used in nuclear cardiology?

The images obtained from a SPECT or PET scan are *transaxial* (i.e., perpendicular to the long axis of the patient's body, which is different from the long axis of the obliquely oriented heart). These transaxial views are oblique section planes and show artifactual differences in thickness and perfusion in the different myocardial segments, owing to the differences in the degree of emitted radioactivity. These transaxial images need to be reprocessed and transformed into short-axis and long-axis images. This is *image reorientation,* which can be performed manually (an operator-dependent process) or in an automated fashion. Incorrect image reorientation between rest and stress may result in artifactual perfusion defects.

117. What is the "step-and-shoot" approach to SPECT imaging?

This is the classic method of image acquisition by SPECT and involves discontinuous image recording, at different angles along the semicircular camera trajectory around the patient (literally, the camera rotates 180° around the patient, "**shooting**" images as it "**steps**" through its course). This method inherently involves "dead periods," while the camera changes position between successive points on the orbit. These dead periods, a potential cause of loss of information, can be avoided by newer imaging systems, which acquire data throughout the duration of the camera rotation around the patient.

118. How many projections are there in a standard SPECT study?

32–64 projections. Views are spaced regularly along the semicircular orbit, and the angle between them should not exceed 6° (corresponding to 30 images over a total span of 180°). The more sampling angles or smaller number of degrees between slices, the higher the image quality.

119. Which imaging angles (slices) are used in a SPECT study?

- Short axis (from base to apex)
- Vertical long axis (displaying the heart as the letter *U,* with the opening toward the left of the person looking at the image; these slices begin at the septum and end at the lateral wall)
- Horizontal long axis (displaying the heart as the letter *U,* with the opening downward; the slices begin at the inferior wall and end at the anterior wall)

These different views are shown in Figure 12.

120. How can you tell, by looking at the nuclear study, if it was done by the planar or the SPECT method?

The presence of numerous series of images, displayed in bright color, correspond to a SPECT study, whereas a series of only three, relatively blurry, black-and-white images represents a pla-

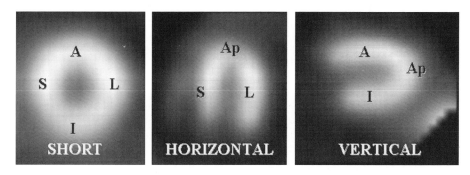

FIGURE 12. The three basic nuclear imaging views. Note that, counterintuitively, the view displaying the heart "lying on its side" (horizontally) is actually called the **vertical** view, whereas the view displaying the heart "standing up" (vertically) is called the **horizontal** view. The SPECT views are different from the planar views, but there is a similarity between the horizontal SPECT view and the LAO planar view and between the SPECT vertical view and the planar anterior view. A = anterior, L = lateral, I = inferior, S = septum, Ap = apex.

nar study. If you are looking at a nuclear scan performed more recently, the chances are it would be a SPECT study, which currently represents the standard of perfusion imaging in nuclear cardiology.

121. What are the sensitivity and specificity of SPECT perfusion imaging for detecting CAD?
Both around 90%.

122. Name the factors influencing the sensitivity of SPECT.
Nuclear perfusion scans have a higher sensitivity in patients with:
- Multivessel disease
- Severe stenosis
- Proximal stenosis

123. What is increased lung uptake of radiotracers, and what is its significance?
In severe exercise-induced ischemia and using thallium-201, there is widespread (often, global) LV dysfunction, which results in an increase in the LV end-diastolic pressure and in the left atrial pressure. This results in extravasation of free water into the lung vasculature and increased thallium uptake and retention. Increased lung uptake indicates severe myocardial ischemia and is an indicator of poor prognosis.

124. What is transient ischemic dilation of the LV, and what is its significance?
Transient ischemic dilation is an increase in the **apparent** LV volume with stress compared with rest and indicates of severe, global LV ischemia (Fig. 13). The pathophysiologic mechanism implied by the name of this finding (i.e., an increase in LV volume owing to widespread ischemia) has been proved, however, *not* to be the cause of transient ischemic dilation. The apparent increased diameter of the LV is caused by the lack of visualization of the endocardial layer of the heart, which, being the farthest away from the epicardial coronary arteries, is the first to experience ischemia. A widespread ("concentric") layer of nonvisualized myocardium is optically "lumped together" with the true LV cavity, creating the false impression of a transient ischemic dilation. An additional important consideration regarding transient ischemic dilation pertains to the radiotracers being used. Technetium images yield a "crisper" visualization of the LV myocardium, with clear delineation of its endocardial border compared with thallium. Technetium images tend to show a larger LV cavity. This is especially relevant in dual isotope protocols, in which the stress images are acquired using technetium, whereas the resting images use thallium. In these patients, transient ischemic dilation should be interpreted with care.

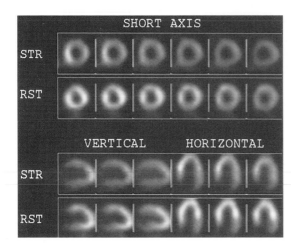

FIGURE 13. Transient ischemic dilatation (TID). STR = stress, RST = rest.

125. What is the 1-year incidence of death or nonfatal MI in patients with negative (normal) SPECT?

< 1%. The negative predictive value of a normal nuclear perfusion scan for coronary ischemia is high.

126. Why is it important to examine the raw data when interpreting a SPECT study?

The final SPECT images are the result of heavy data processing and are only as accurate as the preprocessing (raw) images. Proper quality of a SPECT study is ensured by inspection of these data and ascertaining that proper angles around the 180° orbit were used and that no significant artifact was "factored in" in the final image.

127. How should the heart be segmented for assessment of myocardial perfusion?

There are two main systems of segmentation of the heart, used for perfusion studies: a 20-segment system and a 17-segment system. With both systems, transverse sections through the heart are made at three levels, and several segments are recognized at each of these levels:

- **Distal (apical) short axis**—including the following segments: anterior, lateral, inferior, septal
- **Mid ventricle short axis**—including the following segments: anterior, anterolateral, inferolateral, inferior, inferoseptal, anteroseptal
- **Basal short axis**—including the same segments as the mid ventricle short axis

The **LV apex** represents a segment of its own, visualized longitudinal (vertical) axis cuts. These different segments also may be recognized from longitudinal (horizontal or vertical) sections. The disparity between the two segmentation systems results from the fact that the 20-segment system recognizes two components to the lateral segment (similar to what is seen at the mid ventricle and at the basal level) and divides the apex into two separate segments. The different myocardial segments, as visualized by SPECT, are shown in Figure 13.

128. Which segmentation system is preferable?

Classically, nuclear perfusion studies have used the 20-segment system, whereas the 17-segment system has been proposed more recently. The 20-segment system is better documented. The rationale for introducing a new segmentation system is to facilitate cross-imaging modality comparison (the 17-segment system is more similar, although not completely identical, to the echocardiographic segmentation system) (Fig. 14).

129. Is it possible to "ascribe" a perfusion defect seen on the SPECT scan to stenosis of a specific coronary artery?

Yes, and this is one of the main clinical applications of nuclear perfusion studies.

FIGURE 14. The LV segmentation according to the 17-segment system: 1, basal anterior; 2, basal anteroseptal; 3, basal inferoseptal; 4, basal inferior; 5, basal inferolateral; 6, basal anterolateral; 7, mid anterior; 8, mid anteroseptal; 9, mid inferoseptal; 10, mid inferior; 11, mid inferolateral; 12, mid anterolateral; 13, apical anterior; 14, apical septal; 15, apical inferior; 16, apical lateral; 17, apex.

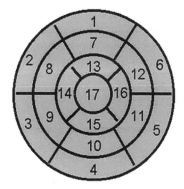

1. The posterior descending coronary artery (most frequently originating from the right coronary artery) supplies the inferior and basal septal segments.

2. The left circumflex artery supplies the lateral segments.

3. The left anterior descending artery supplies the mid and distal septum, and all the anterior wall and, most frequently, the apex (although the apex also can be supplied by the left circumflex or the right coronary artery).

The coronary supply to the different myocardial segments, as visualized by SPECT, is shown in Figure 15.

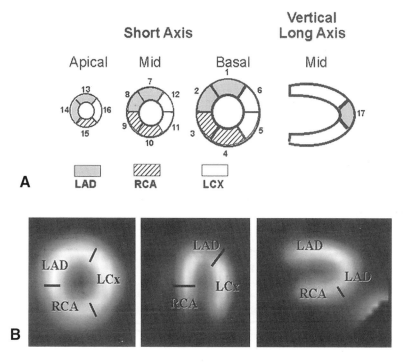

FIGURE 15. Coronary topography (*A*) and the corresponding perfusion segments (*B*) using the 17-segment system. LAD = left anterior descending artery, RCA = right coronary artery, LCx = left circumflex artery.

130. Is it possible to quantify the severity of a perfusion defect seen on a SPECT study?

Although absolute quantification is not possible based on SPECT technology, a semiquantitative severity assessment can be performed easily and has been found to be clinically relevant. Myocardial perfusion can be normal, mildly decreased, moderately decreased, severely decreased, or absent. (These different degrees of radionuclide uptake also can be scored from 0 to 4, with *lower* scores corresponding to *better* perfusion; a score of 0 represents normal perfusion, and a score of 4 represents absent perfusion.)

This perfusion score is based on comparison of the different myocardial segments **in the same patient**. A given segment looks "dark" only in comparison to neighboring, "brighter" segments. As a result, if all the myocardial segments are affected equally by CAD (balanced three-vessel disease), there may not be a substantial difference in brightness among the different segments, potentially leading to a false-negative diagnosis.

131. How is it possible to distinguish patients with balanced three-vessel disease from normals, based on nuclear perfusion studies?

Generally, patients with balanced three-vessel disease show a degree of LV dysfunction commensurate with the extent and severity of myocardial ischemia. This may be observed by nuclear methods (gated SPECT, first-pass; for a discussion of these methods, see Chapter 3) or by other imaging methods, such as echocardiography or MRI. LV dysfunction is an important element in the assessment of these patients. Patients are likely to show transient ischemic dilation, show increased lung uptake, and have a high-risk clinical profile and treadmill ECG stress test.

132. What is the bull's-eye map?

A method of displaying the three-dimensional SPECT perfusion images on a single two-dimensional image, by merging or collapsing together the different short-axis sections (Fig. 16). In this display, the apical slices are placed at the center of the image, and the apical, midcavity, and basal slices are layered sequentially toward the outer rings of the circle. The circumferential orientation of the anterior, lateral, inferior, and septal walls is maintained for each subsequent slice. This image is similar to what theoretically would be obtained if one were able to look at the LV cavity from the base toward the apex, as if looking "down a funnel." Although a bull's-eye map cannot be substituted for the detailed images normally shown by SPECT, it does offer a "balance-at-a-glance" of the myocardial perfusion.

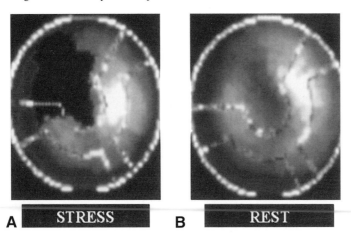

A **STRESS**   B **REST**

FIGURE 16. Bull's eye map. Note the reversible anterior and anteroseptal perfusion defect.

133. What is the next step in the evaluation of a patient with a positive nuclear perfusion scan?

The size and location of the defect helps determine the subsequent management. Patients with small perfusion defects have similar outcome with maximal medical management or referral to cardiac catheterization and revascularization. Patients with high-risk scans should undergo coronary catheterization and revascularization, if necessary.

134. What is the amount of three-dimensional detail provided by PET?

Similar to SPECT, PET provides a high degree of spatial detail concerning regional myocardial perfusion and function.

135. Discuss the basic principles of PET imaging.

PET imaging is based on the radioactive process of *positron annihilation*. The diagnostic radiotracer is energetically unstable and reaches stability only after emitting a *positron* (also called *antielectron*). When the positron encounters an electron, the two particles annihilate each other and produce two high-energy photons orientated in opposite directions (at an angle of 180°). The PET detectors are paired and aligned at 180° from each other and count only the signals impacting simultaneously on two opposite walls of the camera. This "coincidence counting" allows one to discard electronically the background noise (the probability that a pair of noise signals should be simultaneous and oppositely directed being low). With PET, collimation is electronic (for a discussion of collimation, see Chapter 1). This allows elimination of background scatter from the final image, resulting in high-quality images and attenuation correction.

136. What is the main information provided by PET, which cannot be obtained from a SPECT study?

SPECT offers a relative assessment of coronary flow (i.e., considers the brightest myocardial segment as having normal perfusion and displays all the other segments according to their uptake of radioactive tracer compared with the reference segment).

PET can provide relative and absolute quantitative assessment of the capillary blood flow.

137. State the clinical importance of absolute quantification of blood flow, as performed by PET.

Absolute quantification of blood flow rarely is carried out for clinical purposes alone and is at this time mainly of research interest. The most frequent method of interpretation of PET scans is semiquantitative assessment, similar to that performed with SPECT.

138. What are the PET measure units for myocardial perfusion?

Milliliters of blood/minute/gram of myocardial tissue.

139. What is the perfusable tissue index?

An indicator of tissue viability, requiring the use of tracers that are not readily available. Perfusable tissue index is not measured routinely in patients.

140. What are the main types of PET tracers?

- **Flow tracers,** which track with the blood flow
- **Metabolic tracers,** which are similar to certain organic molecules (e.g., glucose) and taken up by cells accordingly

Because of their structural particularities, metabolic tracers cannot be metabolized and become entrapped inside the cells, serving as sensitive markers for various metabolic pathways.

141. Identify the most frequently used PET flow tracers.

The most frequently used flow tracers in the clinical setting are rubidium-82 and N-13 ammonia, whereas O-15 water frequently is used for research purposes. Rubidium-82 has the added advantage of being produced by a generator, whereas the other two compounds require a cyclotron.

142. What is the most frequently used PET metabolic tracer?

The most frequently used PET metabolic tracer is FDG, which serves as a marker for glycolysis. Under normal circumstances, the myocytes use, as a metabolic fuel, free fatty acids and switch to glucose when ischemic. In ischemia, "true" and "fake" (i.e., FDG) glucose is taken up by cells to a greater extent than usual; although glucose can be used for the energetic metabolism, FDG becomes trapped in the cytoplasm. The amount of intracellular FDG is proportional to the intensity of ischemia and can be detected because of the radioactivity it emits.

143. Why is it necessary to perform glucose loading before a PET study?

There are two basic conditions in which myocardial cells preferentially use glucose for their energetic requirements:
- **Physiologic:** after meals, when insulin levels are high
- **Pathologic:** myocardial ischemia

To avoid interpretation of normal glucose uptake into the cells as a sign of ischemia, it is necessary to replenish the intracellular deposits of glucose before a PET study.

144. Is it possible to perform PET scans in diabetic patients?

Approximately 10% of diabetic patients have uninterpretable PET studies, owing to the disturbed glucose metabolism. For this reason, insulin administration together with the glucose-loading dose before a PET study is recommended in diabetic patients.

145. How does the ability of PET to detect radiation compare with that of SPECT?

PET is approximately 100 times more sensitive than SPECT for detection of radiation. This increased sensitivity results in better image definition than is obtained by SPECT imaging (Fig. 17). The image definition obtained by SPECT is sufficient for most clinical decisions, however, so that the clearer images provided by PET do not translate into a clinical advantage.

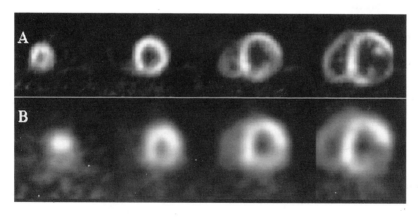

FIGURE 17. FDG PET (*A*) versus SPECT (*B*). Note the texture and detail present with FDG.

146. What is the spatial resolution of PET, and how does it compare with planar and SPECT imaging of conventional single-photon isotopes?

The spatial resolution of PET is 4–6 mm. This means that two points in space, separated by <4–6 mm, would not be distinguished individually. With planar imaging, the resolution is approximately 10 mm, and for SPECT it is 16–18 mm. The poor spatial resolution of SPECT is off-set by the superior contrast resolution, which allows it to identify differences between normal, ischemic, and infarcted areas of myocardium.

147. What is the role of PET in the assessment of coronary circulation?

PET is the most accurate clinically applicable method for the quantitative assessment of blood flow. Its high cost and limited availability compare unfavorably, however, with the characteristics of SPECT.

148. What is the role of PET in clinical practice?

The main clinical application of PET is in the assessment of myocardial viability. By definition, viable myocardium has:
- A decreased resting blood flow, which may be shown by PET perfusion agents
- An energetic metabolism "switched" to glucose, a fact that may be shown by using FDG glucose

Viable myocardial segments show the presence of metabolism, in the face of a decreased blood flow. This is termed *mismatched flow/metabolism pattern* (Fig. 18A), as opposed to:
- Nonviable (scarred) segments, which display significant decreases or absence of flow and metabolism (*matched flow/metabolism pattern*) (Fig. 18B)
- Normal (nonischemic) segments, which also show a match between flow and metabolism, both normal

149. Explain the hybrid PET/SPECT approach.

The main logistical problem with PET assessment of myocardial viability concerns the availability of flow tracers, which require a cyclotron to be produced. These agents have a short half-life and must be produced on the premises (as mentioned earlier, by means of a cyclotron, which, for cost and security reasons, is not widely available). FDG glucose has a much longer half-life (110 minutes), which allows it to be produced in specialized centers then shipped to PET laboratories.

The difficulty regarding PET flow tracers can be circumvented by assessing myocardial perfusion using SPECT, in parallel with metabolic assessment by FDG glucose. This is the *hybrid PET/SPECT approach*. This approach is less well documented than any of its "parent" components (PET, SPECT).

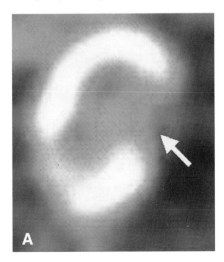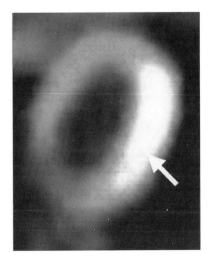

FIGURE 18. *A,* PET study demonstrating a mismatch pattern, diminished perfusion on the left (*arrow*), and enhanced glucose metabolism on the right (*arrow*) indicating viability. (*continued*)

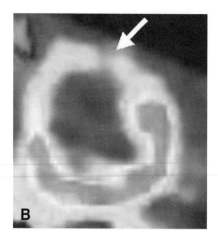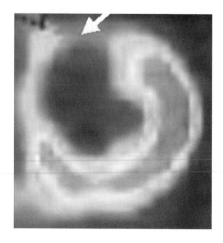

FIGURE 18. (*continued*) *B*, PET study demonstrating a match pattern with diminished perfusion and metabolism indicating an old myocardial infarction. (See also Color Plates, Figure 9.)

Protocols

*Manuel D. Cerqueira, M.D., Dorothea McAreavey, M.D.,
and Gabriel Adelmann, M.D.*

150. Practically, what are the steps involved in performing a nuclear perfusion study?

Regardless of the question being asked (ischemia or viability) or the isotope being used (thallium or technetium), there are two steps in performing a nuclear perfusion study:

1. The rest component, which assesses blood flow at rest.
2. The stress component (exercise or pharmacologic stimulation), which assesses blood flow under stress conditions.

151. Explain the purpose of performing nuclear imaging of the myocardium under conditions of stress.

In many patients, myocardial perfusion at rest may be normal. The myocardial segment supplied with blood by a stenotic artery may not be ischemic under resting conditions and may have the same "brightness" or radiotracer uptake as the other myocardial segments. The ischemic segments are not obvious on a resting study and have to be "brought out" by one of the following methods:

Inducing myocardial ischemia: Under conditions of exercise, the stenotic coronary artery cannot increase coronary blood flow to supply enough blood to the myocardial microcirculation, which becomes ischemic and shows up darker, or even totally black, as opposed to the well-perfused segments, which are bright.

Inducing flow inhomogeneity: Under the influence of vasodilator pharmacologic agents (adenosine, dipyridamole), the normal myocardial microcirculation dilates and increases blood flow fourfold, with correspondingly increased brightness. Dobutamine also may be used as a stress agent for nuclear studies. The microcirculation in the areas supplied by a stenotic coronary artery is already maximally dilated at rest (to meet the metabolic needs of the myocardium), however, and cannot dilate further on administration of a pharmacologic agent. On stress imaging, these segments are seen as dark or black, in contrast to the bright normal segments.

152. Which component (stress or rest) of a nuclear perfusion study is performed first?

When the radiotracer is **thallium-201,** stress is performed first. When the stress study is completely normal, it is not mandatory to perform a resting study. When the stress study is abnormal, the patient is imaged at 3–4 hours, during which time the normal areas lose thallium-201 at a rapid rate, whereas the ischemic areas have a much slower washout and appear to redistribute and look comparable to the normal areas in terms of intensity.

If **technetium** tracers are being used, two separate injections must be done because these tracers do not redistribute. Either the rest or the stress test can be performed first using a low dose of Tc-99m tracer, and after 2–4 hours the second component of the test can be performed using a higher dose.

153. My patient has chest pain, which I suspect to be caused by ischemic heart disease. Should I order a nuclear exercise test or a nuclear pharmacologic test?

Whenever feasible, exercise stress testing is preferable, because of the important additional information offered by the assessment of the patient's exercise capacity and blood pressure and heart rate response. If the patient is unable to exercise (as often happens in elderly patients after orthopedic or neurologic events), pharmacologic nuclear studies are an excellent alternative. Dobutamine can be used as a stress agent in these patients, but for nuclear studies, it usually is reserved in case of a contraindication to adenosine or dipyridamole (most frequently, bronchospasm).

154. What is the diagnostic procedure of choice in patients with left bundle-branch block and why?

Reversible perfusion defects in the anteroseptal segment may be seen in 40% of patients with a normal left anterior descending artery. This finding is thought to be due to abnormal blood flow through the septal perforators at faster heart rates, in the absence of obstructive CAD. When the heart rate is not increased to the extent encountered with dynamic exercise, false-positive results are not present. Pharmacologic myocardial perfusion imaging with vasodilators is the procedure of choice in patients with left bundle-branch block, provided that there is no contraindication (Fig. 19).

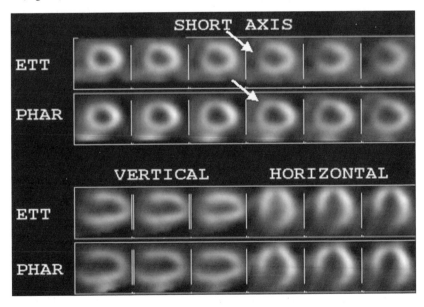

FIGURE 19. LBBB artifact (*arrows*) consisting of a false perfusion defect on an exercise study (*top rows; ETT*) not seen with pharmacologic stimulation (*bottom rows*).

155. What are some differences between rest and stress thallium and technetium scans?

There are major differences in the **timing** of the two components: With either of the tech-netium tracers, following dynamic exercise stress the patient is imaged 15 minutes after injection to allow the radiotracers to be cleared from the liver so that the inferior wall can be seen. Fol-lowing rest injection or pharmacologic stress, imaging is started 45–60 minutes after injection to allow liver clearance. With thallium-201, patients must be imaged within 10–15 minutes after stress, or redistribution occurs, and sensitivity for ischemia is lost. The redistribution studies can be performed at 3–4 hours to identify ischemia and at 18–24 hours to identify viable myocardium

156. Can ischemia be assessed based on one set of nuclear perfusion images only?

Yes. The presence of normal myocardium uptake on an exercise nuclear scan generally signi-fies that the myocardial perfusion is normal, and there is no need for an additional (resting) study.

157. Why are early and delayed imaging of the myocardium performed after a single intravenous resting injection of thallium?

The presence of an area of decreased counts (black area) on the nuclear scan obtained im-mediately after resting thallium injection may have one of the following two meanings:

1. The microcirculation and the myocytes of the area in question have been replaced by fibrous tissue, which can never display significant contractile function, even if the blood flow through the supplying epicardial coronary artery is a re-established (CABG surgery, PTCA).

2. Some of the microcirculation and the myocytes are preserved, but there is diminished blood flow through the microcirculation and slower than normal metabolic activity in the myo-cytes. Simply stated, these areas are able to take up radioactive tracers, but they need time to do so. If nuclear imaging is performed several hours after the initial intravenous injection of radio-tracers, the formerly black areas become bright (in parallel, the well-perfused areas that were bright at rest normally darken on late imaging). This is called *thallium redistribution* and is the basis of viability assessment in the nuclear laboratory. In these patients, myocardial revascular-ization generally results in partial or integral recovery of the myocardial contractile function. Fig-ure 20 illustrates a thallium viability study.

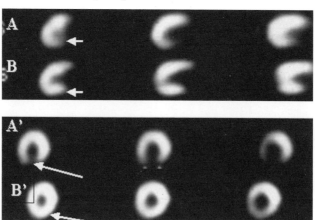

FIGURE 20. Thallium redistribution in the inferior wall (*arrows*), indicating myocardial viability.

158. Can viability be assessed by thallium based on one set of images only?

Yes. As mentioned, the presence of resting thallium uptake abnormalities strongly suggests myocardial scar. It is important to take into account the length of time that this resting study was performed after the initial radiotracer injection, however. It is important to keep in mind "how good of a chance" the radioactive tracer was given to redistribute into the viable myocardial territories. Myocardial segments that are functioning under conditions of severe, prolonged ischemia may need 24 hours for achieving radiotracer uptake.

It is possible to extrapolate this reasoning to a scenario in which one set of images would be taken, under resting conditions, with immediate postinjection imaging. Although segments that would not take up radiotracers even under these conditions ("when they didn't even have to face any ischemia-inducing stress") are probably not viable, there is still a chance that if they were imaged later (giving them the double advantage of "not having to face any ischemia-inducing stress *and* of having plenty of time for radiotracer uptake"), they *would* show uptake after all. Although gross viability assessment is possible based on a single set of images (resting thallium nuclear scan alone), this method may underestimate the extent of viable myocardium. If viability is a serious concern, delayed thallium imaging is essential.

159. Are 2-day protocols ever necessary when using technetium-based tracers?

An important advantage of technetium-based tracers is the possibility of performing a rapid perfusion assessment, minimizing the time requirements imposed on the patient and on the nuclear laboratory. In obese patients, it may be necessary, however, to perform the resting and stress portions of the technetium study on separate days, which provides better image quality because the maximal dose given for each study can be higher.

160. Illustrate the significance of the different radiotracer uptake patterns on rest and stress imaging.

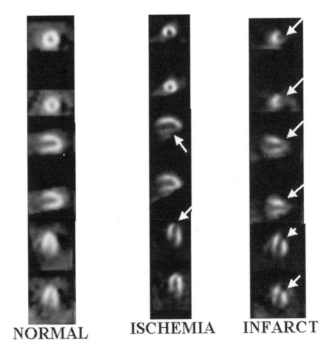

NORMAL   ISCHEMIA   INFARCT

FIGURE 21. The three patterns of stress/rest radionuclide uptake, corresponding to normally perfused myocardium (uptake both at stress and rest), ischemic myocardium (uptake at rest, but not under stress), and infarction (uptake absent at both stress and rest).

*The Patterns of Radiotracer Uptake on the Early and Late Imaging
and Their Clinical Significance*

	EARLY UPTAKE (STRESS)	LATE UPTAKE (REST)	SIGNIFICANCE
Thallium	Present	Not necessary	Normal perfusion
	Absent		Ischemia or scar
	Absent	Absent	Scar
	Absent	Present	Viable myocardium
Technetium	Present	Not necessary	Normal perfusion
	Absent	Absent	Scar
	Absent	Present	Ischemia

161. Discuss the dual isotope technique and its advantages.

This is the technique whereby myocardial perfusion is studied using thallium and technetium and combining the high image quality typical for technetium with the ability of thallium to show myocardial viability.

Here's how it works:

1. **Thallium is injected at rest,** and the patient is imaged a few minutes thereafter. There are two possibilities at this point:
    a. **Normal thallium uptake at rest:** normal perfusion *or* myocardial ischemia that is not evident under resting conditions but possibly will be elicited by stress.
    b. **Perfusion defect at rest:** high probability for irreversible myocardial ischemia or scar; however, this method may underestimate the extent of myocardial viability.
2. **The patient is exercised, and Tc is injected** at peak exercise.
3. **The patient is imaged again,** 15–40 minutes later. There are three possibilities:
    a. **Normal technetium uptake:** normal perfusion.
    b. **Absent uptake, in areas where perfusion was abnormal by resting thallium:** inducible ischemia.
    c. **Absent uptake, only in areas where perfusion was abnormal by resting thallium:** there is no reversible ischemia in addition to the scar shown by thallium.

Figure 22A shows the normal pattern of radiotracer uptake, Figures 22B and C shown reversible ischemia in the anterior and lateral segments, and Figure 22D shows irreversible ischemia in the inferior segment (old infarct).

162. Practically, how is the dual isotope technique different from the single isotope protocols?

The dual isotope technique uses rest imaging before stress imaging, and combines assessment of viability and ischemia with optimal image quality.

Assessment of Left Ventricular Function

*Manuel D. Cerqueira, M.D., Gabriel Adelmann, M.D., and
Evagoras Economides, M.A., B.M., B.Ch.*

163. How is ventricular function assessed using nuclear cardiology techniques?
- Equilibrium radionuclide angiography (ERNA)
- First-pass studies
- Gated SPECT

164. What is the role of LV function assessment in the nuclear diagnosis of ischemic heart disease?

Exercise-induced ischemia results in LV contraction abnormalities, which can be detected by ERNA or first-pass methods. This is the basic method of ischemic heart disease diagnosis based on the systolic function of the LV.

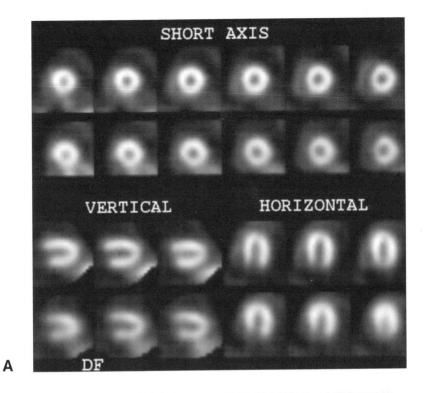

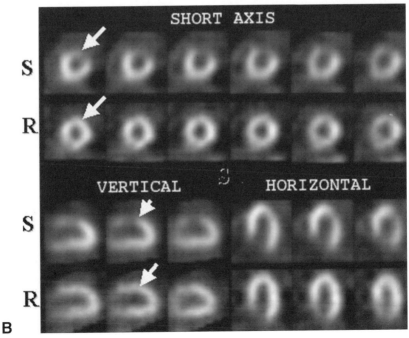

FIGURE 22. Dual isotope studies. *A*, Normal. *B*, Anterior ischemia. (*continued*)

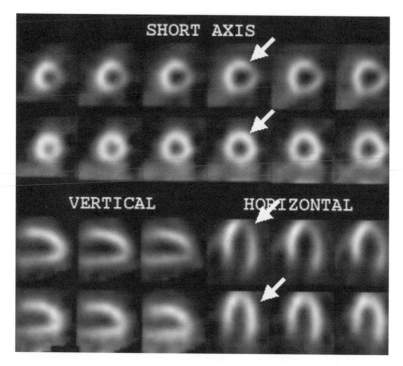

FIGURE 22. (*continued*) *C*, Lateral ischemia. *D*, Inferior infarct with peri-infarct ischemia.

165. How is LV function assessed in the nuclear cardiology laboratory?

LV function can be assessed globally or segmentally and generally is performed on a semi-quantitative basis, which includes the following visually assessed categories: normal contraction, hypokinesis, akinesis, and dyskinesis.

166. Is it possible to assess LV dysfunction quantitatively, using nuclear studies?

Yes, and this is the major strength of the technique because the method is accurate and highly reproducible. The computer algorithms have been validated carefully, and there is a clinical experience of >25 years with this technique.

167. What is ERNA?

ERNA is a method whereby radioactive tracers are injected intravenously, and their presence in the LV and RV cavity is detected based on the emitted radioactivity. By comparing the ventricular volume at end-systole and end-diastole, it is possible to calculate the ejection fraction, a global indicator of the systolic ventricular function. A segmental assessment also is possible, by visualization of the ventricular endocardial borders and demonstration of decreased or absent systolic endocardial motion (hypokinesis or akinesis) in the ischemic segments. These contraction abnormalities can be evident at rest or only under conditions of exercise.

ERNA is synonymous with gated blood pool imaging or MUGA. *Equilibrium* refers to the fact that the tracer has been attached to the red blood cells, which mix uniformly in the blood and circulate throughout the body.

168. Name the methods by which functional assessment is accomplished in practice.

Function may be performed by recording the radioactivity of the intraventricular blood pool:
- Over several hundred heart cycles (ERNA or MUGA)
- Over the first few cardiac cycles corresponding to the first pass of the radionuclide through the RV, pulmonary circulation, and LV

169. What is the main difference between ERNA and first-pass methods?

ERNA is based on the measurement of volume or count changes in the ventricles over time—the so-called time-activity curve. Assuming that the radioactivity is proportional with the volume of blood present at that time in the ventricle, it is possible to calculate the ejection fraction.

To assess the ventricular ejection fraction by this method, it is essential to separate accurately the radioactivity in systole and diastole. ERNA and first-pass methods achieve this in different ways:

1. With **ERNA,** the time-activity is acquired over several hundred beats on several planar views, and ejection fraction is calculated by determining the stroke volume, correcting for the overlying blood pool activity, and dividing the stroke volume by the number of end-diastolic counts.

2. With **first-pass** methods, radioactivity is acquired continuously over a few heart cycles for 25–50 msec images, corresponding to the first pass of the radiotracer through the central circulation, and activity curves are drawn, from which the ejection fraction can be derived.

170. What does the acronym MUGA stand for?

Multiple gated acquisition. This was the brand name of the initial computer program for calculating ejection fraction by ERNA.

171. Name two commonly used nuclear studies for assessing LV function?

1. ERNA
2. ECG-gated perfusion studies using the planar or SPECT methods of acquisition. Figure 11B shows a planar ERNA study, and Figure 23 shows a gated SPECT study.

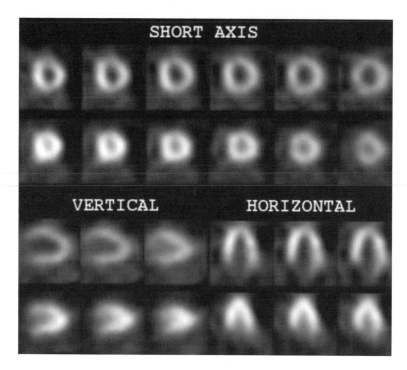

FIGURE 23. Normal ECG gated SPECT perfusion study.

172. What is a *planar ERNA*?

This is the classic method for performing MUGA studies and is based on the comparison of end-systolic and end-diastolic LV volumes, as shown from the anterior oblique and the left anterior oblique views. As opposed to **planar myocardial perfusion** studies, this method visualizes the LV blood pool, rather than the myocardium.

1. With planar MUGA, the LV is displayed as a "black bagel" enclosing a white "filling"; one can infer the diameter of the bagel by measuring how large the filling is.

2. With planar perfusion studies, the LV is displayed as a "white bagel" enclosing a black "filling"; one can measure the bagel directly and identify myocardial perfusion defects as black "bitten-out" areas in the white bagel.

Planar ERNA studies are shown in Figure 11B; Figure 11A shows a thallium perfusion study.

173. What is ERNA SPECT?

This is a tomographic method of imaging the radiolabeled red blood cells using a rotating gamma camera with one or multiple heads. It is seldom used in clinical practice.

174. What is blood pool imaging?

The ECG gated acquisition of the radiolabeled blood cells present in the great vessels or cardiac chambers.

175. Which radiopharmaceutical agents are used for blood pool imaging?

The agent most frequently used for planar ERNA is Tc-99m-pertechnetate attached to red blood cells. Methods for this labeling have been explained previously.

176. Define the beat length acceptance window.

The beat length acceptance window is the acceptable span of R-R interval variation in the heartbeats that are included in an ERNA study. Heartbeats that are too long or too short would al-ter the volume curves artificially and lead to error in the calculation of the ejection fraction. Generally, only beats within ± 10% of the average heart rate sampled before starting acquisition are accepted. The notion of beat length acceptance cannot be applied in the case of patients with atrial fibrillation, in which, by definition, the duration of each heart cycle is different from that of the preceding or the following cycles. The ejection fraction calculated using a wide window is still valid, however.

177. What is gated SPECT?

Classically, SPECT was used for comparing rest and stress myocardial perfusion, with information acquired during systole and diastole being pooled together. Software has been developed to allow acquisition of 8–16 separate images of radioactivity for each beat, and the information from a large number of beats is summed together to obtain accurate edged definition that allows calculation of an ejection fraction. These images may be inspected separately or may be displayed as a digital loop, which allows one to assess the regional and global ventricular function. Gated SPECT is shown in Figure 23. With perfusion and gated SPECT studies, two rows of images are shown for each imaging view. With the two types of nuclear studies, these two rows of images have a different meaning:

1. A perfusion study shows stress images on the upper row and resting images of the same cuts in the lower row.

2. A gated study shows diastolic images on the upper row and systolic images of the same cuts in the lower row (Fig. 24).

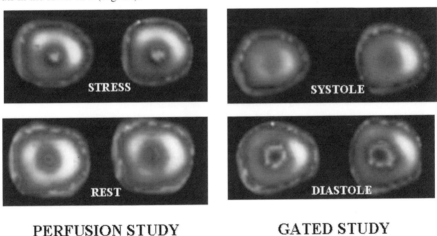

FIGURE 24. Perfusion versus gated study. (See also Color Plates, Figure 10.)

178. Which radionuclides are used most frequently for gated SPECT imaging?

Technetium-sestamibi and technetium-tetrofosmin.

179. Can gated SPECT be performed using thallium?

Gated SPECT first was used with Tc-based tracers. The advent of multidetector cameras has made it possible also to use thallium for this indication. Because of the higher levels of emitted radioactivity (resulting in a higher signal), however, technetium-based tracers remain the diagnostic agents of choice in this setting.

180. What is the spatial resolution of gated SPECT?

Approximately 16–18 mm.

181. List the advantages of gated SPECT perfusion studies.
- High image quality, characteristic for Tc-based tracers
- The ability to evaluate myocardial ischemia and MI
- Measurement of global and regional LV function
- If performed by the dual isotope protocol, information regarding myocardial viability

182. How are SPECT images reconstructed?
Using computerized methods similar to those used for CT.

183. State the main advantage of SPECT.
Greater contrast resolution so that all the segments of the myocardium can be seen without overlap.

184. What is the main difference between gated SPECT and ERNA, in regard to visualization of the myocardial segments?
Although ERNA shows the ventricular function indirectly, by visualization of the intraventricular blood pool (similar to describing a glove by showing the hand that will wear it), gated SPECT shows function by direct visualization of the myocardial segments (the glove itself). Figure 34 in Chapter 2 shows a normal first-pass study, and Figure 23 in this chapter shows a normal gated SPECT study.

185. Is ECG gating a method used with blood pool imaging or with imaging of the myocardium?
ECG gating is used with both.

186. Is ERNA (MUGA) a method used with blood pool imaging or with imaging of the myocardium?
Blood pool imaging.

187. What is the role of first-pass studies in clinical practice?
First-pass studies were described many decades ago. Because of a lack of suitable multicrystal camera systems, these studies seldom are performed today.

188. What radionuclides can be used for first-pass studies?
Virtually all the technetium-based diagnostic agents are suitable for first-pass studies. Sestamibi, tetrofosmin, and teboroxime all have been used for this purpose.

189. How many heartbeats usually are analyzed in a first-pass radionuclide study?
The initial transit of the radionuclide bolus through the central circulation covers an average for 6–10 heartbeats at rest and 4–8 heartbeats during exercise.

190. How long is the acquisition in a first-pass nuclear study?
At rest, the acquisition period is 20–30 seconds, whereas during exercise or pharmacologic stimulation, it is 10–20 seconds.

191. What angiographic views are used for first-pass studies?
For LV determinations, the preferred angiographic view is either the left anterior oblique view or the left lateral view; for RV determinations, the right anterior oblique view is optimal, whereas for intracardiac shunt determinations, the anterior view is preferred. Figure 23B in this chapter and Figure 34 and in Chapter 2 demonstrate normal first pass studies.

192. How is data processing performed in the case of first-pass studies?
The changes in the radionuclide concentration in the intracardiac blood pool are displayed as a time-activity curve. A final representative cycle is generated by averaging all the heartbeats in-

cluded in the study. Premature ventricular beats and the post-premature ventricular contraction beats generally are excluded from the final calculation because these beats have a different LV ejection fraction than the average heartbeats. If there is a small number of heartbeats available for analysis, it may be necessary to include these ectopic and postectopic beats. Data processing also involves background correction methods.

193. Is it possible to calculate LV volumes by first-pass nuclear studies?

Yes. Similar to gated studies, the LV and RV volumes can be calculated based on the number of radioactive counts detected over a period of time.

194. How does irregular heart rhythm affect a first-pass nuclear study?

Similar to gated studies, first-pass studies can provide an accurate assessment of the LV ejection fraction only when the heart rhythm is regular. Premature beats and postextrasystolic beats generally yield an ejection fraction that is substantially different from that seen during regular heart rhythm. If the heart rate variability is small, there are only minor differences.

195. Can PET be used for assessment of LV systolic function?

Similar to SPECT, PET can be performed under ECG gating. Gated PET uses radioactive carbon monoxide for red blood cell labeling and can provide accurate information regarding LV systolic function. Because of the high cost and limited availability of PET, however, this method is not employed widely.

CHEST X-RAY

Curtis E. Green, M.D., and Gabriel Adelmann, M.D.

196. First applied at the end of the 19th century, radiography is the veteran of cardiac imaging techniques. What, if any, is its practical place in the management of ischemic heart disease in the modern age?

The past decades have witnessed an exponential increase in information regarding ischemic heart disease, often leading understanding to the molecular and genetic level. Paradoxically, the *practical* tasks in the management of ischemic heart disease patients have changed very little.

In the hospital, one of the most important everyday problems is to assess the degree of pulmonary congestion in the setting of acute ischemic heart disease. The chest x-ray is ideally suited to provide this information. Radiography is cheap, safe, and fast and can be performed at the bedside of even the most critically ill patient. Although practically every patient hospitalized for ischemic heart disease has at least one additional newer generation test (e.g., echocardiography, cardiac catheterization, nuclear profusion scan), the most **frequently** performed imaging study is the chest x-ray. Typically, at the end of the hospital stay, a patient will have undergone one or two "sophisticated" studies (e.g., nuclear perfusion scan followed by cardiac catheterization) and many more chest x-rays (often on a daily basis, at least during the initial stay in the intensive care unit).

In the outpatient setting, the role of cardiac radiography has diminished with the advent of newer techniques. The chest x-ray is still important in the initial detection of cardiomegaly, aortic or myocardial calcification, or pulmonary congestion, which may point to the possibility of ischemic heart disease.

197. How is the contribution of radiography in the management of heart disease different from that in other fields of medicine?

As mentioned earlier, the most important practical contribution of chest radiography to the management of ischemic heart disease is the assessment of pulmonary congestion and its response to therapy. These clinical problems most often occur in the hospital. This in contrast to the situation in other fields (e.g., orthopedics, pulmonary), in which one of the main assets of radiography is its availability for extensive use in the outpatient setting.

198. When should I order a chest x-ray in a patient with ischemic heart disease?

As with any other decision in medicine, the indication for a chest x-ray should be based on good clinical judgment. The "threshold" for ordering a chest x-ray is much lower, however, than in the case of other imaging modalities.

199. When should I *not* order a chest x-ray in a patient with ischemic heart disease?

There are relatively few instances when obtaining a chest x-ray in a patient with ischemic heart disease may not be a good idea. The most important settings include:

- Acutely ill patients, in whom immediate, lifesaving therapeutic measures take precedence (e.g., extensive acute MI in a patient on the way to the catheterization laboratory, severe arrhythmia)
- Patients in whom the information provided by the chest x-ray would not change the management (e.g., terminal heart failure, unresponsive to therapy)

200. What are the chest x-ray findings in ischemic heart disease?

- Findings showing calcified atherosclerotic plaque (most frequently seen in the aorta, as an indirect marker of CAD; occasionally, chest x-ray may show calcification of the coronary arteries themselves) (Fig. 25)
- Findings showing the effect of ischemic heart disease on the myocardium (focal calcification, aneurysm, cardiomegaly)
- Findings showing the influence of the ischemia-induced LV failure on the pulmonary circulation (pulmonary congestion)

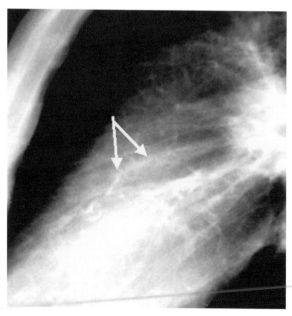

FIGURE 25. Coronary calcification of the left anterior descending coronary artery (*arrows*) in a patient with severe chronic ischemic heart disease.

With the exception of the rare case of evident coronary artery calcification, the radiographic diagnosis of ischemic heart disease is based on indirect signs.

201. What are the chest x-ray findings of LV aneurysm?

LV aneurysm is defined as a localized dilation (*outpouching*) of the LV and is almost always the result of MI, with replacement of the infarcted myocardium with fibrous tissue. LV aneurysm most often involves the cardiac apex and is seen on chest x-ray as an abnormal "bump" on the cardiac contour (Fig. 26). Occasionally the chest x-ray shows bright (white) spots in the area of the LV aneurysm, representing calcium deposition in either the LV wall or blood clots harbored in the aneurysm cavity. The presence of LV aneurysm suggests of ischemic heart disease (old MI). Failure to see an aneurysm on a chest x-ray does not rule out the presence of ischemic heart disease, however.

- Only a few patients with ischemic heart disease actually have MI.
- Only a few MIs are associated with LV aneurysm.
- Even if it is present, an aneurysm occasionally may not be detected by chest x-ray.

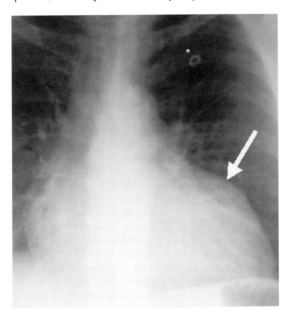

FIGURE 26. Left ventricular aneurysm, evident as a bulge (*arrow*) in the contour of the left ventricle (PA view).

202. What are the chest x-ray signs of cardiac calcification?

Cardiac calcification is represented by isolated small areas of radiopacity (white, bright areas) on the surface of the cardiac shadow. This finding suggests the presence of ischemic heart disease and may result from:

1. Focal areas of calcification in the coronary arteries (coronary artery calcification is studied in detail by electron-beam CT).

2. Calcium deposition in infarcted areas of the myocardium; when caused by MI, myocardial infarction, myocardial calcification becomes evident on the chest x-ray several months or years after the acute event. Although suggestive of an old MI, this finding has little value in establishing the exact time of occurrence of the ischemic event.

3. Calcium deposition in intracardiac thrombus (most often associated with aneurysm).

203. What is the significance of this cardiac calcification on chest x-ray?

Cardiac calcification is not a sensitive sign of ischemic heart disease. It has a high degree of specificity for this diagnosis, however. A common pitfall is the mistaken interpretation of valvular calcification as myocardial calcification.

204. Can chest radiography distinguish acute ischemic syndromes from chronic ischemic heart disease?

Myocardial calcification, aneurysm, or cardiomegaly usually indicates long-standing ischemic heart disease. Conversely, pulmonary congestion associated with a normal cardiothoracic ratio suggests an acute-onset cause of LV failure (most frequently, MI).

5. ISCHEMIC HEART DISEASE AND THE CORONARY ARTERIES

CARDIAC CATHETERIZATION

Gabriel Adelmann, M.D., Andrew E. Ajani, MBBS, FRACP, and Luis Gruberg, M.D.

1. Summarize information obtained from coronary catheterization regarding ischemic heart disease.

Coronary catheterization and angiography is the gold standard in diagnosing coronary artery disease (CAD); it provides information pertaining to:

- The **presence and complexity** of CAD
- The selection of the optimal **therapeutic approach** (balloon angioplasty, stenting, rotablation, directional atherectomy)
- **Assessment after percutaneous intervention**
- Assessment of **CAD progression**
- Assessment of **coronary flow**

2. What is the role of coronary catheterization in the management of patients with ischemic heart disease?

It is the diagnostic procedure of choice to diagnose CAD definitively and allows the performance of percutaneous interventions.

3. Does every patient with suspected or known CAD require coronary catheterization?

No. Most patients with ischemic heart disease do not require coronary catheterization. Noninvasive imaging modalities, such as stress echocardiography and nuclear perfusion scans, have an increasing role as "gatekeepers," for coronary catheterization. For a detailed discussion of the indications for coronary catheterization, see Chapter 1.

4. What elements of information regarding ischemic heart disease are typically *not* obtained by coronary angiography?

Coronary angiography is a luminogram—that is, it is able to show pathologic changes that involve the coronary lumen only, not the coronary artery wall itself. It may underestimate significantly the severity of coronary disease, especially in cases of concentric, diffuse atherosclerotic disease involving the entire lumen circumference and not causing focal luminal stenosis. Coronary angiography does not allow assessment of pathologic processes that are confined to the vessel wall, such as intramural hematoma; such an assessment requires intravascular ultrasound (IVUS).

5. Which terms are used to describe a coronary stenosis?

Based on their structural characteristics, coronary artery stenosis is classified as either **simple** or **complex**. This classification is based on:

- **Length** (Fig. 1A and B)
- **Location** (proximal, mid, or distal; in addition, lesions located at the coronary ostium or at the site of an important coronary branch [bifurcation lesions] are noted)
- **Lesion morphology,** noting the presence of "hazy" (i.e., inhomogeneous, low-density) or calcified areas
- The type of coronary segment involved **(native versus graft or in-stent stenosis)**

Figure 1D shows a normal saphenous vein graft, whereas Figure 1E shows stenotic vein grafts of different complexity.

- **Calcification**
- The presence or absence of **total vessel occlusion**
- The presence or absence of **coronary thrombus**

A coronary stenosis with one or more of the characteristics listed is complex. These coronary lesions are associated with plaque rupture or acute thrombosis (or both) with development of acute ischemic events (unstable angina, myocardial infarction [MI]).

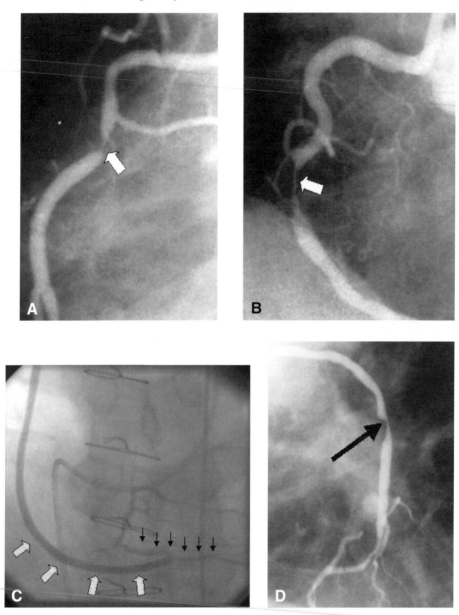

FIGURE 1. *A,* Discrete (short) coronary stenosis. RCA stenosis distal to acute marginal branch (*arrow*). *B,* Long stenosis in the mid-RCA (*arrow*). *C,* Normal saphenous vein graft (*large arrows*) anastamosed to PDA (*small arrows*). *D,* Stenotic saphenous vein graft (*arrows*). (*continued*)

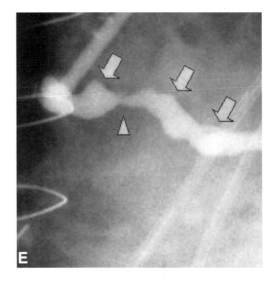

FIGURE 1. (*continued*) *E*, Degenerated saphenous vein graft (SVG). Note the "bead string" irregularities of the vessel lumen, demonstrating an alternation of aneurysmal vessel dilatations (*arrows*) and stenotic lesions (*arrowhead*).

6. Why is it important to identify if a lesion is a complex coronary stenosis?

Percutaneous interventions on a complex lesion are more technically demanding. Certain morphologic characteristics of the stenosis may indicate the utility and necessity of special therapeutic approaches, such as rotablation for a calcified lesion.

7. State the practical importance of coronary calcification.

Diagnostic: The identification of coronary calcification on chest x-ray, fluoroscopy, or external-beam computed tomography (CT) is virtually pathognomonic for CAD.

Therapeutic: Percutaneous interventions on a calcified coronary lesion frequently require the use of the rotablator, an abrasion device that removes the coronary calcium before balloon dilation or stent implantation.

8. What are coronary aneurysms?

Localized dilations of the coronary arteries, with a diameter ≥ 1.5 times that of adjacent healthy coronary segments (Fig. 2). Coronary aneurysms often are associated with atherosclerosis but may be congenital.

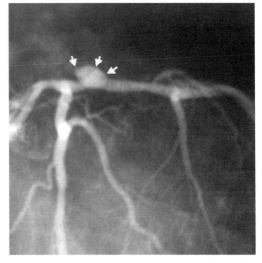

FIGURE 2. Coronary aneurysm, visualized as a discrete bulging of the vessel lumen (*arrows*).

9. Describe the angiographic appearance of a coronary aneurysm.

Saccular—a localized, "abrupt" outpouching of the coronary wall

Fusiform—a local dilation of the coronary artery gradually increasing to its maximum diameter, then gradually tapering off

10. What are the angiographic characteristics of coronary thrombus?

Coronary thrombus is a hypodense area in the coronary lumen ("intracoronary mass" that does not fill with contrast material) (Fig. 3).

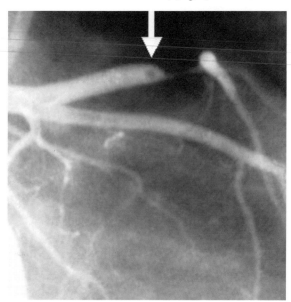

FIGURE 3. Occlusive intracoronary thrombus. Note the "cutoff" of the artery, as well as the nonhomogenous, opaque clot (*arrow*).

11. Where are the coronary artery bypass graft (CABG) attachments to the aorta?

Saphenous vein grafts generally originate as follows:

- To the **right coronary artery:** from the anterolateral aorta, 2–3 cm cranial to the native right coronary ostium
- To the **left anterior descending and left circumflex arteries:** from the anterior wall of the aorta

Arterial grafts generally originate as follows:

- The **left internal mammary artery** and **right internal mammary artery:** not attached to the aorta because they originate from the inferior side of the left and right subclavian arteries
- The **gastroepiploic artery:** originates from the hepatic artery
- **Free radial grafts:** have a similar aortic attachment as a saphenous vein graft

12. What are the angiographic characteristics of coronary pseudoaneurysms?

Coronary pseudoaneurysms may look like aneurysms on angiography but are an area of coronary vessel perforation sealed off with blood clot or contained by the adventitia. Pseudoaneurysms are usually a complication of percutaneous interventions.

13. What is the difference between a true coronary aneurysm and a pseudoaneurysm?

True aneurysm is an expansion of the vessel wall and lumen (all the layers of the vessel wall expand). **Pseudoaneurysm** is a sealed perforation of the wall, contained by a thrombus or the adventitia (or both) and extravasation of blood (contrast with an intracoronary injection of contrast material) into a pocket outside the vessel wall.

14. How is an angiogram different in a patient with an acute coronary syndrome and in a patient with stable angina?

Patients with **acute coronary syndromes** have, by definition, intracoronary thrombosis, generally superimposed on a complex plaque; this thrombus may or may not be appreciated and may or may not be there at the time of angiography (because patients with acute coronary syndromes are treated immediately with anticoagulation).

Patients with **stable angina** generally have nonulcerated, cholesterol-poor, fibrotic, nonthrombosed coronary stenosis.

15. How can coronary artery flow be assessed in the catheterization laboratory?

The invasive assessment of coronary artery flow can be performed semiquantitatively by the Thrombolysis in Myocardial Infarction (TIMI) flow classification or quantitatively using flow and intracoronary Doppler studies. For a discussion of these methods, see Chapter 11.

16. What is POBA?

Plain **o**ld **b**alloon **a**ngioplasty, or balloon dilation of a stenotic vessel without a stent. Beyond its humorous nature, this acronym implicitly reveals the immense popularity of stents in current practice (>80% of interventions); *not* using stents in a coronary intervention has become a fact worthy of a special designation.

17. List the main complications of POBA.
- Spasm
- Thrombosis
- Dissection (separation of a portion of the endothelium from the media)
- Aneurysm
- Pseudoaneurysm (coronary rupture, sealed by a blood clot)
- Restenosis

18. What are coronary stents?

Cylinders of meshlike synthetic material, meant to "scaffold" a coronary segment after balloon dilation (Fig. 4). Coronary stents are mounted on the outside of a balloon, at the tip of a catheter. The tip of the catheter is positioned in the stenotic coronary segment, and the balloon is inflated, "deploying" the stent. Stents can be deployed after preliminary balloon dilation or directly in the stenotic coronary segment ("primary" stenting). Because of their relatively rigid structure, stents do not allow the coronary artery to become occluded. Coronary stents sometimes may be visible by fluoroscopy and coronary angiography, but most stents are not seen by fluoroscopy.

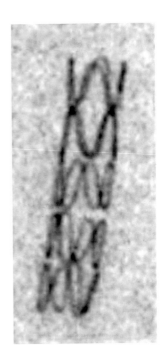

FIGURE 4. Coronary stent.

19. List indications for a coronary stent.
- Medium-diameter or large-diameter vessels (> 2.75 mm)
- Lesions < 25 mm in length
- Total occlusions
- Lesions responsible for an acute coronary syndrome (MI, unstable angina)
- Restenosis lesions
- Ostial lesions

20. For which coronary lesions is there still controversy whether or not a stent should be used?
The following lesions may or may not be aided by using a stent:
- LMCA stenosis interventions (in general) are controversial (there is increasing experience with stenting of these lesions, but this is generally limited to tertiary care, specialized centers)
- Diffuse atherosclerotic disease when stenting would have to cover (almost) the entire length of the vessel
- Atherosclerosis in very small vessels
- Bifurcation lesions

21. List the main complications of coronary stenting.
- Stent thrombosis (Fig. 5A)
- Coronary artery dissection
- Coronary artery perforation (vessel rupture) (Fig. 5B)
- Intramural hematoma

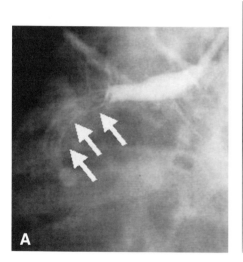 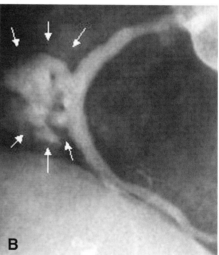

FIGURE 5. *A,* Thrombosed stent (*arrows*) in the proximal RCA, completely occluding the coronary blood flow. *B,* Coronary artery perforation after stenting, with massive extravasation of contrast material (*arrows*).

22. What is rotational atherectomy, and when is the use of the rotablator indicated?
Percutaneous intervention may be problematic in patients with calcified coronary stenosis, owing to increased vessel rigidity. The rotablator, a device consisting of a rapidly rotating abrasive head, is effective in removing the calcific deposits of chronic stenosis and in making these lesions amenable to percutaneous transluminal coronary angioplasty (PTCA) and stenting.

23. What is directional coronary atherectomy?

PTCA with or without stenting does not excise the atherosclerotic plaque, but rather compresses it and moves it, altering its distribution throughout the vessel. Directional coronary atherectomy is a method of coronary plaque removal, by means of a cutting device, which captures the cut plaque and removes it from the vessel.

24. What is the role of directional coronary atherectomy in current practice?

This method is not widely employed, owing to the technical expertise necessary and controversy as to its incremental value compared with PTCA with stent deployment.

25. What is coronary bridging?

Coronary bridging occurs when a portion of an epicardial coronary artery (usually the left anterior descending) penetrates into the myocardium, then re-emerges on the surface of the epicardium. This results in systolic squeezing of the coronary artery and is occasionally the cause of ischemia. In these patients, the myocardium is said to be "bridging" the abnormal segment (Fig. 6).

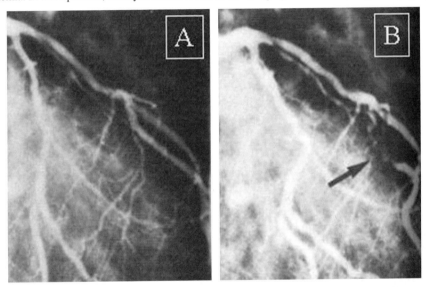

FIGURE 6. Coronary bridging in the LAD. *A*, Diastolic frame, showing unimpeded blood flow through the artery. *B*, Systolic frame, demonstrating complete cessation of flow in the mid-LAD, at the level of the intramyocardial course of the artery (*arrow*).

ECHOCARDIOGRAPHY

Gabriel Adelmann, M.D., and Neil J. Weissman, M.D.

26. When can echocardiography visualize the coronary arteries?

The ostium of the left main and right coronary arteries can be seen by transesophageal echocardiography in adults and children and by transthoracic echocardiography (routinely) in children. The main parameters that can be assessed are the location of the origin of the coronary ostia and the ostial involvement with other processes, such as aortic dissection.

27. What is the role of echocardiography in the visualization of coronary stenosis?

It is possible to show by echocardiography the left and right coronary ostium (Fig. 7) and the coronary blood flow, by means of Doppler studies. Normally the blood flow in the left coronary system is mainly diastolic, whereas the blood flow in the right coronary artery is approximately equal in systole and diastole. A blunting of the diastolic component of coronary blood flow in the left coronary system is evidence of significant coronary stenosis. Owing to the small diameter of the coronary arteries and to the difficulty in aligning accurately the Doppler interrogation line with the long axis of the coronary arteries, this assessment is difficult.

Overall, the role of echocardiography in the visualization of the coronary arteries is modest at present (with the exception outlined in question 26). The main importance of ultrasound in the assessment of coronary arteries resides in the IVUS approach.

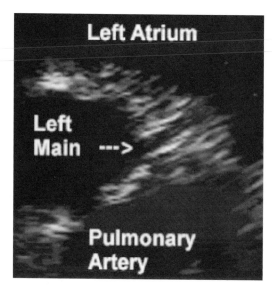

FIGURE 7. The left main coronary artery, as seen from a transesophageal short axis view.

INTRAVASCULAR ULTRASOUND

Marco T. Castagna, M.D., Gabriel Adelmann, M.D., Jun-ichi Kotani, M.D., and Neil J. Weissman, M.D.

28. How does IVUS work?

IVUS uses a miniaturized ultrasound transducer attached to the tip of a catheter and inserted into the coronary artery. The ultrasound is directed toward the vessel wall, and the returning echoes are captured by the same transducer and converted into ultrasound images. The images are displayed as a cross-sectional image of the coronary artery so that all the layers of the arterial wall are displayed (see later). In general, the higher the tissue density (atherosclerotic plaque), the more intense the echo it produces. For a discussion about the principles of ultrasound imaging, see Chapter 1.

29. How is IVUS different from classical echocardiography?
- Its **invasive nature** because the transducer is inserted during a cardiac catheterization, as opposed to the noninvasive character of transthoracic echocardiography and to the semi-invasive character of transesophageal echocardiography
- The **high ultrasound frequency** used (20–40 MHz), which is 10 times higher than that of classic echocardiography

30. What is the advantage of using a high-frequency transducer?

The higher the transducer frequency used, the greater the image quality. Higher frequency also has lower penetration, however. With high-frequency transducers, one can see clearly, but only a relatively thin layer of tissue. Because of the direct contact between the transducer and the vessel wall (absence of any interposing tissue), IVUS works well with high frequencies (obtaining clear images), while still imaging all the layers of the artery.

31. What is the spatial resolution of IVUS?

The spatial resolution (the ability of discriminating two points in space) of a 40-MHz IVUS catheter is 80–100 μ axially (parallel to the beam) and 150–200 μ laterally (perpendicular to the beam and the catheter). Of note, 100 μ = 0.1 mm.

32. Which vessels can be imaged by IVUS?

The tip of current IVUS catheters can be as small as 2.9 Fr (Fr stands for *French*, which is the unit of measure for the diameter of catheters; 1 Fr = 0.33 mm), reaching all major epicardial coronary arteries and their medium-sized branches, and as large as 10 Fr for the assessment of the aorta, and carotid arteries, aorta, and iliac and femoral arteries or intracardiac assessment.

33. What are the smallest vessels that can be examined by IVUS using current technology?

A lumen diameter slightly > 1 mm.

34. Can IVUS be used for assessment of venous disease?

The only venous disease currently studied by IVUS refers to saphenous vein grafts (SVGs) used during a CABG. IVUS is an important tool in the assessment of these structures.

35. List the main layers of the arterial wall, all imaged with IVUS.

The vessel wall has the following components (working from the inside out):

1. The lumen where the blood flows—appears dark on an IVUS image.
2. The intima (endothelium) where atherosclerotic disease is deposited.
3. The media (present in muscular-type vessels, such as the peripheral arteries or the coronaries, and absent in elastic arteries, such as the carotid arteries), which is a layer of homogeneous smooth muscle cells (and outlines the size of the artery if there is no atherosclerotic thickening of the intima).
4. The adventitia, which provides external support to the vessel.

36. What information about the atherosclerotic plaque is obtained by IVUS?

- The **presence** of coronary stenosis
- The **size and shape** of the atherosclerotic plaque
- The **morphology** of the atherosclerotic plaque
- The dimensions of the **adjacent** unaffected coronary **segments**
- The presence of **complications after percutaneous interventions** (dissection, hematoma, pseudoaneurysm)

37. How do these structures appear when seen by IVUS?

The normal coronary artery has a three-layer appearance (Fig. 8):

1. **External layer:** The adventitia is visualized as an echogenic, bright layer.
2. **Middle layer:** The media is visualized as a thin clear (dark) layer.
3. **Internal layer:** The internal elastic lamina and the endothelium are visualized together, as a relatively echogenic layer; atherosclerotic plaque, when present, is incorporated into this internal layer and may protrude into the vessel lumen.

In patients with *no* atherosclerotic disease deposited into the intima (i.e., young children), the intima is not visualized (being < 100 μ thick), and the artery wall appears as a monolayer.

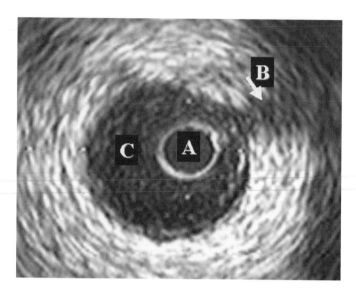

FIGURE 8. General aspect of an IVUS image: IVUS catheter (A), catheter artifact (B), and vessel lumen (C).

38. What are the plaque morphologies identified by IVUS?

The different types of plaque morphology have different densities and histologic composition:

1. **Fatty-fibrotic (soft) plaque** is the least dense atherosclerotic plaque. These structures appear as hypoechoic (i.e., "not very bright white") (Fig. 9).

2. **Fibrotic and fibrocalcific plaque** is rich in fibrin, collagen, and elastin; these plaques are echogenic and at least as dense ("bright white") as the adventitia.

3. **Calcified plaque** reflects most of the ultrasound back to the transducer, resulting in echogenic ("bright white") images; no ultrasound waves penetrate beyond the calcium, resulting in a dark cone of shadow (acoustic shadow) (see Figure 12B).

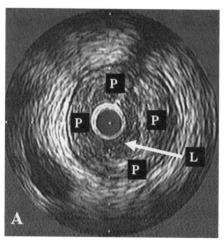
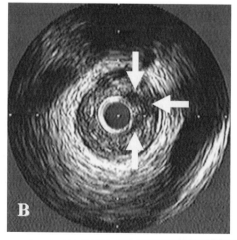

FIGURE 9. *A,* IVUS image of stenosis A from the previous figure, demonstrating significant atherosclerotic plaque (P). L = lumen. *B,* IVUS image of stenosis B in Figure 10. As opposed to stenosis A, stenosis B would have been missed without IVUS; the remanent lumen of the artery is delineated by the white arrows. Both stenoses are composed of soft plaque.

39. Summarize the limitations of IVUS.
- Visualization is of only one artery at a time.
- Only arteries large enough to accommodate the IVUS catheter may be examined.
- IVUS delineates the thickness and echogenicity but not the true histology of the plaque.
- IVUS has a relatively low sensitivity and specificity for coronary thrombus.
- IVUS is more costly than angiography (however, if performed in patients with a true indication, IVUS has been shown to be cost-effective).

40. Describe the most common IVUS artifacts.

Ring-down artifact: This is a bright halo surrounding the catheter, produced by acoustic oscillation in the housing of the transducer and obscuring the area immediately adjacent to the catheter. As a result, the catheter is displayed as having larger dimensions than in reality.

Blood speckle: The intensity of the blood speckles increases at high transducer frequencies and low blood flow velocity. This can limit the ability to differentiate the wall components, especially soft plaque, neointima (tissue proliferation inside coronary stents), and thrombus.

NURD (nonuniform rotational distortion): This artifact occurs when a mechanical catheter system is passed through areas of sharp bends or tortuosity in the course of the artery and results in a distorted image of the vessel.

Catheter angulation artifact: This makes the vessel section appear elliptical, rather than round.

Off-center position of the catheter in the lumen: This makes structures closer to the catheter appear brighter than structures situated in the far field.

41. What are the main complications of IVUS?
- Coronary spasm (in 2.9% of patients)
- MI (0.1%), described in the setting of IVUS use for guidance of interventional procedures

42. What are the advantages of using IVUS compared with angiography for CAD assessment?

Although angiography is still the gold standard for CAD assessment, it has several limitations, which are overcome by IVUS. Angiography is only a projection of the lumen contour and does not allow visualization of the layers of the artery. In addition, angiography:
- Underestimates lesion severity, especially in complex lesions (Figs. 10–12; see also Fig. 9)
- Underestimates lesion length

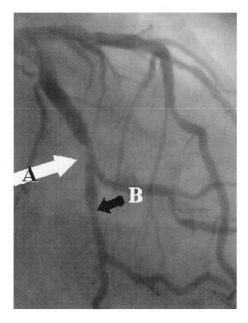

FIGURE 10. Two coronary stenoses of the LAD, by classical angiography: one stenosis is obvious (*A*), whereas the other is a barely detectable (*B*).

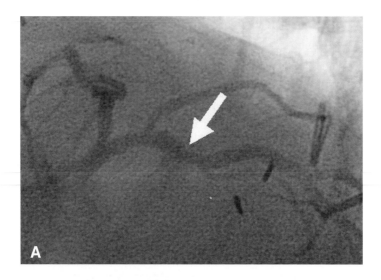

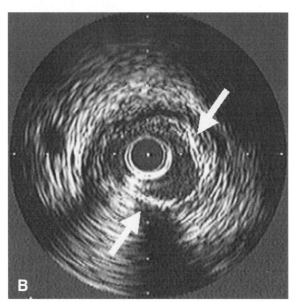

FIGURE 11. *A,* Mid-LAD stenosis, appearing "mild" by classical angiography (this type of stenosis is often described as "vessel irregularities"). *B,* Fibrocalcific, significant coronary stenosis detected by IVUS at the same site as *A.*

- Has limited ability to assess plaque distribution (concentric versus eccentric)
- Is unable to assess for vascular remodeling (enlargement of the vessel to accommodate the plaque and preserve the lumen size)

Correct assessment of these characteristics is important in:

- Selecting the most appropriate device for interventions on a given lesion

Figure 12 shows a calcified coronary stenosis that was not appreciated on classic angiography; coronary rotablation was used before PTCA in this patient, based on the IVUS information.

- Assessing the risk of restenosis after percutaneous intervention

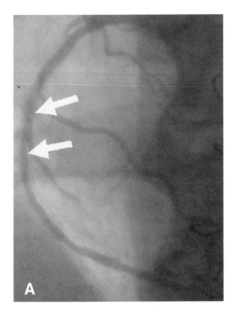
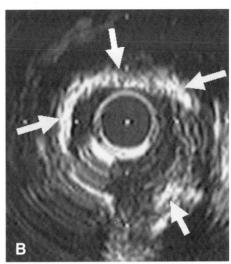

FIGURE 12. *A,* Apparent normal RCA by classical angiography. However, this diagnosis was not considered satisfactory because of the high pretest probability of an RCA lesion (ischemic ECG changes in the inferior leads, unstable angina, hypokinetic inferior myocardial wall by echo); therefore, IVUS was performed. The white arrows pointing at the mid RCA represent the sites of coronary stenosis, as revealed by IVUS (see *B*). *B,* In the same patient, IVUS demonstrated concentric coronary calcification (*arrows*), unsuspected by classical angiography.

43. State the principle on which IVUS quantitative measurements of coronary stenosis are based?

As in the case of QCA, IVUS measurements are based on a comparison of the stenotic segments to the proximal and/or distal normal (unaffected) segments, located within 10 mm from the lesion.

44. How does the IVUS image of a coronary stenosis compare with its angiographic aspect?

Because of its increased ability to visualize the vessel wall, IVUS generally shows a higher degree of stenosis than is possible to appreciate based on angiography. Occasionally, coronary stenoses suspected based on angiography are ruled out by IVUS. Figures 9–12 show angiograms and the IVUS images obtained in the same patients.

45. If IVUS is vastly superior to classic angiography for definition of vessel anatomy, should it be performed in every patient undergoing coronary catheterization?

No. IVUS is used whenever the information provided by angiography (1) is suspected to be incomplete, (2) is discrepant with the clinical scenario, or (3) is not sufficient for performing an optimal coronary intervention.

46. What are the indications for IVUS in clinical practice?

To date, there are no class I indications for IVUS in the American Heart Association guidelines for management of CAD, but this method is gaining popularity rapidly and often is carried out in the following settings:

1. **Preinterventional assessment of the coronary lesion and selection of the optimal interventional device**

   Assessing the degree of coronary stenosis that is not apparent on angiography

   Detection of presence and distribution of coronary calcium in patients in whom rotational atherectomy is considered

Determination of plaque location and distribution in patients in whom directional atherectomy is considered

Determining the length of a plaque and the size of the artery to size stents properly

Detection of vulnerable plaque (i.e., plaque prone to rupture and to cause acute coronary syndromes; this indication remains investigational)

Detection of coronary aneurysm or pseudoaneurysm

2. **Immediate postintervention assessment**

Assessment of adequacy of coronary stent deployment

Identification of complications, such as coronary dissection, intramural hematoma, and stent thrombosis

Assessment of suboptimal results by angiography after percutaneous cardiac intervention. (e.g., the significance of vessel haziness or impaired TIMI flow after percutaneous intervention)

Assessment after high-risk procedures (e.g., multiple stents)

Obtain information about likelihood of restenosis

3. **Follow-up after coronary intervention**

Determination of the mechanism of in-stent restenosis (insufficiently deployed stent [Fig. 13] versus stent restenosis); this information is important for selection of appropriate therapy (balloon expansion versus plaque ablation)

Assessment of vessel remodeling

4. **Diagnosis and management of CAD after cardiac transplant** (see question 54)

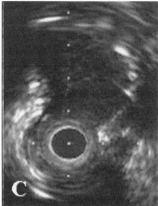
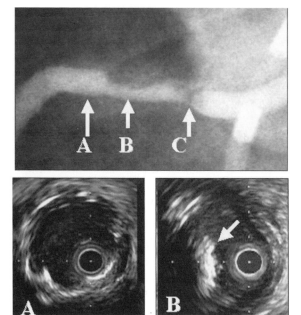

FIGURE 13. *A,* Normal proximal segment. *B,* Incorrectly deployed coronary stent, masquerading as coronary stenosis, and shown by IVUS as an echogenic structure "crowded" to one side of the vessel. *C,* The "real" coronary stenosis was virtually "untouched" by the interventional procedure.

47. Discuss vulnerable plaques, their importance, and the role of IVUS in their identification.

Plaques prone to rupture and thrombosis (resulting in acute coronary syndromes) are turned *vulnerable*. Generally, these plaques are characterized by a high fatty-to-fibrous tissue ratio, a thin fibrous cap, and macrophage infiltration. Most of these vulnerable plaques occur in areas of mild-to-moderate ($<$ 70%) coronary stenosis, and their importance for patient prognosis generally is not detected by angiography. IVUS may help assess overall plaque morphology but has not yet been able to identify reliably which plaques are vulnerable.

48. What is the remodeling process of the coronary arteries, and what are its implications?

For many years, atherosclerotic disease has been perceived as gradual narrowing of the vessel lumen, culminating with total vessel occlusion. In this classic model, the vessel is a passive conduit, not much different from the inert pipes of a building gradually becoming clogged with deposit from the water they carry. The concept of vascular remodeling, introduced by Glagov, has revolutionized the understanding of atherosclerosis. The artery is not an inert conduit for blood flow, but rather a living structure that accommodates for the plaque by expanding and maintaining the lumen size. This response is termed *vascular remodeling,* and includes the following:

1. **Positive remodeling** consists of vessel dilation, with preservation of the total vessel lumen area, despite the presence of atherosclerotic plaque. Positive remodeling is seen in vessels in which the atherosclerotic plaque occupies $\leq$ 40% of the artery.

2. **Negative remodeling** consists of *vessel shrinkage,* seen with older plaques, and is less common than positive remodeling.

Because of its ability to detect plaque morphology and to differentiate the adventitia from the media and intima, IVUS is uniquely suited to identify remodeling, whereas angiography is limited to the assessment of the vessel lumen and completely misses the remodeling phenomenon.

49. Summarize the IVUS findings with a coronary aneurysm.
- **True coronary aneurysm**—a localized dilation of the vessel (involving the lumen, media, and adventitia), generally defined as having a diameter at least 1.5 times greater than the normal adjacent segments; the media encompasses the full perimeter of the aneurysm
- **False coronary aneurysm**—a rupture in the vessel wall contained by the adventitia or blood clot (or both); in the damaged part of the vessel wall, the media is absent

50. What are the IVUS characteristics of an intracoronary thrombus?

There are no IVUS findings pathognomonic for intracoronary thrombus. An intraluminal mass, often with a layered, lobulated, or pedunculated appearance, echolucent or showing a pattern of "speckling" (scintillation), should raise the suspicion of coronary thrombus.

51. What is the main IVUS artifact simulating thrombus?

Stagnant blood flow. Injection of saline or contrast material disperses the stagnant flow and clears the vessel lumen.

52. What are the IVUS findings in patients with coronary dissection?
- The **dissection flap** (Fig. 14)
- The **false lumen,** which results from accumulation of blood or a hematoma between the media and the intima, owing to the intimal tear

53. Name the IVUS characteristics of intramural hematoma.

Intramural hematoma is seen as an echodense accumulation of material (blood) in the media.

54. What is the use of IVUS in the follow-up of patients after cardiac transplant?

IVUS is important not only for detecting classic atherosclerosis, but also for showing the so-called cardiac allograft vasculopathy. This condition is different in nature from coronary athero-

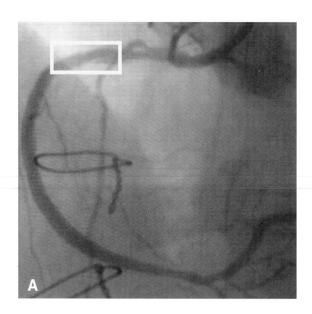

FIGURE 14. *A,* Coronary dissection, seen as a faint "white spur" by classical angiography. The area enclosed in the white rectangle is shown close up in *B. B,* Coronary dissection (*arrows*) (magnification of *A*). *C,* IVUS demonstration of the coronary dissection shown on the previous figures (*arrows*). Although the dissection itself was identified by classical angiography, IVUS provides information regarding the exact location, morphology and length of the dissected area. This information is essential for selection of the optimal stent to be deployed.

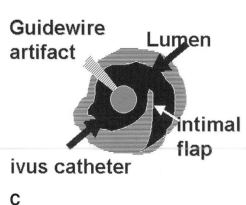

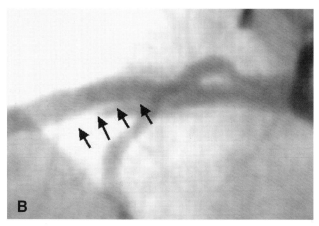

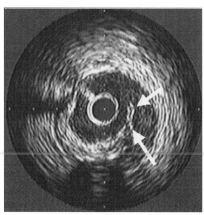

sclerosis and may be viewed as a form of chronic graft rejection. Cardiac allograft vasculopathy has the following characteristics:

- It is diffuse and concentric, usually without associated ulceration or calcification.
- There is no development of collateral circulation.
- It involves smaller branches and the large epicardial vessels (as opposed to classic atherosclerosis, which affects only epicardial vessels).
- Because of cardiac denervation, the patients do not have the benefit of the "alarm system" represented by angina pectoris.
- Noninvasive tests are much more useful for ruling it *out* (negative predictive value > 85%) than for ruling it *in* (positive predictive value 25%).
- It is difficult to detect by coronary angiography, owing to its diffuse and concentric nature, which makes "totally normal" (reference) coronary segments virtually absent.

The current approach to follow-up in transplant patients involves yearly catheterization and IVUS.

55. What is IVUS elastography?

This is a newly introduced technology aimed at assessment of the mechanical properties of the vessel wall, which depend on the histopathologic characteristics of the atherosclerotic plaque. IVUS elastography is an indirect method of assessing vessel wall morphology.

56. Summarize some of the foreseeable *future* developments of IVUS.

- **Imaging guidewires:** Instead of using a separate and sometimes bulky IVUS catheter, the guidewires used for introduction of the catheters into the coronary arteries may be equipped with an ultrasound imaging device.
- **Therapeutic IVUS:** Applying ultrasound to coronary occlusion that cannot be crossed readily by a usual guidewire may create "channels" in the occlusion, allowing one to cross and perform PTCA.
- **Tissue characterization:** The ultrasound backscattered by the vessel wall has different properties, depending on the histologic composition of the wall. Efforts are under way to establish a reliable histologic correlation of the different backscatter patterns.
- **Forward-viewing catheters:** Currently, it is necessary to cross an atherosclerotic lesion to image it by IVUS, potentially causing plaque rupture, distal embolization, or coronary spasm; forward-viewing catheters are devices aimed at viewing atherosclerotic plaques from a distance, avoiding the above-mentioned complications.
- **Three-dimensional reconstruction:** This technique aims to reconstruct reliably the three-dimensional image of the visualized vessel, rather than displaying a series of slices (transverse sections).

57. What is intracardiac ultrasound imaging?

As its name implies, this technique is aimed at visualization of the heart by an IVUS catheter introduced into the right or left ventricle.

58. List potential applications of intracardiac ultrasound.

- Evaluation and monitoring of left ventricle function
- Assessment of the valvular morphology
- Monitoring device deployment, such as patent foramen ovale or atrial septal defect occluders, or balloon dilation of a stenotic mitral valve
- Monitoring of electrophysiology radiofrequency ablation

59. What is optical coherence tomography?

An intracoronary imaging technique that uses light in the same manner as ultrasound. The use of infrared laser light has a much higher resolution than IVUS (at least 20 μ) and someday may allow identification of the vulnerable plaque. Early experience with OCT is promising (Fig. 15).

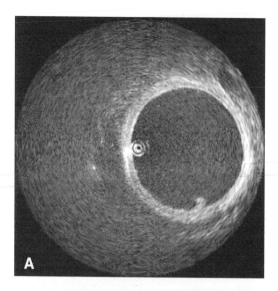

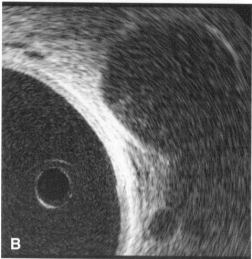

FIGURE 15. *A,* High-resolution OCT (1-Fr imaging catheter in vivo). *B,* High-resolution OCT (zoomed LAD). (Images courtesy Lightlab Imaging, LLC.)

MAGNETIC RESONANCE IMAGING

Anthon R. Fuisz, M.D., and Gabriel Adelmann, M.D.

60. What is the current role of MRI on the diagnosis of coronary artery stenosis?

The use of MRI in the diagnosis of coronary artery stenosis is developing rapidly. An article published in the *New England Journal of Medicine* in 2002 reported excellent results of MRI visualization of coronary stenosis compared with the gold standard of coronary angiography carried out in the catheterization laboratory. MRI was especially sensitive for detecting and ruling out three-vessel and left main coronary artery disease. Figure 16A was taken from a series of MRI images showing an essentially normal coronary artery tree (figure shows a normal left anterior descending artery). Additional coronary structural problems, such as coronary aneurysms, can be shown accurately by MRI (Fig. 16B and C).

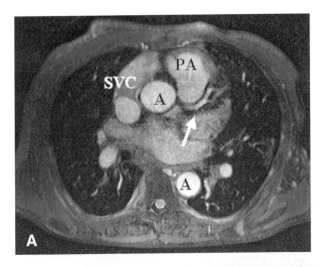

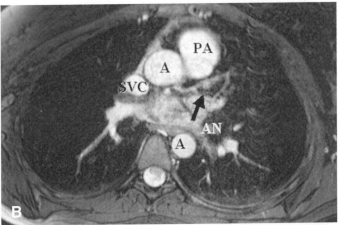

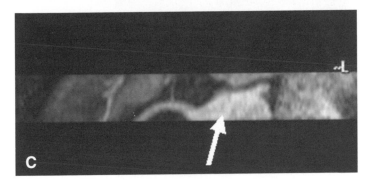

FIGURE 16. *A,* Large and patent LAD (*arrow*) in a patient with moderate renal insufficiency, severe left ventricular dysfunction, and a history of severe allergic reaction to iodine contrast agents. Magnetic resonance coronary angiography is the only diagnostic alternative to cardiac catheterization in these patients. *B* and *C,* Aneurysm of the LAD, visible as a localized "bulge" (*arrow*) measuring 7.3 mm in diameter. (The LAD is visualized as a thin structure, originating from the aortic root.) This finding was confirmed by coronary angiography. A = aorta, PA = pulmonary artery, SVC = superior vena cava, An = aneurysm

61. In view of these exciting developments, can I start referring my patients to coronary MRI, rather than cardiac catheterization, for diagnosis of suspected ischemic heart disease?

Not yet. The excellent results reported in the literature were obtained in tertiary centers with substantial experience in MRI and only for the proximal portion of the coronary arteries. Even if these results are validated in other centers, MRI is costly and is not widely accessible. Its widespread practical application for diagnosis of CAD is still a thing of the future.

62. Does MRI allow visualization of CABGs?

Similar to native coronary arteries, MRI can be used to establish the potency of CABGs by two methods:

1. Direct visualization of the CABG at multiple levels
2. Evaluation of blood flow in the graft

63. What is the main problem with MRI visualization of CABGs?

The presence of metallic graft anastomosis markers can create an artifact that makes MRI images difficult to interpret.

64. Is the presence of a coronary stent a significant problem in the context of coronary artery visualization by MRI?

MRI has been proved safe in patients with coronary stents. It is difficult to visualize in-stent restenosis, however, owing to the field defect produced by the stent. Although active research is aimed at solving this problem, current assessment of in-stent restenosis is based on myocardial perfusion studies, using adenosine or dipyridamole.

65. What is the current role of MRI in the diagnosis of anomalous coronary arteries?

MRI is currently the gold standard and has been shown to be more accurate than angiography in establishing the proximal trajectories of the coronary arteries (Fig. 17).

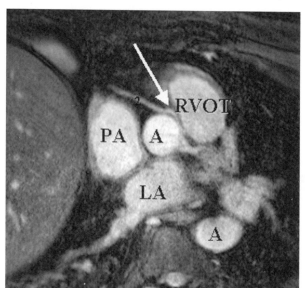

FIGURE 17. Anomalous ostium of the RCA (*arrow*).

66. Can MRI provide information leading to characterization of the atherosclerotic plaque?

MRI has been used to separate plaque components within the lumen of midsize and large-size vessels *in vivo*. Specialized equipment and sequences allow noninvasive assessment of the plaque cap and core in the carotid artery.

67. What is a practical indication for MRI of the coronary arteries whereby it is the procedure of choice?

Visualization of coronary artery anomalies.

68. Discuss the main practical problems concerning coronary MRI that still have to be solved before this technique can become widely used in clinical practice for the diagnosis of CAD.

Some important problems that still have to be solved include shortening the time needed to image the complete arterial tree and development a blood pool MRI contrast agent (i.e., a substance that optimally would resonate in a magnetic field, without diffusing into the tissues); this would make coronary imaging much faster and would minimize motion artifact, one of the primary technical limitations. Also, if coronary MRI is integrated into the interventional angiographic laboratory (at present, MRI is performed in a dedicated suite, separate from the catheterization laboratory), it would have the potential to be used to guide interventions.

6. VALVULAR HEART DISEASE

CARDIAC CATHETERIZATION

Gabriel Adelmann, M.D., Andrew E. Ajani, MBBS, FRACP, and Benjamin Kleiber, M.D.

1. Summarize information that cardiac catheterization can provide in patients with valvular disease.

1. **Fluoroscopy** may show calcification of native or bioprosthetic valves or obstruction of mechanical prosthetic valves.

2. **Ventriculography** may show different degrees of hypertrophy, dilation, or dysfunction (hypokinesis) and reflux of contrast material from the ventricles into the atria (mitral regurgitation [MR] or tricuspid regurgitation [TR]).

3. **Injection of contrast material into the great arteries** (aortography or pulmonary arteriography) allows assessment of the degree of aortic or pulmonic regurgitation

4. **Invasive measurement of pressures** in the heart chambers and great vessels allows calculation of pressure gradients and valvular area, in the case of stenotic valves; in addition, the pulmonary capillary artery wedge tracing may show findings (v wave) suggestive of MR.

5. **Coronary angiography** shows the presence of significant coexistent coronary disease, which may require surgical therapy at the time of valvular surgery.

2. Of the different parameters mentioned in question 1, which generally has the most importance?

Coronary angiography. For all the other parameters listed in question 1, echocardiography is usually the procedure of choice. Performing revascularization at the time of valvular surgery significantly diminishes the frequency of acute ischemic events (perioperative myocardial infarction [MI]).

3. Is coronary angiography indicated in every patient before valvular surgery?

According to the American Heart Association guidelines for coronary angiography, there is a class I indication (expert agreement in favor of the test) in the following categories of patients with valvular heart disease scheduled for surgical therapy:

- Patients with **chest discomfort, ischemia by noninvasive imaging, or both**
- Patients free of chest pain but of substantial age or with multiple **risk factors** for coronary disease
- Patients with infective **endocarditis with** evidence of **coronary embolization**

Coronary angiography also may be appropriate in younger patients scheduled for valvular surgery if there is a concern about coexistent coronary malformation associated with the valvular disease.

4. What is the preferred angiographic view for visualization and semiquantification of MR in the catheterization laboratory (cath lab)?

The left anterior oblique projection allows optimal visualization of the left ventricle (LV), left atrium (LA), and mitral valve. This is the preferred projection for demonstration of contrast regurgitation from the LV into the LA in systole.

5. Name the hallmarks of MR on cardiac catheterization.

- Reflux of contrast from the LV into the LA (Fig. 1A)
- A large v wave on the pulmonary capillary wedge tracing in patients with significant MR and normal (i.e., nonincreased) LA compliance (Fig. 1B)

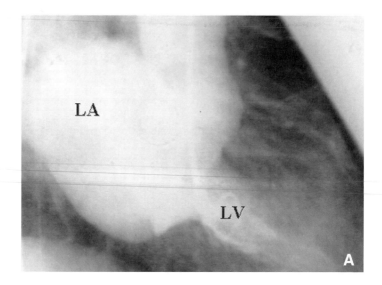

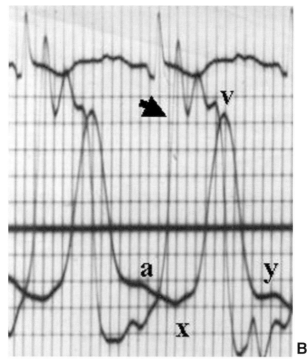

FIGURE 1. *A,* Chronic severe (4+) MR. Complete left atrium (LA) opacification was observed on the first beat after contrast injection, and the contrast material did not clear from the LA, but became more intense with every beat. Note the substantial LA dilatation. *B,* V wave in MR. Pulmonary capillary wedge pressure in a patient with severe MR. Note the significant increase in v wave amplitude, as a result of blood regurgitation from the LV into the LA, with consequent increase in left atrial and pulmonary capillary wedge pressure. a = atrial systole; v = ventricular systole; x = x descent; y = y descent; arrow = LV pressure tracing.

6. **How can the severity of MR be graded in the catheterization laboratory?**
   - Semiquantitative, based on assessment of contrast regurgitation from the LV into the LA
   - Quantitative, based on cine angiography

7. **What are the degrees of severity of MR, as assessed semiquantitatively in the cath lab, and what are their respective definitions?**
   Semiquantitative assessment of MR in the cath lab is based on the:
   - Amount of contrast material returning from the LV into the LA in systole
   - Degree of LA opacification with contrast regurgitating from the LV
   - Persistence of LA opacification from beat to beat

   Taking these elements in consideration, MR is graded from 1+ to 4+, as follows:

   1+ (mild): The contrast material clears with each beat and never opacifies the entire LA.

   2+ (moderate): The contrast material does not clear with each beat but generally does not opacify the entire LA, and opacification of the LA is less intense than that of the LV.

   3+ (moderate-to-severe): Opacification of the LA is complete and equal to that of the LV.

   4+ (severe): Opacification of the entire LA occurs with one beat and becomes progressively more dense with each beat, with reflux of contrast material into the pulmonary veins during LV systole (see Figure 1A).

8. **To what extent does interobserver variability affect the accuracy of semiquantitative MR assessment in the cath lab?**
   Interobserver variability is a common problem in this setting and may change the assignment of MR severity to one lower or higher grade. (For example, there is general agreement among different readers in distinguishing mild from severe regurgitation, but there is substantially more variability in separating a moderate-to-severe jet from a severe one.) This variability may be significant clinically, insofar as it may create the false impression of progression in severity between successive studies, when, in fact, all that has changed is the person performing the assessment. Also, in eligible patients, severe MR is often an indication for surgery, whereas lesser degrees of MR generally are treated conservatively; interobserver variability may affect patient management significantly.

9. **What is the role of semiquantitative assessment of MR in clinical practice?**
   Because of its ease of performance and wide availability, semiquantitative assessment is the most frequently used method of MR severity assessment **in the cath lab.** The imaging method of choice for MR (and for any valvular disease) remains echocardiography.

10. **What is the correlation between the severities of MR as assessed invasively (in the cath lab) and noninvasively (by echocardiography)?**
    Generally, the correlation is good. Occasional discrepancies between the two methods may reflect:
    1. **True differences in the degree of MR because of the different settings in which the measurements are taken;** common clinical settings include:
       a. Changes in loading conditions: Increases in afterload (arterial hypertension) or decreases in preload (dehydration) may cause transient increases in the severity of regurgitation.
       b. Assessment of the MR at the time of acute ischemia, when regurgitation may be more severe.
       c. In patients with VVI pacemakers; periods of pacing sometimes cause significant MR that may subside when "native" heart rhythm resumes.
    2. **Improper technique of MR assessment,** including:
       a. Incorrect contrast material injection; MR underestimation resulting from an insufficient volume of contrast material is the most frequent pitfall in this setting.

    b. Positioning of the catheter across the mitral valve, with creation of transient MR or increase of preexisting regurgitation.
    c. Using an insufficient number of views in the echocardiography laboratory, with underestimation of the regurgitant jet.

11. Do all patients with angiographic signs of MR need echocardiographic confirmation?

No. Patients with mild or mild-to-moderate degrees of MR generally *do not need* echocardiographic confirmation because:

1. It is improbable that these patients should have severe regurgitation missed in the cath lab (the concordance between invasive and noninvasive assessment of MR is highest for "extreme" degrees of regurgitation).

2. Less than severe degrees of MR generally are treated conservatively, and "accurate" classification would not affect patient management.

Echocardiography **is generally indicated:**

1. In patients with moderate-to-severe regurgitation by invasive assessment, to ascertain whether or not the regurgitation is truly less than severe in degree.

2. In patients with severe regurgitation, for assessment of the underlying mechanisms of MR and for identification of pathologic changes in the other valves; the mechanism of MR may dictate the type of surgery needed to repair the valve (versus replace the valve).

12. Define quantitative cine angiography.

This is a method that allows calculation of the regurgitant volume, based on the following formula:

$$RF = (TSV - FSV)$$

where RF = regurgitation flow; TSV = total stroke volume, representing the total volume of blood expelled from the LV in each systole, calculated by Simpson's rule; and FSV = forward stroke volume, representing the volume of blood expelled from the LV into the aorta in each systole, calculated by Fick's method (thermodilution). For a discussion of Simpson's rule and of the thermodilution principle, see Chapter 1.

13. If the regurgitant volume in a patient with MR can be assessed by quantitative cine angiography, why is the semiquantitative assessment more common?

Quantitative cine angiography is a good example of a technique that holds great intuitive appeal but that is rarely carried out in real life. This is due to several factors:

1. The accuracy of the measured regurgitant flow is only as high as the quality of the endocardial border tracing. Classically, this tracing is performed by the technician processing the images and is operator-dependent. Newer systems include software able to generate automatic endocardial border tracings, but even in this case the quality of the tracing depends directly on the quality of the image. Despite the appealing designation *quantitative* with its inherent suggestion of precision, this method still may be fraught with error.

2. Quantitative cine angiography is tedious and time-consuming, especially when using older systems, in which the endocardial border tracing is manual.

3. The ultimate test of usefulness of a diagnostic method is the degree to which the information it provides changes patient management. This incremental value has not been shown conclusively for quantitative cine angiography, and semiquantitative assessment remains the most frequently used method in clinical practice.

14. In a patient with MR, what is the significance of a tall v wave on right heart catheterization?

A tall v wave reflects a significant increase in LA systolic pressure. The LA systolic pressure depends on the **regurgitant volume** and the **ability of the LA to accommodate this increased blood volume:** A highly compliant LA is able to "stretch" (dilate) so that the higher volume of blood does not cause an increase in chamber pressure. Conversely, even moderate degrees of acute MR (chordal rupture, valvular perforation owing to endocarditis) can cause tall v waves because, in these patients, the LA is not accustomed to high blood volumes (see Figure 1B).

15. Is a tall v wave suggestive of acute or chronic MR?

Patients with **acute MR** universally have tall V waves, owing to the disparity between the normal LA compliance and the unusually high volume of blood filling the LA in systole. Patients with chronic MR have different degrees of LA compliance increase, and v waves may be present or absent in this population.

16. Explain the relationship between v waves and the severity of the underlying MR.

The presence of v waves is neither sensitive nor specific for severe MR. They can be absent in patients with severe degrees of chronic regurgitation, and they can be present in patients with mild MR and severely decreased LV and LA compliance (and consequent increases in LV end-diastolic and LA pressure), even in the absence of significant MR.

17. What information can be obtained in the catheterization laboratory in patients with mitral stenosis (MS)?

- Transvalvular **gradients,** measured directly
- Mitral valve **area**
- **Pulmonary artery pressure**
- Degree of **LA enlargement** (Figure 1A shows significant LA enlargement in a patient with chronic severe MR)
- Degree of associated **MR**

18. How can the LA pressure be measured in the cath lab (necessary for assessment of transvalvular gradients in a patient with MS)?

1. Indirect measurement, by assuming the LA pressure is equal to the mean pulmonary capillary wedge pressure; this is the most commonly used method

2. Direct measurement, by accessing the LA from the right atrium (RA), using a transseptal puncture

19. How can mitral valve area be assessed in the cath lab?

Mitral valve area can be assessed by means of **Gorlin's formula,** which combines the following parameters:

- Cardiac output (obtained by right heart catheterization, using the thermodilution principle)
- Diastolic filling period
- Pressure gradient across the mitral valve (obtained using simultaneous catheterization of the LV and of the pulmonary capillary wedge) (Fig. 2)
- Heart rate

20. What is the role of cardiac catheterization in the assessment of MS?

Usually, echocardiography is sufficient for complete assessment of MS. In MS patients, cardiac catheterization is reserved for:

- Assessment of coexistent significant coronary artery disease, which may necessitate surgical intervention at the time of mitral valve replacement
- Assessment of discrepancies between the clinical symptoms and the echocardiographically determined severity of MS

21. What are the pitfalls of invasive assessment of MS severity?

- Poor technique of cardiac output and transmitral pressure gradient determination
- Coexistent significant TR, leading to inaccurate assessment of cardiac output by the thermodilution method

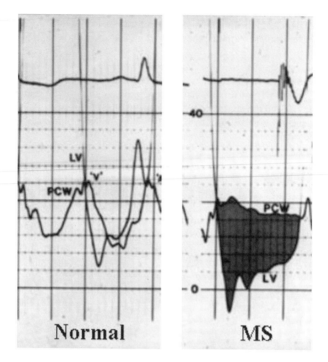

FIGURE 2. Mitral stenosis pressure tracing. In both normals and mitral stenosis (MS) patients the diastolic LA pressure (reflected by the PCWP) is higher than the left ventricular (LV) pressure. However, in patients with mitral stenosis, this gradient (area colored in black) is greatly increased. PCW = wedge pressure, LV = left ventricular pressure.

- Using a damped pulmonary artery pressure rather than a true wedge pressure (pulmonary artery pressure "damping" is an acquisition artifact that results in incorrect pressure tracings, bearing a superficial resemblance to the wedge pressure tracing). Because damped pulmonary artery pressure tracings are generally higher than true wedge pressures, LA pressure may be overestimated, leading to overestimation of the transvalvular pressure gradient and consequent underestimation of the mitral valve area

22. What is the correlation between the severity of MS as assessed invasively (in the catheterization laboratory) and noninvasively (by echocardiography)?

If meticulous technique is used, there is good correlation between invasive and noninvasive assessment of MS severity.

23. What is the role of catheterization in the diagnosis of mitral valve prolapse?

Mitral valve prolapse usually can be observed by left ventriculography, but echocardiography is essential for assessment valve morphology. Coronary catheterization is performed routinely in surgical candidates.

24. What is the role of left ventriculography in the assessment of aortic stenosis (AS)?

Echocardiography is the first method of choice for AS assessment but may be difficult in some patients. The "usual" remedy to a suboptimal transthoracic study (i.e., transesophageal echocardiography [TEE]) may not be helpful in the setting of AS, because of the difficulty in aligning the TEE Doppler beam with the direction of blood flow through the aortic valve. Invasive assessment may be the only alternative in these patients. Additionally, coronary angiography is performed routinely before the surgical correction of AS.

25. Summarize the catheterization findings in patients with AS.

Fluoroscopy, often performed in the catheterization laboratory before the catheterization procedure, may reveal aortic valve calcification, especially in patients with degenerative AS. The invasive assessment may reveal the following:

On left ventriculography: typically, LV hypertrophy, with a normal LV ejection fraction. In the late stages of AS and in patients with significant associated aortic insufficiency (AI), there may be significant LV dilation and systolic dysfunction.

On the invasive pressure tracings: a systolic gradient between the LV and the aorta (Fig. 3).

On the coronary angiogram: the presence and degree of coexistent coronary artery disease (frequent in elderly patients with degenerative AS)

26. Discuss the correlation between the severity of AS as assessed by cardiac catheterization and echocardiography.

The transaortic pressure gradient (peak-to-peak), as assessed in the cath lab, is usually lower than the peak gradient assessed by echocardiography. There are several reasons for this discrepancy:

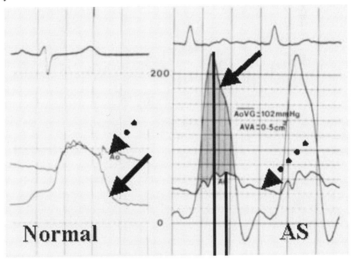

FIGURE 3. Invasive assessment of valvular gradient in a patient with aortic stenosis. The catheter-derived transvalvular aortic gradient is calculated off-line as the difference between the peak pressure in the LV (*continuous arrows*) and the aorta (*dotted arrows*). Note the systolic LV-aortic gradient (*shaded area*) and the time lag between the two peak pressures (between the two vertical lines).

1. **The two methods measure different entities.** The catheter-derived transaortic gradient is calculated off-line as the difference between the peak aortic pressure and the peak LV pressure. The peak of the aortic pressure does not occur at the exact same time as the peak of the LV pressure. Conversely, Doppler echocardiography measures the maximum instantaneous transaortic pressure gradient, which is consistently higher than the peak-to-peak gradient.

2. **Catheterization may underestimate the transaortic gradient** as a result of the phenomenon of pressure recovery. Pressure recovery is an expression of the principle of conservation of energy. Blood possesses kinetic energy, expressed as a blood velocity, and potential energy, expressed as intracavitary pressure. The total energy of blood leaving the LV is equal to the energy of blood in the aorta. What changes, however, is the division of this total energy into kinetic and potential energy. As blood passes through the stenotic aortic valve, some of its potential energy is converted to kinetic energy (velocity increases as blood approaches, then crosses, the aortic valve).

This conversion of potential energy into kinetic energy continues for a few millimeters into the aorta and reaches a maximum at a point called the ***vena contracta.*** At this point, the velocity of the blood flow is maximal, and the intracavitary (i.e., aortic) pressure is minimal. Beyond the vena contracta, some of the kinetic energy is reconverted to potential energy, and the intracavitary aortic pressure increases (blood velocity decreases). Measuring the LV-aortic gradient based on the pressure at the vena contracta yields the maximal LV-aortic gradient. Echocardiography performs this measurement. It may be difficult to place (and to keep) the tip of a catheter at the precise point of the vena contracta, however. Even a slight displacement of the catheter tip distal to this point results in measuring an aortic pressure that is higher (i.e., partly "recovered ") than at the site of the vena contracta, which results in measuring a less-than-maximal gradient.

   3. **Doppler techniques can overestimate the transaortic gradient,** because of several factors:

   a. Doppler assessment of transaortic gradients is based on the continuity equation, which is an expression of the principle of conservation of matter. The continuity equation states that the volume of blood per unit of time (i.e., flow) in the LV and in the proximal aorta are equal. Blood flow is calculated as the product of blood flow velocity and of the section area of the LV and the aorta. Generally, the blood velocity in the LV is much lower than in the aorta, and can be neglected in the pressure-gradient calculations. In patients with high-output states or with AI, in whom the proximal velocity is increased, not taking this velocity into account leads to an overestimation of the peak transaortic gradient.
   b. The high-velocity jet of coexistent MR can be misinterpreted as the jet through the aortic valve. The usual velocity of an MR jet is approximately 5 m/sec; a similar blood velocity through the aortic valve corresponds to critical AS. Mistaking an insignificant jet of mild MR for critical, surgery-requiring AS is a serious error.
   c. Nonparallel alignment of the Doppler beam may result in underestimation of the proximal velocity and consequent overestimation of the transvalvular gradient by continuity equation.

27. What are the angiographic findings in patients with AI?

The angiographic hallmark of AI is reflux of contrast material from the aorta into the LV. There also is a variable degree of LV dilation and systolic dysfunction (decreased ejection fraction). The severity of AI can be assessed semiquantitatively, in a manner similar to that used for assessment of MR. Simultaneous assessment of the pressure in the LV and in the aorta shows rapid equalization of the pressures in diastole between these two chambers (Fig. 4).

28. Can chronic and acute AI be distinguished in the cath lab?

In acute AI, there is no LV dilation, whereas this finding is the hallmark of chronic AI. Also, the LV end-diastolic pressure in these patients generally is severely elevated.

29. What is the correlation between the severities of AI as assessed invasively (in the cath lab) and noninvasively (by echocardiography)?

If meticulous technique is used, the correlation is excellent, especially in patients with moderate or severe regurgitation.

30. List are the main angiographic findings in tricuspid stenosis (TS).

- A marked reduction in the resting cardiac output
- A diastolic tricuspid valve gradient ≥ 3 mmHg
- A large a wave on the central venous pressure tracing in patients in sinus rhythm

31. State the main pitfall of angiographic assessment of tricuspid stenosis.

Patients with TS almost always have associated TR, which makes blood flow determinations through this valve inaccurate, leading to error in the calculation of the transvalvular gradient and the valve area.

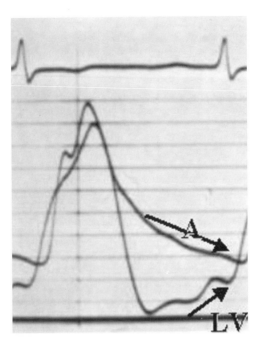

FIGURE 4. AI pressure curves. In aortic regurgitation, there is a rapid decrease in diastolic aortic pressure and a parallel rapid increase in the left ventricular pressure). The arrows indicate the evolution of the diastolic pressures (A, LV).

32. What is the role of angiography in the assessment of the severity of TS?

Angiography is not the diagnostic method of choice. Echocardiography is the best diagnostic method.

33. List the angiographic findings in patients with TR.

Similar to MR, TR causes:
- Reflux of contrast material into the atrium in systole
- A tall v wave on the central venous pulse tracing
- Right ventricle (RV) dilation

34. What is the role of right ventriculography in the assessment of TR?

Angiography is not the diagnostic method of choice for assessment of TR, owing to several potential problems:
- **Overestimation of TR** because of the presence of a catheter across the tricuspid valve, which can increase falsely the degree of regurgitation or create regurgitation despite a normal tricuspid valve.
- **Underestimation of TR:** Patients undergoing cardiac catheterization usually are dehydrated as a result of diuretic therapy and of the fasting conditions. These factors can lead to underestimation of the severity of TR.

As with other valvular conditions, echocardiography is the imaging modality of choice.

35. Describe the angiographic findings in patients with prosthetic valvular dysfunction.

Fluoroscopy is a useful (albeit neglected) imaging modality for visualizing the valvular ring and struts and, in the case of mechanical prosthesis, visualizing the tilting disk. Fluoroscopy may show dehiscence or "stuck" valves (absence or decrease of occluder device motion). In patients with a degenerative valvular bioprosthesis, significant valvular calcification frequently is seen.

Ventriculography may reveal (1) normal LV function or, more frequently, LV dilation and dysfunction and (2) reflux of contrast material, in the case of valvular regurgitation.

36. Can left ventriculography be performed in patients with a valvular prosthesis?

In patients with mitral valve prosthesis, ventriculography is not a problem because the retrogradely placed LV catheter does not have to cross the mitral prosthesis. In patients with a mechanical aortic prosthesis, retrograde catheterization of the LV may be hazardous because the catheter may become entangled between the different parts of the mechanical valve. In the case of bioprosthetic aortic valves, LV catheterization is possible, but special care should be exercised in patients with severe valvular degeneration, in whom the catheter may damage the valve further or produce embolic phenomena (or both). Although occasionally feasible, left ventriculography generally should be avoided in patients with aortic valvular prosthesis. In these patients, assessment of LV function and valvular gradients should be performed by echocardiography.

ECHOCARDIOGRAPHY

Overview

Gabriel Adelmann, M.D., Kenneth Horton, RDCS, and Neil J. Weissman, M.D.

37. Summarize the role of echocardiography in the assessment of valvular disease.
- Identification of the valvular disease
- Assessment of the severity of regurgitation or stenosis
- Assessment of the mechanism of valve disease
- Assessment of the impact of the valve disease on the structure and function of the ventricles and atria
- Determination whether surgical correction or other mechanical interventions are necessary
- Assistance in the determination of the optimal surgical or interventional technique (e.g., mitral repair versus replacement)
- Intraoperative assessment in patients undergoing valvular surgery
- Postoperative follow-up

38. List the principal components of an echocardiographic evaluation of valvular stenosis.
- Direct visualization of leaflet mobility and measurement of valvular area (planimetry)
- Doppler assessment of transvalvular pressure gradient, using the Bernoulli equation (the Doppler method is the cornerstone of valvular evaluation in the echocardiography laboratory (echo lab)
- Assessing the impact of valvular stenosis on the size, thickness, and function of the ventricles and atria

39. What are the principal components of an echocardiographic evaluation of valvular regurgitation severity?

1. Semiquantitative assessment using the jet area or width using color Doppler; this assessment usually classifies valvular regurgitation as trace/physiologic, mild, moderate, or severe.

2. Quantitative methods using a combination of two-dimensional and Doppler measurements, which allow calculation of the regurgitant orifice area or the regurgitant volume of blood.

3. The impact of valvular disease on the size and function of the ventricles and atria (e.g., otherwise unexplained significant LV dilation in a patient with MR suggests severe regurgitation).

Aortic Stenosis

Steven A. Goldstein, M.D., Gabriel Adelmann, M.D., Kenneth Horton, RDCS, and Neil J. Weissman, M.D.

40. What is the role of echocardiography in the evaluation of AS?

It is the mainstay of noninvasive evaluation of AS. It allows identification of all parameters listed in question 37.

41. How can AS be identified by echocardiography?

1. **M-mode echocardiography** shows a decreased systolic separation of the aortic valve leaflets.

2. **Two-dimensional echocardiography** shows structural changes of the aortic valve (fibrosis, calcification, bicuspid aortic valve) or of the subaortic or supra-aortic regions (membranes, muscular stenosis, septal hypertrophy) and the adaptive mechanisms of the LV to the increased afterload (LV hypertrophy).

3. **Doppler echocardiography** shows increased blood flow velocity through the aortic valve, representing an increased pressure gradient between the LV and the aorta (blood flow obstruction).

The different echocardiographic techniques in isolation (planimetry by two-dimensional, gradient calculation by Doppler) are complementary and give added data in combination (aortic valve area calculation by combining two-dimensional and Doppler information).

42. When is AS considered to be present?

The normal aortic valve area is 3.0–4.0 cm^2 in adults. In principle, an area < 3 cm^2 is abnormal. An aortic valve area < 2 cm^2 is clinically important and is considered to represent AS.

43. Name the different types of AS.

Valvular, subvalvular, and supravalvular.

44. Summarize the most frequent causes of AS.

Etiology of Aortic Stenosis

TYPE OF AS	CAUSE
Valvular	Degenerative fibrosis, sclerosis, and calcification of a previously normal trileaflet valve (the **most frequent cause of AS in adults**)
	Bicuspid aortic valve
	Rheumatic valvular disease
Subvalvular	Fixed obstruction by a subvalvular membrane
	Fixed muscular obstruction
	Dynamic obstruction (HOCM)
Supravalvular	Supravalvular membrane
	Localized fibromuscular thickening
	Diffuse hypoplasia of the ascending aorta

HOCM = hypertrophic obstructive cardiomyopathy.

45. Name the echocardiographic characteristics of degenerative AS.

Leaflet thickening, leaflet calcification, and commissural fusion from sclerosis at the base of the leaflets (Fig. 5).

46. What are the two-dimensional echocardiography characteristics of a bicuspid aortic valve?

A bicuspid aortic valve has only two leaflets, as opposed to the three leaflets present in normal subjects. A bicuspid aortic valve is the most frequent congenital abnormality in the general population. The two-dimensional echocardiography characteristics include:

1. The **morphology** of the leaflets, best appreciated from the parasternal short-axis view. Typically the two leaflets are unequal in size. Bicuspid valves often have a raphe in the larger leaflet, which may be mistaken for a third commissure.

2. The **opening pattern** of the leaflets in systole. The **parasternal short-axis view** has a football-shaped (oval contour) opening pattern. Normally the leaflets open along three convergent lines, representing the three commissures; this normal opening pattern often is compared with the trademark of the Mercedes Benz company and is casually called the *Mercedes Benz sign*. In the **parasternal long-axis view,** systolic leaflet appears bowing ("doming") into the aorta (Fig. 6).

47. What are the M-mode characteristics of a bicuspid aortic valve?

An eccentric closure line of the valve leaflets on M-mode echocardiography is the hallmark of a bicuspid aortic valve.

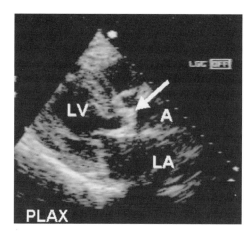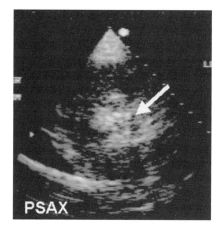

FIGURE 5. Degenerative AS. Valvular aortic stenosis in parasternal long axis (PLAX) and parasternal short axis (PSAX) views. The valve itself is heavily thickened and dense (*arrows*). Note the associated left ventricular hypertrophy.

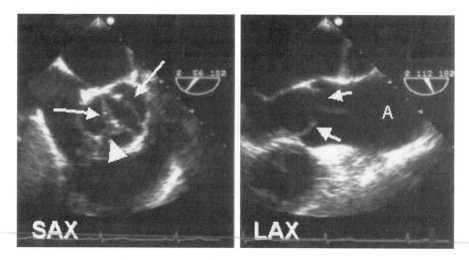

FIGURE 6. Bicuspid aortic valve. Note the football-shaped opening (*arrows*) and the raphe (*arrowhead*), best visualized from the short-axis view (SAX), and the typical leaflet "doming," seen in long axis (LAX). Although the images were obtained by TEE, similar images may be obtained by high-quality transthoracic echo (TTE).

48. If a bicuspid aortic valve is detected on an echocardiogram, what other associated conditions should come to mind and be excluded?
- Aortic coarctation
- Aneurysmal dilation of the ascending aorta
- AS or AI or both
- The Shone complex, a rare condition associated with a bicuspid valve and several additional cardiac abnormalities (subaortic stenosis, valvular AS, supravalvular AS, coarctation, parachute mitral valve).

49. What are the echocardiographic characteristics of rheumatic AS?
Similar to degenerative AS, rheumatic AS can cause thickening and calcification of the valvular leaflets and leaflet fusion leading to obstruction of blood flow. In contrast to degenerative disease, leaflet fusion starts *at the tips* and causes a "doming" motion in systole similar to that seen with bicuspid aortic valves.

50. Describe the echocardiographic appearance of a subaortic membrane.
A subaortic membrane is a crescent-shaped fibrous structure extending from the interventricular septum to the anterior mitral leaflet (Fig. 7). These membranes can cause stenosis, regurgitation, or a combination of both. They are identified best on two-dimensional studies from the apical views (in the parasternal long-axis view, the ultrasound beam is approximately parallel to the membrane, and multiple transducer angulations are necessary for optimal visualization). Often they are not visible by two-dimensional echo but are suspected based on the presence of otherwise unexplained turbulent subaortic flow and subaortic gradient. In these patients, TEE should be performed to confirm the diagnosis.

51. What is the echocardiographic appearance of muscular subaortic stenosis?
The spectrum of severity ranges from discrete stenosis to a tunnel-like diffuse muscular stenosis. Muscular subaortic stenosis is rarely seen in adults.

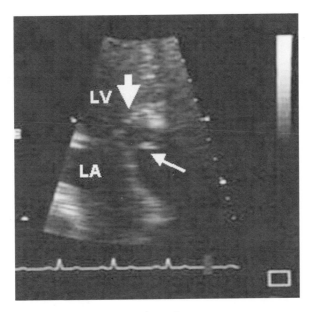

FIGURE 7. Subaortic membrane. LV = left ventricle, LA = left atrium, thick arrow = subaortic membrane, thin arrow = aortic valve.

52. What is the mechanism of dynamic subaortic obstruction in patients with hypertrophic obstructive cardiomyopathy?

In these patients, blood flow through the LV outflow tract (LVOT) is unimpeded at the beginning of systole; however, during mid- and late systole there is dynamic obstruction to flow caused by the close proximity between the anteriorly displaced anterior mitral valve leaflet and the hypertrophic interventricular septum.

53. How is the mechanism of dynamic subaortic obstruction detected by echocardiography?

On the echocardiogram, there is systolic anterior motion of the mitral leaflet and a "dagger shape" of the LVOT Doppler profile, corresponding to the rapid, late-systolic increase in LVOT flow velocity. This characteristic flow profile is important for distinguishing subvalvular from valvular stenosis (Fig. 8). See Chapter 3 for further discussion of hypertrophic obstructive cardiomyopathy.

54. What are the echocardiographic characteristics of supravalvular AS?
- A discrete membrane
- A localized fibromuscular thickening, producing a typical hour glass aspect of the aorta, generally at the sinotubular junction
- Diffuse hypoplasia of the ascending aorta

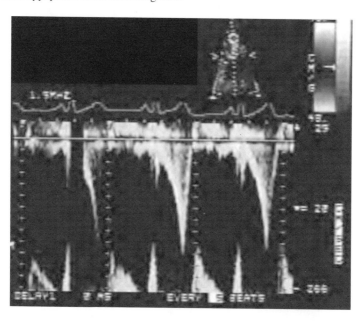

FIGURE 8. CW Doppler study of the LVOT in HOCM. Note the specific shape of the LVOT pressure tracing.

55. Which age group is predominantly affected by supravalvular AS?
Pediatric population.

56. Define the degrees of severity of valvular AS.
- **Mild:** valvular area > 1.5 cm².
- **Moderate:** valvular area 1.0–1.5 cm².
- **Severe:** valvular area < 1.0 cm². In severe AS, the peak transvalvular gradient is usually >

50 mmHg, and the mean gradient is usually > 30 mmHg, under conditions of normal cardiac output. When the aortic valve area is < 0.8 cm^2, it is considered **critical** AS.

57. Does a normal aortic valve area rule out obstruction to blood outflow into the aorta?
No. Besides valvular stenosis, the obstruction to blood flow may be subvalvular or supravalvular.

58. List the echocardiographic methods of assessing AS severity.
- Doppler assessment—mean and peak transvalvular gradients
- Two-dimensional assessment—planimetry
- Combined Doppler and two-dimensional assessment—continuity equation to calculate aortic valve area

59. What is the role of transvalvular gradient assessment in patients with AS?
In patients with a normal cardiac output, there is a direct relationship between the severity of AS and the mean transvalvular pressure gradient. In general, a mean pressure gradient > 50 mmHg corresponds to severe AS (Fig. 9).

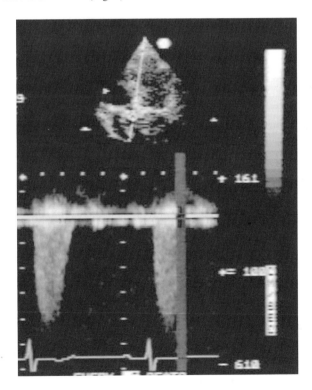

FIGURE 9. CW Doppler flow through the aortic valve (AS patient), with peak velocity of at least 4 m/sec corresponding to a peak gradient of at least 64 mmHg. Note the early-peaking transaortic velocity as opposed to the late-peaking gradients of HOCM.

60. Summarize the influence of cardiac output on the pressure gradient through the aortic valve.
1. In patients with increased cardiac output (hyperdynamic syndrome, AI), there may be increased transvalvular gradients in the absence of severe AS.
2. In patients with irregular heart rhythm, the heartbeats following a prolonged diastole have a

higher stroke volume with an increase in gradient; in these patients, 10 consecutive beats should be averaged.

3. In patients with decreased cardiac output (significant LV dysfunction), transvalvular pressure gradients may not be elevated, even in the presence of severe AS.

61. When should dobutamine echocardiography be used to help assess the severity of AS?

Patients with severe LV dysfunction may have a low transvalvular pressure gradient despite severe AS. In addition, the continuity equation may underestimate the aortic valve area in this situation (see later). Administration of a low dose of dobutamine in these patients elevates the cardiac output, allowing one to distinguish between truly severe AS from pseudosevere AS:

- In patients with truly severe AS, there is equal increase in the peak blood velocity in the LVOT and through the aortic valve, so the calculated aortic valve area remains small.
- In patients in whom the apparently severe AS is due to the low cardiac output, dobutamine increases the LVOT flow velocity and opens the aortic valves further, so there is no increase in the transaortic velocities and a decrease in the assessed degree of "AS."

62. What is the dimensionless index?

The ratio between the LVOT flow velocity and the aortic valve flow velocity. Generally, variations in cardiac output affect both velocities equally; the dimensionless index may serve as a cardiac output–independent indicator of AS severity. The most frequent use of the dimensionless index is to follow patients with prosthetic aortic valves.

63. What is the role of planimetry in the assessment of AS severity?

Although the primary echocardiographic method of assessing the severity of AS is a combination of Doppler and two-dimensional measurements to calculate aortic valve area (see the continuity equation next), it is sometimes possible to trace the aortic valve area directly by planimetry. This is rarely possible from the parasternal short-axis view on transthoracic echocardiography (TTE) but commonly is performed by TEE. Planimetry may be difficult in patients with severe aortic valve calcification because of reverberation and shadowing.

64. What is the continuity equation?

The mathematical formula used for calculation of aortic valve area in the echocardiography laboratory. The continuity equation uses the concept that blood flow in the LVOT is equal to the blood flow through the aortic valve ("what comes in must go out").

The general equation for calculating the flow rate (volume per unit of time) of a fluid flowing through a tube is:

$$\text{Flow rate} = \text{cross-sectional area of the tube} * \text{flow velocity}$$

Thus:

$$\text{Blood flow through the LVOT} = \text{area (LVOT)} * \text{velocity of blood (LVOT)} \textit{ and}$$

$$\text{Blood flow through the aortic valve (AV)} = \text{area (AV)} * \text{velocity of blood (AV)}$$

In other words:

$$\text{Area (LVOT)} * \text{velocity (LVOT)} = \text{area (AV)} * \text{velocity (AV)} \textit{ or}$$

$$\text{Area (AV)} = \text{area (LVOT)} * \text{velocity (LVOT)/velocity (AV)}$$

The area of the LVOT can be measured from the two-dimensional parasternal long-axis view (the diameter is measured, then the area is calculated), the velocity in the LVOT can be measured by pulse wave Doppler from the apical window, and the velocity in the aortic valve can be measured by continuous wave Doppler from the apical window. The equation is solved for the aortic valve area (Fig. 10).

65. Discuss the limitations of the continuity equation.

Obtaining an accurate measurement of the LVOT diameter is the greatest potential source of error. This measurement can be especially difficult in patients with a highly calcified aortic annulus, in whom reverberations do not allow precise identification of the LVOT borders, or with an upper septal bulge ("sigmoid septum"), which distorts the LVOT contour; this is seen especially in elderly patients.

When performing echocardiographic follow-up of a patient with AS, it is extremely helpful to have the prior LVOT measurement because this diameter rarely changes over time to any significant degree. Any apparent change may introduce an error in the aortic valve calculation.

Additional problems with the continuity equation include:

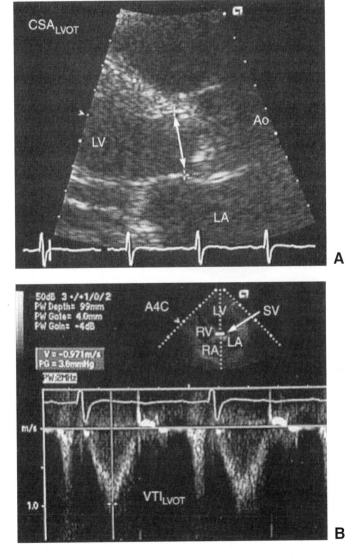

FIGURE 10. Continuity equation aortic valve area (AVA) calculations require measurement of left ventricular outflow tract diameter on the parasternal long-axis view for circular cross-sectional area calculation (*A*), pulsed Doppler recording of the left ventricular outflow tract velocity-time integral (VTI) from an apical approach (*B*), and continuous-wave Doppler recording (*continued*)

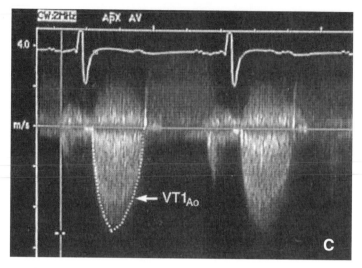

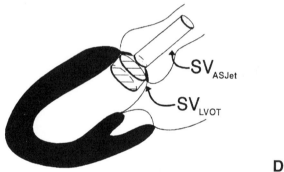

$$SV_{LVOT} = SV_{AS\text{-}Jet}$$

$$CSA_{LVOT} \times VTI_{LVOT} = AVA \times VTI_{AS\text{-}Jet}$$

E $$AVA = (VTI_{LVOT} \times CSA_{LVOT})/VTI_{AS\text{-}Jet}$$

FIGURE 10. (*continued*) (*C*) of the aortic stenosis velocity-time integral (VTI-AS jet; (*D*) from whichever window gives the highest-velocity signal. (From Otto CM: Textbook of Clinical Echocardiography, 2nd ed. Philadelphia, W.B. Saunders, 2000, p 241, with permission.)

- Obtaining the maximum aortic velocity, which requires sampling from several locations
- Beat-to-beat variations in blood flow secondary to atrial fibrillation or premature beats (10 consecutive beats should be averaged)
- Confusion of other pathologic cardiac blood flows for the transvalvular aortic jet (see next question)

66. Name other pathologic cardiac blood flows that may be mistaken for the AS jet.

Several cardiac conditions are associated with systolic jets in a similar direction as the AS jet: **MR, TR,** and **subaortic stenosis.**

67. How can the AS jet be distinguished from the MR jet?

Compared with the AS jet, the MR jet has the following characteristics:

1. A longer duration spanning the entire systole (holosystolic) compared with the AS jet, which is limited to the ejection period.

2. MR starts "within" the electrocardiographic QRS complex, whereas AS starts at the end of the QRS (there is no transaortic flow during the isovolumic contraction period).

3. Jet velocity consistent with a typical LV-LA pressure gradient during systole (110 mmHg in the LV − 10 mmHg in the LA, i.e., 100 mmHg) would be approximately 5 m/sec (if $4 v^2 = 100$, then $v = 5$). Only in situations with critical AS would jets attain 5 m/sec.

4. In patients with combined AS and MR, the MR jet velocity is always the higher of the two (i.e., aortic diastolic pressure is higher than LA pressure).

5. MR jet (in systole) is associated with a diastolic pattern of mitral inflow (in diastole), whereas AS jet either has no diastolic profile associated with it or has an associated diastolic profile of AI.

68. How can the jet of AS be distinguished from that of TR?

The same principles as stated in question 67 apply to TR; in addition, the TR jet may show respiratory variation.

69. How can the jet of AS be distinguished from that of subaortic obstruction?

The jet of subaortic obstruction:

- Has a characteristic dagger shape on Doppler
- Is associated with subvalvular turbulence on color Doppler, as opposed to the valvular turbulence with AS
- Increases with specific maneuvers (Valsalva)
- Is associated with typical two-dimensional findings (systolic anterior motion, septal hypertrophy)

70. What are the echocardiographic measurements needed for the aortic valve area calculation using the continuity equation?

The **LVOT diameter** is measured in a systolic frame from the parasternal long-axis view as the distance between the insertion site of the anterior aortic leaflet on the interventricular septum and the junction between the posterior aortic leaflet.

The **LVOT blood velocity** is measured from the apical long-axis view (three-chamber view) just below the aortic valve (at the level of the aortic annulus), using pulse wave Doppler. It is important to avoid being too close to the aortic valve, which is achieved by stepping back from the valve with the sample volume. Using a falsely elevated LVOT flow velocity in the continuity equation results in an overestimation of the aortic valve area.

Maximal flow velocity through the aortic valve is obtained using continuous wave Doppler. It is essential to search for the highest blood velocity by using multiple views (apical, right parasternal, suprasternal notch).

71. Summarize the echocardiographic characteristics of severe AS.

- An aortic valve area $< 0.8–1.0$ cm^2
- A mean pressure gradient > 50 mmHg

72. How does the LV adapt to the presence of AS?

AS causes pressure overload, and the LV develops hypertrophy. This is evident on echocardiography as a thickening of the LV walls. The LV cavity dimensions and volume remain normal until late in the disease, when they may increase.

73. How is echocardiography helpful in selecting the optimal therapy for a patient with AS?

Echocardiography is crucial to deciding if a patient with AS needs surgery. A detailed list of the indications for surgery in patients with AS is beyond the scope of this text. The most important echocardiographic parameters are:

- The **severity of AS** (at least moderate or moderately severe AS is usually present before even considering surgery; alternatively the presence of severe AS in itself is not an indication for surgery)
- **LV dysfunction** (especially worsening LV dysfunction noted by an increase in end-systolic dimensions is usually an indication for surgery)

74. What is the role of TEE in the assessment of AS?

TTE, *not* TEE, is the procedure of choice for the diagnosis and assessment of AS severity. TTE obtains good alignment of the Doppler beam with the AS blood flow and accurately measures the peak gradient. TEE may be required:

- In patients with suboptimal images on TTE
- For assessment of MR (frequently present in AS patients even in the absence of structural mitral valve disease)
- For intraoperative assessment and guidance in patients undergoing aortic valve repair or replacement

75. How has echocardiography changed the need for an invasive assessment of patients with AS?

Catheterization of AS patients was once the mainstay of the AS evaluation but rarely is required today. The main role of cardiac catheterization in AS patients is to assess for concomitant coronary artery disease.

76. What is the role of echocardiography in the follow-up of a patient with AS?

Echocardiography permits serial assessments of patients with AS and follow-up of the transvalvular gradient, aortic valve area, and hypertrophic response of the LV. Although the American Heart Association guidelines do not mention definitive indications concerning the frequency of echocardiographic follow-up in asymptomatic AS patients, many suggest that such follow-up be performed:

- At least yearly—in patients with severe AS
- Every 1–2 years—in patients with moderate AS
- Every 3–5 years—in patients with mild AS

Aortic Insufficiency

Gabriel Adelmann, M.D., M. Therese Tupas-Habib, B.S., RDCS, and Neil J. Weissman, M.D.

77. List general causes of AI.

- Disorders affecting the valve leaflets (intrinsic valve disease)
- Disease affecting the aortic root (dilation or deformity or both), which leads to an external deformation of the aortic valve leaflets
- A combination of intrinsic and extrinsic mechanisms

78. Name specific common causes of AI.

Common Causes of Aortic Insuffficiency

INTRINSIC DISEASE	AORTIC ROOT DISEASE
Bicuspid aortic valve	Hypertensive aortic root dilation
Infective endocarditis	Annuloaortic ectasia (Marfan syndrome)
Rheumatic heart disease (postinflammatory scarring)	Syphilitic aortitis
	Aortic dissection
Myxomatous valve disease	Ankylosing spondylitis
	Giant cell aortitis

79. What is the role of echocardiography in the assessment of patients with AI?

As with the other valvular disorders, echocardiography provides information on all the entities listed in question 37.

80. Summarize the echocardiographic signs of AI.

1. **Color Doppler,** the mainstay of the echocardiographic assessment of AI, shows the characteristic regurgitant jet from the aorta into the LV in diastole.

2. **Pulse and continuous wave Doppler** shows the AI jet and allows assessment of its severity; Doppler may show flow reversal in the aorta (see question 85).

3. **Two-dimensional echocardiography** shows structural abnormalities of the aortic valve leaflets and the LV response (LV dilation).

4. **Color M-mode echocardiography** can be useful to confirm the diastolic timing of a jet through the aortic valve, which may be helpful with a patient with tachycardia, and jet width.

81. What are the Doppler methods of AI assessment?

Doppler Methods of Aortic Insufficiency Assessment

Color flow mapping (color Doppler)
   Regurgitant jet width
   Regurgitant jet area
Continuous wave Doppler
   Signal intensity of the spectral pattern
   Pressure half-time of the aortic regurgitation jet
Aortic diastolic flow reversal in descending aorta
Calculation of the volume of regurgitant flow

82. Discuss the color Doppler signs of AI.

Color Doppler shows the **presence** of the characteristic regurgitation jet from the aorta into the LV. The best views for color Doppler assessment of AI are the parasternal long-axis and short-axis views.

The **severity** of regurgitation can be assessed by several methods:

1. Calculation of the ratio between the regurgitant jet width at its base and the width of the LVOT (parasternal long-axis view).

2. Calculation of the ratio between the regurgitant jet area at its base and the area of the aortic valve (parasternal short-axis view at the level of the aortic valve).

3. Calculation of effective regurgitant orifice (i.e., the area of the hole in the aortic valve during diastole). This method is not as frequently used in clinical practice.

83. How is AI graded semiquantitatively?

- Trace (minimal area and width of regurgitant jet) (Fig. 11A)
- Mild
- Moderate
- Severe (Fig.11B)

84. How important is the AI jet length into the LV for the assessment of regurgitation severity?

AI jet length is the least reliable indicator of regurgitation severity. This is especially important for beginner echocardiographists who are often overly impressed by a long jet and may interpret incorrectly it as severe AI. The width or area of the jet should always be assessed and used for determining severity.

85. Discuss the signs of AI on pulse and continuous wave Doppler.

Doppler allows the identification of the *presence* of AI and the assessment of the *severity* of regurgitation by several methods:

1. The **pressure half-time method,** based on analysis of the continuous wave Doppler tracing. This method measures the time it takes the diastolic gradient between the aorta and the LV to decrease to half its initial value; the more severe the AI, the more rapid the aorta-LV pressure equalization and the shorter the pressure half-time. A pressure half-time > 400–600 msec represents mild AI and < 250 msec represents severe AI.

2. **Identification of diastolic aortic flow reversal.** Diastolic reversal in the descending thoracic aorta is consistent with at least moderate AI. Diastolic reversal in the abdominal aorta is consistent with severe AI.

3. Assessment of the spectral Doppler AI signal intensity is a crude indicator of regurgitation severity: the "brighter" the jet on spectral Doppler, the more severe the AI.

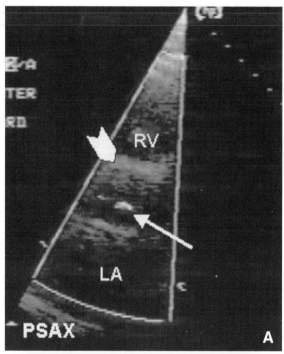

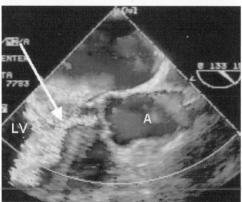

FIGURE 11. *A,* Trace AI Minimal flow on color Doppler in a patient with mild aortic insufficiency (*arrow*). Parasternal short axis view at the level of the aortic valve (*arrowhead*). (See also Color Plates, Figure 11.) *B,* Severe AI (*arrow*). LV = left ventricle, A = aorta. (See also Color Plates, Figure 12.)

4. Assessment of the regurgitant fraction (the percentage of systolic flow through the aortic valve that returns to the LV in diastole). In the absence of MR and AI, the total aortic outflow is equal to the mitral inflow. In the absence of MR, aortic regurgitant flow can be determined by calculating the mitral inflow and subtracting it from aortic outflow (because aortic outflow is the outflow of blood that came into the LV through the mitral valve and through the aortic regurgitation).

86. What are the two-dimensional echocardiography signs of AI?

Abnormalities of the aortic valve or of the aortic root and the adaptive response of the LV (chamber dilation) to the valvular abnormality. The different causes of AI are given in questions 77 and 78.

87. What are the M-mode echocardiography signs of AI?

1. Anatomic abnormalities of the aortic valve and aortic root
2. The effect of the AI jet on the anterior mitral valve leaflet (impeded leaflet motion due to the regurgitant jet):
    a. Impaired leaflet opening causing "functional MS" (Austin-Flint murmur)
    b. Coarse fluttering of the anterior mitral leaflet in diastole
    c. Increased early diastolic distance between the anterior mitral leaflet and the interventricular septum (E-point septal separation)
3. The adaptive LV response (dilation) caused by the presence of AI

88. List the echocardiographic criteria of severe AI.

Color Doppler criteria
A ratio between AI jet width and LVOT width > 60%
A ratio between the AI jet surface and the surface of the aortic valve > 60%
Regurgitation fraction > 60 mL
Spectral Doppler criteria
AI jet pressure half-time < 250 msec
Diastolic flow reversal in the abdominal aorta

89. Can echocardiography provide information to distinguish acute from chronic AI?

The following characteristics suggest an **acute onset** of AI:
- A decrease in the mitral E wave deceleration time, in the absence of other explanations (rapid LA-LV pressure equalization)
- Premature closure of the mitral valve (same mechanism)
- The absence of LV dilation in a patient with severe AI (LV dilation is an adaptive mechanism in these patients; its absence suggests an acute onset of the AI and a "lack of time" for the LV to mount an adaptive response)

90. What are the pitfalls of echocardiography for the assessment of AI severity?

A **false-negative** diagnosis of severe AI (i.e., mistakenly classifying severe AI as mild) can occur whenever the true extent of the regurgitant jet is not appreciated. This occurs whenever the operator does not locate the maximal regurgitant jet, which happens more often if the jet is eccentric or if the patient is tachycardic.

A **false-positive** diagnosis of severe AI (calling mild AI severe) can be due to inappropriately using the regurgitant jet length to determine severity, confusing AI with other pathologic jets (most frequently, MS), or having the color gain set too high.

91. How can the jet of AI be distinguished from that of MS?

1. The jet of AI is **holodiastolic,** as opposed to the MS jet, which is absent during isovolumic relaxation. Simultaneously displaying the LVOT jet and the AI jet on the Doppler examination clarifies that the jet is truly AI if it begins immediately after cessation of the LVOT flow. If there is a pause between the cessation of the LVOT flow and the beginning of the jet, it is probably MS.
2. The jet of AI has a much higher velocity than the MS jet.
3. The jet of AI originates from the aortic valve.

92. Give examples that illustrate the higher velocity jet of AI compared with MS.

Example 1

A patient with AI and a diastolic blood pressure of 64 mmHg. Assuming a negligible LV early diastolic pressure, the aorta-LV gradient can be calculated as the aortic pressure - LV pressure = 64 mmHg. Using the Bernoulli equation, this translates into an AI peak velocity of 4 m/sec (if 4 v^2 = 64 mmHg, then v = 4 m/sec)

Example 2

A patient with MS and severely increased LA pressure (20 mmHg). Assuming a negligible early diastolic pressure, the LA-LV gradient can be calculated as LA pressure − LV pressure = 20 mmHg. Using the Bernoulli equation, this translates into a peak MS flow velocity of approximately 2.2 m/sec.

93. What is the LV response to AI?

The chronic volume overload of severe AI leads to:

- Progressive LV dilation. Extreme LV dilation is termed *cor bovinum* (Latin for "cow's heart") (Fig. 12).
- Increased sphericity of the LV (i.e., near-equalization of the LV long and short axes). Increased sphericity is an adaptive mechanism allowing a higher stroke volume for a given degree of LV dilation and dysfunction.

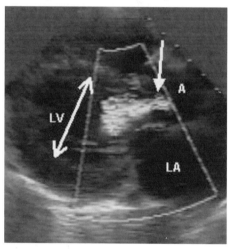

FIGURE 12. Cor bovinum. Severe dilatation of the left ventricle (LV, double arrow approximately 7 cm [*double arrow*]) in a patient with aortic regurgitation (*small arrow*). LA = left atrium, A = aorta. (See also Color Plates, Figure 13.)

94. What is the role of TEE in the assessment of AI?

The preferred diagnostic modality for diagnosis of AI is TTE because it can obtain optimal alignment between the Doppler beam and the AI jet. TEE is necessary, however, in patients with suboptimal TTE images and aortic root disease–related AI.

95. How is echocardiography used to select the optimal therapeutic strategy in a patient with AI?

A detailed list of the indications for surgery in patients with AI is beyond the scope of this text. The most important echocardiography parameters that, in the proper clinical setting, are an indication for surgery include severe, symptomatic AI and LV dysfunction. Severe LV dilation is defined as end-diastolic diameter 70–75 mm or end-systolic dimension 50–55 mm.

96. What is the role of echocardiography in the follow-up of patients with AI?

In patients with severe AI in whom there are no immediate indications for surgery (asymptomatic with a normal LV), echocardiographic follow-up every 4–6 months is indicated to monitor for development of LV dilation or dysfunction.

In patients after aortic valve replacement, echocardiographic follow-up is indicated:
- Before patient discharge or at the first follow-up visit, a few weeks after surgery, for a baseline assessment
- Yearly after surgery
- At any time during follow-up when questions arise regarding the function of the valvular prosthesis or concern about LV systolic dysfunction

97. Can echocardiography assess the prognosis of patients after aortic valve replacement?

Echocardiography can provide important prognostic indicators after aortic valve replacement. The best indicator of a good prognosis is a reduction in LV size after surgery. Approximately 80% of the total reduction in LV size occurs within the first 10–14 days after aortic valve replacement and correlates well with the degree of improvement in the LV ejection fraction. A reduced LV ejection fraction or a decrease in ejection fraction is an indicator of poor prognosis after surgery.

Mitral Stenosis

Gabriel Adelmann, M.D., M. Therese Tupas-Habib, B.S., RDCS, Benjamin Kleiber, M.D., and Neil J. Weissman, M.D.

98. Name the main cause of MS.

Rheumatic heart disease.

99. What is the role of echocardiography in making the diagnosis of MS?

Echocardiography is ideally suited to identify rheumatic MS as well as the rare cases of non-rheumatic MS (e.g., degenerative calcification, vegetation).

100. List some relatively uncommon conditions that may mimic rheumatic MS on clinical examination but can be distinguished from MS by echocardiography.
- LA myxoma (see Chapter 8)
- Cor triatriatum
- Parachute mitral valve

101. What is cor triatriatum?

This anomaly is a membrane in the LA that divides the LA into two chambers: (1) a superior chamber receiving the pulmonary vein flow and (2) an inferior chamber associated with the atrial appendage and the mitral valve. This relatively uncommon condition can be considered a form of supravalvular MS.

102. What is a parachute mitral valve?

A relatively uncommon congenital abnormality that is characterized echocardiographically by:
- Insertion of both mitral valve leaflets onto a single papillary muscle
- Restricted leaflet excursion
- Valvular and subvalvular thickening and fusion
- Occasionally, presence of a supravalvular mitral ring, representing an additional obstacle to LV filling

103. Summarize the two-dimensional echocardiography signs of MS.
1. Structural changes of the mitral valve and the subvalvular apparatus (Fig. 13A):
   a. Valvular thickening (leaflet thickness > 5 mm in diastole is considered abnormal)
   b. Valvular calcification
   c. A typical "hockey-stick" appearance of the anterior mitral valve leaflet in diastole
   d. Thickening of the subvalvular apparatus (chordae tendineae)

e. Decrease in the mitral valve area, as measured by planimetry
    f. A typical "fish-mouth" appearance of the mitral valve orifice in short axis (i.e., the orifice is rounded, rather than oval)
    2. Restricted (doming) valvular motion, resulting from rheumatic involvement of the leaflet tips (Fig. 13B).
    3. Immobility of the posterior mitral valve leaflet.
    4. LA dilation, owing to the chronic increase in LA pressure.

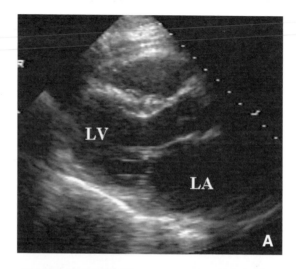

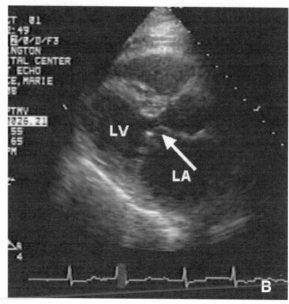

FIGURE 13. *A,* Parasternal long axis in a patient with MS. Systolic frame. LA = left atrium; LV = left ventricle. *B,* Two-dimensional study of MS (diastole). Note the "doming" of the anterior MV leaflet (*arrow*) and the thickened MV leaflets and subvalvular apparatus. LA = left atrium; LV = left ventricle.

104. What are the Doppler signs of MS?

MS affects the LV filling in diastole. Pathophysiologically, MS has two characteristics:

1. An increased LA-LV pressure gradient in diastole.

2. A decreased rate of LV filling and slower gradient decay, resulting from the narrowing in the mitral valve; in other words, it takes a longer time for the LA and LV diastolic pressures to equalize because of the narrower "passage" between the two chambers.

Because the E wave represents diastolic filling, the presence and severity of MS are reflected mainly in E wave changes:

> The increased LA-LV pressure gradient translates into an increased velocity of the mitral E wave (high flow velocities at the time of mitral valve opening owing to the significant gradient between the atrium and the ventricle).

> The decreased rate of pressure equalization between the atrium and the ventricle results in an increased mitral E wave deceleration time (slope of the descending arm of the E wave). The LV of a patient with MS fills more slowly in diastole. In patients with severe MS, diastasis (i.e., the interval between the mitral E and A waves when transmitral flow almost stops) is abolished, and the A wave begins before the descending slope of the E wave reaches the baseline.

105. Describe the M-mode echocardiogram of MS.

- A characteristic flattened descending slope of the early diastolic anterior mitral leaflet motion, which parallels the increased E wave deceleration time seen on Doppler (Fig. 14)
- Leaflet thickening and calcification
- A typical motion of the posterior leaflet of the mitral valve, parallel to the anterior leaflet (as opposed to the normal situation, when the two valve leaflets have a "mirror-image" motion in respect to each other)

106. What is the normal mitral valve area?

4–6 cm^2.

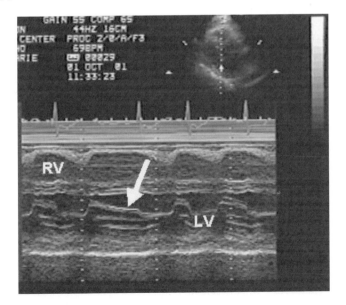

FIGURE 14. M-mode study of a stenotic mitral valve. Note the decreased slope of the anterior motion in diastole (*arrow*) corresponding to the decreased deceleration time of the transmitral Doppler E wave. RV = right ventricle, LV = left ventricle.

107. When is MS considered to be present?

In principle, any decrease in mitral valve area $< 4\ cm^2$ represents MS. However, Narrowing of the MV orifice is important only at $< 2\ cm^2$.

108. List the degrees of severity of MS.

- Mild MS—mitral valve 1.6–2.0 cm^2
- Moderate MS—mitral valve area 1.1–1.5 cm^2
- Severe MS—mitral valve area ≤ 1.0 cm^2

109. If MS is not severe (by mitral area criteria), does that mean that the MS is not clinically significant?

No. There are at least two groups of patients who may complain of severe dyspnea as a result of "nonsevere" MS:

1. Patients with exercise-induced transmitral gradient increases and pulmonary artery pressure elevations

2. Patients with a disproportionate degree of pulmonary hypertension, owing to a highly reactive pulmonary vasculature (pulmonary vasoconstriction)

110. How is MS assessed using Doppler?

By calculating:

- The MV area, by one of the following methods: (1) pressure half-time (most commonly used), (2) continuity equation (rarely used), or (3) the PISA method (rarely used)
- The transmitral diastolic pressure gradient (commonly used)

111. What is the pressure half-time method for MS?

The mitral valve area can be calculated from the Doppler by tracing the descending slope of the transmitral E wave, using the following equation:

$$MVA = 220/PHT$$

where, MVA = mitral valve area and PHT = pressure half-time.

Contemporary echocardiography machines contain software that calculates the pressure half-time and the mitral valve area when the operator traces the mitral E wave descending slope (Fig. 15).

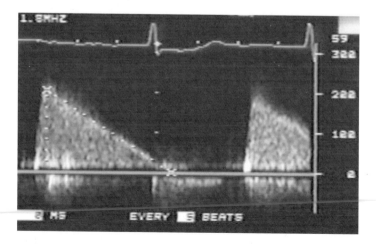

FIGURE 15. MV area by PHT. CW Doppler tracing of the transmitral blood flow in a patient with mitral stenosis. Tracing the descending slope of the E wave yields the MV area (in this patient, 1.2 cm^2).

112. What are the pitfalls of mitral valve area assessment using the pressure half-time method?

Although it is convenient to use the pressure half-time for calculating the mitral valve area, the mitral valve orifice in diastole is not the sole determinant of LA-LV pressure equalization. Additional determinants include:

1. Factors that tend to decrease mitral valve flow and pressure half-time, causing an underestimation of MS severity, such as:

    a. A decreased LV distensibility (compliance) (i.e., a limited ability to accommodate blood inflow into the LV because of the LV properties); in these patients, the mitral E wave velocity is not increased as it is in MS.

    b. Coexistent aortic insufficiency, which represents an alternative source of LV filling in diastole, causing an increase in LV chamber pressure with blunted transmitral flow.

2. Factors that tend to increase mitral valve flow and pressure half-time, causing an overestimation of MS severity, such as coexistent MR, which causes an increased blood flow through a fixed mitral valve orifice.

3. Other factors that can affect pressure half-time, such as:

    a. Beat-to-beat variability in patients with atrial fibrillation; in these patients, 10 cycles (and no less than 5) should be averaged.

    b. The presence of an eccentric MS jet (color Doppler guidance is helpful in these patients).

113. How do you calculate mitral valve area using the continuity equation?

The continuity equation is based on the fact that the blood flow through the mitral valve is equal to that through the LVOT (in the absence of MR or aortic regurgitation):

$$\text{LVOT area} * \text{LVOT TVI} = \text{MV area} * \text{MV TVI}$$

so

$$\text{MV area} = \text{LVOT area} * \text{LVOT TVI}/ \text{MV TVI}$$

where TVI = time-velocity integral and MV = mitral valve.

Calculation of the mitral valve area requires:

1. Calculation of the LVOT area, using the LVOT diameter (D-LVOT), measured from a systolic freeze-frame in the parasternal long-axis view

2. Measurement of the LVOT TVI measured by pulse wave Doppler from the apical view

3. Measurement of the mitral valve TVI using continuous Doppler wave from the apical view

114. Can mitral valve area be assessed by the continuity equation in the presence of MR?

In the presence of significant MR, flow through the mitral valve exceeds the flow through the LVOT, leading to an underestimation of the mitral valve area.

115. Explain the importance of significant AI on the assessment of mitral valve area using the continuity equation.

In the presence of significant AI, flow through the LVOT exceeds flow through the mitral valve, leading to an overestimation of the mitral valve area.

116. How can the mitral valve area be calculated using the PISA method?

PISA is an acronym for proximal isovolumic surface area. Similar to the continuity equation, the PISA method is based on the principle of flow conservation ("what comes in must go out"). The difference between the two methods is that:

- The continuity equation uses the flow through the mitral valve and through the LVOT
- The PISA method uses the flow from the LA through the mitral valve

The PISA method is used more often for quantification of MR.

117. How can transmitral pressure gradients be calculated by Doppler echocardiography, and what are the role and limitations of this determination in clinical practice?

There is a direct relationship between the pressure gradient from the LA to the LV during diastole and the velocity of blood flow through the mitral valve. The **mean** pressure gradient through the mitral valve is related to the integral under the curve of the velocity of blood from the LA to the LV during diastole (the mitral time-velocity integral) (Fig. 16). Gradients are calculated rapidly using software on the echocardiography machine when the mitral velocity contour is traced by the operator. Generally the more severe the MS, the higher the mean transvalvular pressure gradient. A mean gradient > 10 mmHg usually is associated with severe MS. Pressure gradients are influenced strongly by the magnitude of flow, however, and coexistent MR or hyperdynamic conditions (causing tachycardia) may result in increased pressure gradients, even in patients with nonsevere MS. Conversely, low cardiac output can be associated with low pressure gradients, even in patients with severe MS.

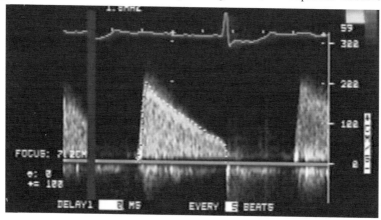

FIGURE 16. MV mean gradient by CW Doppler. By tracing the contour of the MV flow CW Doppler envelope, the mean transmitral gradient is obtained (in this patient, 6 mmHg).

118. Explain the importance of direct planimetry in the assessment of MS.

Although the most frequently employed methods of echocardiographic measurement of aortic valve area are based on Doppler technology (see previous questions), planimetry of the mitral valve has been shown to correlate well with invasive determinations in the catheterization laboratory (Fig. 17). The main pitfall of planimetry is the inability to trace accurately the mitral valve contour because of poor images.

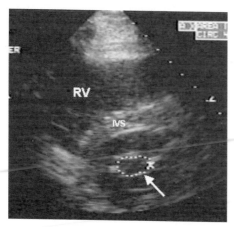

FIGURE 17. MV planimetry. The MV area (*arrow*) can be directly measured by planimetry from a TTE or TEE short-axis view (in this MS patient, area = 1.90 cm^2). Note the markedly dilated right ventricle (RV). IVS = interventricular septum.

119. List the echocardiographic characteristics of severe MS.
- A mitral valve area < 1.0 cm^2
- Pressure half-time ≥ 220 msec
- Resting mean pressure gradient ≥ 10 mmHg

120. How does the echocardiographic assessment of MS severity correlate with the invasive assessment of MS in the catheterization lab?

The **echocardiography** based assessment of mitral valve area generally yields a **similar or slightly larger area** than the catheterization-based assessment. This discrepancy is sometimes due to the overestimation of LA pressure by using pulmonary capillary wedge pressure as a surrogate for LA pressure. If pulmonary capillary wedge pressure is higher than LA pressure (i.e., not a good "wedge"), there is an overestimation of the LA-LV pressure gradient (i.e., underestimation of mitral valve area). Echocardiographic assessment of MS severity is considered to be accurate and does not usually need confirmation in the catheterization laboratory.

121. What is the importance of pulmonary artery pressure in the setting of MS?

1. Pulmonary hypertension contributes to the pathogenesis of MS-associated dyspnea.

2. The presence of pulmonary artery systolic pressures > 50 mmHg at rest or 60 mmHg with exercise is a class IIa indication for mitral valvuloplasty in asymptomatic patients with moderate or severe MS; a class IIa indication is considered controversial, with the weight of evidence slightly in favor of the indication.

3. In symptomatic patients with severe MS who are not candidates for valvuloplasty, severe pressure half-time (pulmonary artery pressure > 60–80 mmHg) is a class IIa indication for surgery.

122. What is the role of exercise echocardiography in the assessment of MS?

Occasional patients with mild or moderate MS present with exercise-induced dyspnea. In these patients, treadmill exercise is helpful to determine if the transmitral pressure gradient and the pulmonary artery pressures increase with exercise and explain the exercise-induced dyspnea.

123. How is echocardiography helpful to the cardiologist selecting the optimal therapeutic strategy for a patient with MS?

A detailed list of the indications for surgery or percutaneous mitral valvuloplasty is beyond the scope of this text. In the presence of symptoms, the echocardiographic parameters of moderate or severe MS or MS causing pulmonary hypertension is an indication for surgery.

124. When the decision for surgery or valvuloplasty has been made, how can echocardiography help select the best candidates for percutaneous valvuloplasty?

Valvuloplasty is opening up the valve with a large balloon introduced percutaneously. Echocardiography can help assess the chances of successful percutaneous mitral valvuloplasty by using the *mitral valve score*. The elements of this score include valvular and subvalvular thickening, valve mobility, and valve calcification. The less calcium, the more mobile the leaflets, the thinner the leaflets, and the less subvalvular thickening all are predictors of a good outcome from percutaneous mitral valvuloplasty. Each component is scored on a 1- to 4-scale, and an overall score < 8 predicts a good outcome with a high accuracy. A score < 10–12 has a fair chance of a good outcome.

125. What is the role of echocardiography during percutaneous mitral valvuloplasty?

Some form of echocardiography (usually TTE but sometimes TEE or intracardiac echocardiography) is recommended to ensure:
- An accurate calculation of the echocardiography score
- Reliable identification and quantification of coexistent MR
- Intraprocedural guidance (crossing of the interatrial septum, assessing the optimal position of the balloon before inflation, and assessing the MR after each balloon inflation) (Fig. 18)

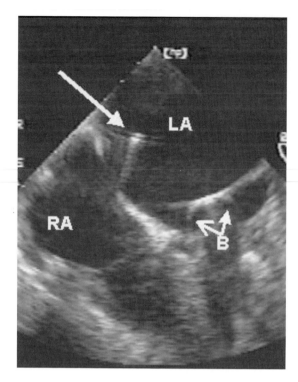

FIGURE 18. PTMV. Balloon (B) dilatation of a stenotic mitral valve. RA = right atrium, LA = left atrium; arrow = LA guiding wire.

126. Besides the components of the mitral valve score, what else is an important predictor of percutaneous mitral valvuloplasty outcome?

The degree of commissural fusion (the degree of adherence of the two mitral valve leaflets at their medial and lateral points of insertion on the mitral valve annulus) has been shown also to predict the lack of success of percutaneous mitral valvuloplasty; a higher risk for tearing the mitral valve leaflets with the balloon inflation may lead to more MR.

127. When should the new mitral valve area be assessed after a percutaneous mitral valvuloplasty?

During the procedure, the operators usually can determine the degree of success of a percutaneous mitral valvuloplasty. Formal reassessment of valve area should be carried out > 72 hours after the procedure to allow for changes in LA and LV compliance in the new hemodynamic setting.

128. Are all MS patients with an echocardiography score < 8 and a low degree of commissural fusion candidates for percutaneous mitral valvuloplasty?

No. There are two absolute contraindications for percutaneous mitral valvuloplasty: (1) coexistent moderate or severe MR and (2) the presence of a known LA thrombus.

129. What is the difference between a high mitral score and severe MS?

Although there is a general concordance between these two concepts (i.e., severe MS usually is associated with a high degree of valvular and subvalvular structural changes), many patients with severe MS are good candidates for percutaneous mitral valvuloplasty. **Mitral score** is a description of the mitral anatomy and candidacy for percutaneous mitral valvuloplasty, whereas **severity of MS** refers to the "tightness" of the mitral opening.

130. What is the role of echocardiography in the follow-up of MS patients after an intervention?

Follow-up is indicated for reevaluation of MS patients who become symptomatic.

Mitral Regurgitation

Gabriel Adelmann, M.D., and Neil J. Weissman, M.D.

131. What is the role of echocardiography in the assessment of MR?
It is the imaging procedure of choice for assessment of MR. As with other valvular diseases, echocardiography provides essential information on MR:
- Presence
- Cause
- Severity
- Adaptive responses of the heart (LV and LA)
- Necessity for surgical intervention
- *Type* of surgical intervention most likely to treat the valvular problem successfully (mitral valve repair vs. replacement)
- The success of the surgical procedure (intraoperative assessment and long-term follow-up)

132. What is the role of TEE in the assessment of MR?
When TTE images are suboptimal, TEE is the most accurate method of assessing MR.

133. Is TEE necessary in every patient with MR?
No. Most MR cases seen in clinical practice are mild or moderate and generally are well assessed by TTE. TEE is indicated in:
- Patients in whom TTE is not able to establish confidently the severity of MR (suboptimal studies, eccentric jets)
- Surgical candidates (to assess valve morphology, MR severity, and optimal surgical strategy)

134. What are the color Doppler signs of MR?
Color Doppler shows a turbulent systolic jet from the LV into the LA (Fig. 19). The MR color Doppler jet is characterized further by:
- The jet size (as ratio of the jet area to the LA area)
- Direction of flow (central versus eccentric jets)
- The "thickness" of the regurgitant jet at its origin (vena contracta)
- The radius of the *convergence zone* (the hemispheric flow velocity as it enters the mitral valve from the LV)
- Backflow of blood into the pulmonary veins (indicates severe MR)

135. Summarize the two-dimensional echocardiography signs of MR.
The signs are related to anatomic changes of the mitral valve and adaptive changes of the cardiac chambers. **Anatomic** changes that may cause MR include:
1. **Increased** leaflet mobility
    a. Mitral valve prolapse
    b. Flail mitral valve caused by ruptured chordae tendinae or papillary muscles)
2. **Restricted** leaflet mobility
    a. Rheumatic fibrosis
    b. Papillary muscle dysfunction after MI causing tethering of the leaflets (after MI)
3. **Disturbed** leaflet motion
    a. Vegetation (endocarditis) that interferes with normal leaflet closure in systole
    b. Annular dilation with decreased coaptation of the leaflets; the more severe the MR, the more severe the LV and annular dilation, establishing a vicious circle whereby "MR begets more MR"
4. **Loss of leaflet integrity**
    a. Leaflet perforation due to endocarditis
    b. Cleft MV

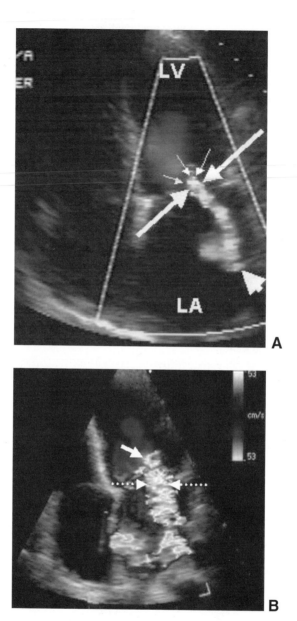

FIGURE 19. *A,* Mild-to-moderate MR by color Doppler *(arrowhead).* PISA = proximal acceleration of blood flow velocities into the mitral valve from the LV *(thin arrows)*; vena contracta *(between thick arrows)*; LV = left ventricle; LA = left atrium. (See also Color Plates, Figure 14.) *B,* Severe MR by color Doppler on a TEE echo. Note the mosaic, severely eccentric jet, the large PISA *(arrow),* and the wide vena contracta *(between dotted arrows).* (See also Color Plates, Figure 15.)

Adaptive changes of the heart chambers resulting from MR include:
1. LV and LA dilation
2. LV dysfunction
3. RV dilation and dysfunction due to pulmonary hypertension from MR

136. What are the M-mode signs of MR, and what is the role of M-mode echocardiography in the diagnosis of MR?

In current practice, M-mode echocardiography has a limited role in the assessment of MR. On M-mode echocardiography, there are signs corresponding to the different entities shown by two-dimensional echocardiography. The most important M-mode echocardiography sign, still occasionally sought in contemporary practice, refers to systolic billowing of one or both mitral valve leaflets into the LA (not in all MR patients, only in patients with underlying mitral valve prolapse).

137. List the most common causes of MR.

   Mitral valve prolapse
   Ischemic MR
   Dilated cardiomyopathy
   Endocarditis

138. What are the echocardiographic characteristics of mitral valve prolapse?

Mitral valve prolapse is diagnosed by two-dimensional echocardiography, based on the characteristic systolic buckling of the anterior mitral valve leaflet into the LA at least 2 mm behind the plane of the mitral annulus (this is the main two-dimensional finding) (Fig. 20) with associated thickening and redundancy of the mitral valve leaflets.

139. What is the best echocardiographic view to assess for mitral valve prolapse?

The parasternal long-axis view.

140. How does mitral valve prolapse cause MR?

Mitral valve prolapse causes poor coaptation of the mitral valve leaflets in systole. In addition, myxomatous degeneration and potential rupture of the chordae tendineae cause a flail mitral leaflet. This results from a vicious circle whereby the thinner the chordae tendineae (owing to intrinsic myxomatous disease), the more severe the valvular prolapse. The more severe the prolapse, the greater the tension on the chordae tendineae, which increases chordal thinning. Ultimately the increased tension exerted on the thinned chordae tendineae may lead to chordal rupture, flail mitral leaflet, and severe MR. The tip of a flail leaflet points toward the LA (Fig. 21).

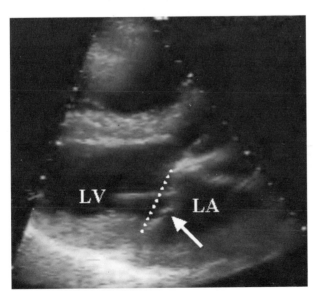

FIGURE 20. Mitral valve prolapse (*arrow*). In this patient, both the anterior and the posterior mitral valve leaflets protrude into the LA, beyond the annular plane (*dotted line*). LA = left atrium, LV = left ventricle.

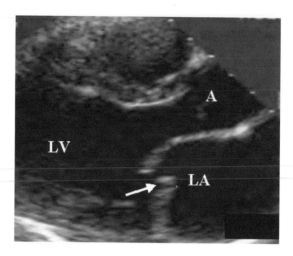

FIGURE 21. Mitral valve prolapse with a partially flail posterior leaflet causing mitral regurgitation. A = aorta, LV = left ventricle, LA = left atrium.

141. For many years after its initial clinical description, mitral valve prolapse was grossly overdiagnosed by echocardiography (high rate of false-positive studies). Why did this happen, and how do we prevent it from happening today?

The mitral valve annulus has a characteristic saddle shape (see Chapter 2). As a result of the saddle shape, the mitral leaflets appear to be "above" the annular plane from the apical four-chamber view and "prolapse" into the LA. If viewed in a plane 90° from the four-chamber view (i.e., in the parasternal or apical long-axis view), the leaflets are "below" the annular plane and do not prolapse into the LA. It is essential that mitral valve prolapse be diagnosed only from the long-axis view.

142. Define ischemic MR.

As its name implies, this is MR that results from myocardial ischemia, either acute or chronic. The most common mechanisms include:

1. **Papillary muscle dysfunction or posterior wall motion abnormalities.** The papillary muscles are an integral part of the mitral subvalvular apparatus, and failure of the papillary muscle to contract normally results in deficient mitral valve closure with secondary MR.

2. **Ruptured papillary muscles.** This is a severe complication of an MI. Complete papillary muscle rupture leads to severe, acute MR and fulminant pulmonary edema. This can lead quickly to a fatal outcome in the absence of immediate surgery.

3. Global **LV dilatation** (ischemic cardiomyopathy) with consequent annular dilation and decreased mitral leaflet coaptation.

143. What are the mechanisms of MR in patients with dilated cardiomyopathy?

Annular dilation and poor leaflet coaptation and **abnormal geometry of the subvalvular apparatus** secondary to changes in shape of the LV (LV aneurysm, increased sphericity of the LV) with consequent decreased leaflet coaptation.

144. What is the mechanism of MR in patients with endocarditis?

Bacterial endocarditis can cause MR by destruction or perforation of the mitral valve or the subvalvular apparatus or both and interference of leaflet coaptation.

145. If there is no MR, does that mean that the valve is not infected and there is no endocarditis?

No. Endocarditis is a clinical diagnosis and can exist in the absence of any valvular regurgitation.

146. What is the mechanism of MR in patients with a cleft mitral valve?

In these patients, the structural deficiency of the mitral valve (i.e., the presence of a valvular "slit") is directly causing the valvular regurgitation. This condition mainly affects the anterior mitral valve leaflet and occasionally is associated with other cardiac abnormalities (endocardial cushion defects).

147. What is the mechanism of MR after percutaneous mitral valvuloplasty for MS?

Direct mechanical trauma to the mitral valve during the procedure.

148. List the color Doppler methods for assessing MR severity.

- Jet area and its ratio to the LA area
- Vena contracta method
- PISA method
- Regurgitant volume method

149. How can MR severity be assessed by jet area?

1. Frame-by-frame analysis of several systolic frames from multiple views
2. Selection of the frame that displays the greatest MR jet
3. Planimetry of the jet and of the LA
4. Calculation of the ratio between the two jet areas; a ratio > 40% is considered to represent severe MR

In clinical practice, gross visual assessment of the MR-to-LA ratio is performed, without actual planimetry measurements. MR is classified as:

- Trivial or physiologic (a brief regurgitant jet is seen just behind the leaflets)
- Mild (MR-to-LA ratio < 20%)
- Moderate (MR-to-LA ratio 20–40%)
- Severe (MR-to-LA ratio > 40%)

150. What are the pitfalls of the jet area method?

The MR jet area depends strongly on:

- Echocardiography machine settings (e.g., color gain, image depth, pulse repetition frequency)
- The direction of the jet (concentric or eccentric)—for the same regurgitant volume, an eccentric jet has a smaller area than a concentric jet
- The echocardiographic view that is used—the same jet may have different areas when imaged from different views; in this situation, the largest jet area should be used
- The hemodynamic conditions, especially the afterload (the greater the afterload, the more severe the regurgitation); these factors cause *true* variations in MR severity

151. What is the vena contracta method for assessing MR severity?

The vena contracta represents the thinnest portion of a fluid jet as it progresses between two chambers. In the case of MR, the passage of blood from the LV into the LA occurs through an area where there is no leaflet coaptation. This area is called the *regurgitant orifice*. The larger the regurgitant orifice, the more severe the MR. The dimensions of the regurgitant orifice are reflected by the diameter of the regurgitant jet immediately after it enters the LA (i.e., at the site of the vena contracta).

152. How do you assess MR using the vena contracta?

1. Frame-by-frame systolic analysis of several heart cycles in the "zoom" mode in the parasternal long-axis view
2. Selection of the frame that displays the widest vena contracta
3. Measurement of the vena contracta

At the usual settings of the echocardiography machine (color scale, aliasing velocity), a vena contracta > 5 mm in diameter usually is considered to represent severe MR.

153. What are the pitfalls of the vena contracta method?

The vena contracta method is not useful for multiple jets, and intermediate values (3–5 mm) require confirmation with another method.

154. What is the PISA method for assessing MR severity?

The PISA method is based on the principle of flow conservation: The volume of blood that regurgitates through the mitral regurgitant orifice is equal to the volume of blood converging toward the LV side of the mitral valve in systole. The PISA method is based on analysis of the jet in the LV, as it converges toward the mitral regurgitant orifice.

155. Name the units of regurgitation that the PISA method provides.
- The area of the regurgitant mitral valve orifice
- The volume of blood regurgitating from the LV into the LA (regurgitant volume, LV-LA)

156. How does the systolic blood flow on the LV side appear echocardiographically?

Before entering the regurgitant mitral orifice, the blood moving from the LV to the LA converges toward the regurgitant orifice (like a funnel) and assumes a hemispheric shape with the center of the hemisphere at the center of the regurgitant orifice. These *convergence hemispheres* can be seen easily by Doppler echocardiography (see Figure 19B).

157. What are the echocardiographic steps for calculation of the regurgitant orifice area using the PISA method?

MR volume = volume of blood converging from the LV toward the mitral valve

Blood volume = velocity * cross-sectional area of the blood column, *so*

Regurgitant orifice area * MR velocity = convergence flow area * convergence flow velocity,

or

Regurgitant orifice area = convergence flow area * convergence flow velocity/MR velocity

The elements necessary for computing this equation are readily accessible from the Doppler study:

1. The convergence flow area is measured as $3.14 * r^2$, where r is the radius of the hemisphere measured on a systolic freeze-frame.
2. The convergence flow velocity is equal to the color aliasing velocity.
3. The MR velocity is measured from continuous wave Doppler.

A regurgitant orifice area > 50 cm^2 is considered to represent severe MR. The regurgitant orifice area is often referred to as **effective regurgitant orifice area.**

158. Why is the convergence flow velocity equal to the color aliasing velocity?

The *aliasing velocity* is the maximal velocity of blood flow that still can be displayed by Doppler as pure color. The convergence hemisphere is precisely the area where blood flow velocities attain the aliasing threshold: Convergence low velocity = color aliasing velocity.

Before setting out to apply the PISA method, the echocardiography operator sets the color aliasing velocity at lower values than for the general color Doppler examination; this displays a larger convergence hemisphere, making the radius easier to measure. These manipulations have no influence on the final calculated regurgitant orifice area because there is an inverse relationship between the aliasing velocity and the measured radius.

159. How can the MR regurgitant volume be calculated by echocardiography?

This calculation is based on the fact that the volume of blood passing through an orifice = area of the orifice * time velocity integral of the blood flow through the orifice.

In the case of MR:

Regurgitant volume = regurgitant orifice area * time velocity integral of MR flow

In turn:

1. Regurgitant orifice area is calculated as shown in question 157.
2. Time velocity integral of MR flow is calculated from continuous wave Doppler.
A regurgitant volume > 60 mL is considered severe MR.

160. Some of the previous calculations relate to *flow* and others to *flow rate*. What is the difference?

Flow rate represents the amount of flow per unit of time (second).

161. At what point in systole should the radius of the convergence zone be measured?

At midsystole.

162. Is there any simpler way to use PISA in clinical practice?

Yes, although some do not think it is substantially easier or accurate. If the peak MR velocity is assumed to be 500 cm/sec (i.e, LV-LA gradient of 100 mmHg) and if the color aliasing velocity is set at 30 cm/sec, the formula for regurgitant orifice area becomes: area = $r^2/2$. Because of the assumptions involved, this method is rarely used.

163. What role does the PISA method have in clinical practice?

Most clinical centers do not routinely use the PISA method. Although the validity and accuracy of this method (if correctly performed) are accepted, its incremental value over simple visual semi-quantitative assessment is not clear, especially with clear cases of mild or severe MR. The most convincing clinical application of the PISA method is with moderate degrees of regurgitation.

164. What are the pitfalls of MR assessment by the PISA method?

- Failure to decrease adequately the aliasing velocity, resulting in a small convergence area and substantial error measuring the radius (which becomes even worse because this value is squared when carrying out the calculations)
- Difficulty in visualizing the convergence zone in patients with an eccentric jet
- The need for substantial operator experience before this method can be applied confidently

165. What is the volumetric method of assessing MR?

The effective forward blood flow through the mitral valve (i.e., the total volume of blood crossing the mitral valve in diastole − the volume of blood that regurgitates into the LA in systole) is identical to the blood flow through the LVOT:

$$\text{Mitral valve diastolic blood flow} - \text{MR regurgitant volume} = \text{LVOT blood flow } or$$

$$\text{MR regurgitant volume} = \text{mitral valve diastolic blood flow} - \text{LVOT blood flow}$$

The elements necessary for calculation of this equation are readily available from the combined two-dimensional and Doppler examination:

$$\text{MV diastolic blood flow} = \text{MV TVI (from CW Doppler)} * \text{MV area} = \text{MV TVI} * 3.14 * (\text{MV annulus diameter}/2)^2$$

$$\text{LVOT blood flow} = \text{LVOT area} * \text{LVOT TVI}$$

where MV = mitral valve and TVI = time velocity integral. A regurgitant volume > 60 mL represents severe MR.

166. What is the regurgitant fraction?

The regurgitant fraction (RF) is the percentage of the total stroke volume regurgitating into the LA and can be calculated as follows:

$$\text{RF} = \text{mitral valve regurgitant flow/mitral valve flow in diastole}$$

A regurgitant fractuion > 60% is considered severe MR.

167. Is the volumetric method of MR assessment used in clinical practice?

These calculations are rarely carried out in clinical practice because of the difficulty of accurately measuring the MV annulus diameter.

168. How do the hemodynamic conditions affect the severity of MR?

In patients with MR, the LV may be considered a two-outlet chamber, injecting blood into the aorta (normal) and into the LA (abnormal). The volume of blood ejected into the LA (i.e., the regurgitant volume) is determined by the interplay among:

- The area of the regurgitant orifice
- The resistance to blood being ejected into the aorta (i.e., afterload, determined mostly by systemic blood pressure)
- The resistance to blood being ejected into the LA (least important factor)

The MR regurgitant volume is increased in patients with an increased afterload, such as high systolic blood pressure or AS. Therapeutic manipulations of the afterload (i.e., management of blood pressure, aortic valve replacement) are an important component of MR management. Because systemic blood pressure affects MR severity to a great degree, it should always be documented at the time of echocardiographic assessment of MR.

169. What are the indicators of MR severity on spectral Doppler studies?

1. **Dense continuous wave Doppler tracing.** There is a direct relationship between the number of echocardiography reflectors in a blood flow jet and the density of the spectral Doppler tracing of that jet (i.e., homogeneity and brightness of the white color). In patients with severe MR, the higher number of red blood cells included in the regurgitant jet is responsible for an increased density of the continuous wave Doppler tracing. This method offers only a crude assessment of MR severity.

2. **Increased mitral E wave velocity.** The E wave represents the flow velocity from the LA into the LV at the beginning of diastole. The higher the LA-LV pressure gradient, the higher the E wave velocity. In patients with MR, the LA pressure is increased, due to a dual filling of the atrium from the pulmonary veins (normal) and from the LV (abnormal); consequently, there is "torrential" LV filling in early diastole resulting in an increased E wave velocity.

3. **Flow reversal in the pulmonary veins.** The normal pulmonary vein flow has two components (S and D) corresponding to systole and diastole (see Chapter 2). Both components are directed toward the LA. In patients with severe MR, there is substantial increase in the LA systolic pressure with consequent blunting, abolishment, or even reversal of the systolic component of pulmonary blood flow (Fig. 22). This sign should always be interpreted in the context of other echocardiographic and clinical findings because it lacks specificity.

170. In patients with severe MR, what is the catheterization finding corresponding to systolic flow reversal in the pulmonary veins shown by echocardiography?

The v wave on the pulmonary artery catheter tracing.

171. Can echocardiography distinguish between acute and chronic MR?

Acute MR causes a rapid increase in the LA pressure because it is almost always severe and because LA compliance is not increased, as it would be with chronic MR. The rapid increase in LA pressure results in a rapid decrease in the LA-LV pressure gradient and a characteristic early peaking continuous wave Doppler envelope. In addition, the LA may not yet be dilated with acute MR.

172. What important information about LV function can be made by analysis of the MR Doppler tracing?

In patients with severe LV dysfunction, there is an abnormally slow LV pressure increase in systole: It takes a longer time for a dysfunctional ventricle to reach its peak systolic pressure. The peak LV-LA pressure gradient is reached later in systole. This is seen in the continuous wave Doppler tracing of the MR jet (most patients with severe LV dysfunction have associated MR).

The peak velocity of the MR jet is attained in late systole, and consequently the spectral Doppler envelope has a characteristic late-peaking appearance.

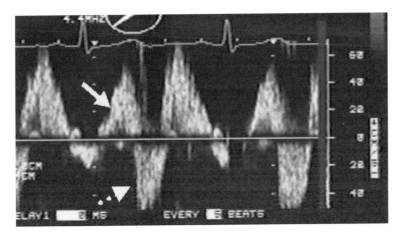

FIGURE 22. Pulmonary vein flow reversal in severe MR. In this patient there is blunting of the blood flow through the pulmonary veins during the first half of systole (*short continuous arrow*) and frank reversal during the latter half (*short dotted arrow*).

173. Outline the two-dimensional echocardiography indicators of MR severity.
1. The mechanism of MR:
   a. The presence of flail mitral leaflet
   b. Severe annular dilation
   c. Severe mitral valve prolapse
   d. Visible lack of leaflet coaptation (normally the mitral leaflet tips overlap in systole over a distance of a 0.8–1.2 cm)
2. The adaptive response of the LV and LA to the valvular regurgitation:
   a. LV dilation
   b. LV dysfunction
   c. LA enlargement (LA diameter > 5.5 mm in the absence of alternative explanations suggests chronic, severe MR)

174. A patient with severe MR has an LV ejection fraction of 50%. Does this patient have normal LV function?
It is essential to understand the meaning of *normal LV function* in a patient with MR. An ejection fraction of 50% usually is considered the lower limit of normal in most situations. The physiologic response of the LV to significant MR is to increase the ejection fraction to > 60%, however. The "normal" LV of a patient with severe MR should have a higher ejection fraction than the "normal" LV of a normal subject. In the case of the patient in this question, there is evidence of LV dysfunction.

175. What is severe MR?
Doppler signs
- A regurgitant orifice area > 0.5 cm²
- A regurgitant volume > 60 mL
- A regurgitation fraction > 60%
- Pulmonary vein flow reversal
- Color flow area > 40% of LA surface area
- Eccentric MR jet reaching the posterior wall of the LA

Two-dimensional signs*
- Flail mitral leaflet
- Severe annular dilation
- Leaflet malcoaptation
- Severe mitral valve prolapse, involving more than one cusp of the mitral valve
- LV systolic diameter > 7 cm
- LA diameter > 5.5 cm

*Signs on two-dimensional echocardiography consistent with but not independently diagnostic of severe MR.

176. What is the difference between the concept of severe MR and clinically significant MR?

Severe MR is almost always clinically significant (even in the absence of symptoms, severe MR requires treatment of some form). **Nonsevere MR** can be clinically significant or not, depending on cardiac comorbidity (asymptomatic, moderate MR in a patient with a hyperdynamic LV is not causing clinical problems and may just need to be monitored, whereas the same degree of MR in a patient with an abnormal ventricle usually needs intervention).

177. What is the role of echocardiography in establishing the indication for surgery in a patient with MR?

A detailed list of the indications for surgery in patients with MR is beyond the scope of this text. The most important echocardiography parameters that, in the proper clinical setting, are indications for surgery, include:
1. LV ejection fraction < 50%
2. LV end-systolic diameter > 50 mm
3. Pulmonary hypertension
4. Acute MR resulting from mechanical failure (ruptured chorda or papillary muscle)

178. Explain the importance of echocardiography assessment of LV ejection fraction in patients with severe MR.

In MR patients, LV function is one of the most important factors to be taken into account in determining the indication for surgery and the prognosis after surgery. Although the classic approach has been to indicate surgery in patients with a falling ejection fraction, many centers are moving toward an aggressive strategy of early surgical intervention in patients with severe MR and fully normal LV function (55–60%), to prevent the onset of potentially irreversible LV dysfunction.

179. The management of patients with severe MR and severely decreased LV function (ejection fraction < 30%) is problematic because in this setting conservative medical and surgical approaches have a high morbidity and mortality. How can echocardiography help establish the candidacy for mitral valve replacement among these patients?

It is important to distinguish between the following two possibilities:
1. MR resulting from intrinsic mitral valve disease (e.g., prolapse) with secondary LV dysfunction
2. LV dysfunction resulting from primary or secondary cardiomyopathy with secondary MR from annular dilation

Patients belonging to the first group (primary mitral valve disease, secondary LV dysfunction) are generally better surgical candidates, especially if mitral valve repair is feasible. Echocardiography can help answer these questions.

180. What is the role of echocardiography in the selection of the best surgical technique in a patient with MR (i.e., replacement versus repair)?

Perhaps the highest predictor of success of mitral valve repair is the degree of expertise of the surgeon. There are many patient-related factors to be taken into account, however. The following groups of patients are *generally* poor candidates for mitral valve repair (mitral valve replacement surgery *generally* indicated):

- Patients with rheumatic MR (extensive valvular and subvalvular fibrosis and calcification often make repair impossible)
- Patients with severe prolapse of the anterior mitral leaflet (mitral valve repair is technically easier in case of posterior leaflet prolapse)
- Patients with a limited extent of leaflet prolapse (as a rough indicator, prolapse of > 50 % of the leaflet length may be associated with less chances for successful repair)
- Patients with extensive valvular calcification

181. What is the role of echocardiography in intraoperative assessment of patients with MR?

Intraoperative TEE in MR patients is important for:

- Assessment of the mechanism of severe MR (this assessment ideally should be carried out before surgery)
- Assessment of the quality of mitral valve repair, before discontinuation of the extracorporeal circulation; generally, more than mild degrees of MR after mitral valve repair are unacceptable, and additional repair or valve replacement may be indicated.

182. What is the role of echocardiography in the follow-up of MR patients?

- In patients with known MR and changes in the symptomatic status
- In patients with moderate or severe MR in which surgery is being delayed (meticulous echocardiographic follow-up of the LV function is essential)
- In follow-up of patients after MV surgery, for detection of complications (prosthesis dysfunction or degeneration, thrombosis, pannus formation, recurrent MR despite initially successful repair)

Tricuspid Regurgitation

Gabriel Adelmann, M.D., Benjamin Kleiber, M.D., Ellen Burton, R.N., B.S.N., and Neil J. Weissman, M.D.

183. What are the two-dimensional echocardiography signs of TR?

TR is diagnosed with Doppler, not two-dimensional, echocardiography; however, two-dimensional echocardiography may have findings related to the cause of the TR such as:

- LV failure causing pulmonary hypertension
- Rheumatic disease (thickened, retracted leaflets and subvalvular apparatus)
- Tricuspid valve prolapse (often associated with mitral valve prolapse)
- Annular dilation
- RV infarction or enlargement
- Ebstein's anomaly (apical displacement of the tricuspid valve, atrial septal defect)
- Tricuspid valve damage caused by trauma or endocarditis
- Carcinoid disease (leaflet thickening)
- Iatrogenic (e.g., valve perforation or obstruction to leaflet mobility by a pacemaker wire or right heart catheter)

184. What is the role of echocardiography in the assessment of TR?

Doppler echocardiography is the imaging procedure of choice for assessing TR. Multiple views are necessary for this assessment:

- Right ventricular inflow view
- Apical four-chamber view
- Short-axis view at the aortic valve level
- Subcostal view

185. What are the Doppler signs of TR?

The Doppler signs of TR are similar to the ones described for MR except the jet goes from the RV to the RA (Fig. 23). A complete Doppler examination in a TR patient includes:

- Color Doppler assessment of the tricuspid valve
- Continuous wave Doppler assessment of the tricuspid valve velocity
- Pulse wave Doppler assessment of the hepatic veins

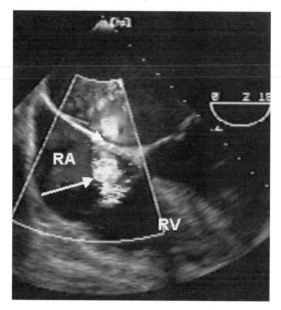

FIGURE 23. Mild to moderate TR jet on color Doppler (*arrow*). RV = right ventricle; RA = right atrium. (See also Color Plates, Figure 16.)

186. List the Doppler signs of severe TR.

1. TR jet area > 30% of the RA surface area.

2. Systolic flow reversal in the hepatic veins: Throughout the cardiac cycle, blood should flow toward the RA. Severe TR causes a significant increase in the RA and the inferior vena cava (IVC) pressure with systolic flow reversal in the hepatic veins.

Supportive findings consistent with severe TR are:

Dense continuous wave Doppler signal

Annular dilation > 4 cm

Increased tricuspid E wave velocity (> 1 m/sec)

187. Why is it necessary to perform Doppler assessment of the hepatic vein flow, instead of simply assessing the flow in the IVC?

On TTE, the subcostal view is generally the only view that shows the IVC and the hepatic veins. Systolic flow reversal in the IVC is less specific for severe TR than systolic flow reversal in the hepatic veins.

188. Why perform color Doppler and continuous wave Doppler assessments of TR?

Color Doppler assesses the severity of TR, whereas continuous wave Doppler assesses the velocity of the TR jet. The TR velocity is used to estimate the pulmonary artery pressure using the Bernoulli equation (see Chapter 10). If the TR velocity is 3 m/sec, the gradient between the RV and RA in systole is 36 mmHg ($4 v^2$). If we assume the RA pressure is 10 mmHg, the the RV pressure during systole is 46 mmHg (10 + 36). If there is no pulmonary stenosis, the pulmonary artery systolic pressure is also 46 mmHg (Fig. 24).

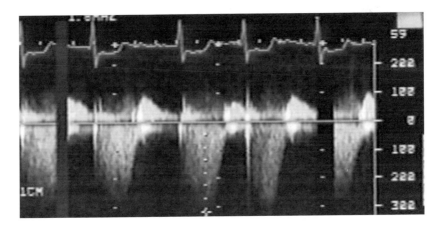

FIGURE 24. CW Doppler of a TR. Application of Bernoulli's equation jet in this patient yielded a PA pressure of 46 mmHg (assuming an RA pressure = 10 mmHg).

189. What is the difference between *TR severity* and *TR jet velocity*?

TR severity refers to the volume of blood regurgitating from the RV into the RA in systole. **TR jet velocity** is determined by the gradient between the RV and RA and is a measure of RV systolic pressure. Severe TR can have low velocity if the RV and pulmonary artery pressure are not high, and, conversely, a mild TR jet can have high velocity in a patient with pulmonary hypertension.

190. What are the echocardiographic indicators of severe TR?

The color Doppler, spectral Doppler, and two-dimensional indicators of severe TR are similar to those of severe MR. Practically, TR severity assessment is almost always semiquantitatively assessed by the color Doppler jet area.

191. How is TR classified on echocardiography?

Trace/trivial/physiologic (these terms are synonyms)
Mild
Moderate
Severe

192. What is severe TR?

- TR jet area > 30% of that of RA area
- Annular dilation > 4 cm
- Increased tricuspid E wave velocity (> 1 m/sec)
- Systolic slow reversal in the hepatic veins

193. How can echocardiography help determine if a patient with TR needs surgery?

A detailed list of the indications for surgery is beyond the scope of this text. Surgical interventions on the tricuspid valve generally are performed in conjunction with other valve surgery. The most important echocardiographic parameters that, in the proper clinical setting, are indications for surgery include severe TR and **absence** of severe, irreversible pulmonary hypertension.

194. What is the role of echocardiography in selecting the optimal surgical therapy in a patient with severe TR (tricuspid valve replacement versus repair)?

The presence of intrinsic tricuspid leaflet distortion, as is seen in rheumatic disease, precludes the possibility of repair. Conversely, in patients in whom severe TR is due to tricuspid annular dilation, implantation of a tricuspid ring may decrease significantly the degree of regurgitation.

Tricuspid Stenosis

Gabriel Adelmann, M.D., Benjamin Kleiber, M.D., and Neil J. Weissman, M.D.

195. What is the most frequent cause of TS?
Rheumatic disease, characterized by leaflet thickening and retraction; although this is the most common cause of TS, it is a rare finding today.

196. List some uncommon causes of TS.
- Carcinoid disease
- Endocarditis (bulky vegetations can interfere with the closure of the tricuspid valve)
- Obstruction of the tricuspid valve by tumor

197. What are the Doppler characteristics of TS?
Increased pressure gradient across the tricuspid valve and increased tricuspid E wave velocity.

198. What is the Doppler hallmark of severe TS?
A pressure gradient across the tricuspid valve > 7 mmHg.

Pulmonic Stenosis

Gabriel Adelmann, M.D., Kenneth Horton, RDCS, and Neil J. Weissman, M.D.

199. Describe the main causes of pulmonic stenosis (PS).
PS may occur in isolation or as part of a complex congenital heart syndrome. According to the site of blood flow obstruction, PS can be **valvular** (congenital, carcinoid, endocarditis), **subvalvular** (tetralogy of Fallot, extrinsic compression by tumor), or **supravalvular** (continuum of lesions ranging from discrete stenosis to diffuse hypoplasia of the pulmonary artery, extrinsic compression by tumor).

200. What should the echocardiography detection of PS be followed by?
The detection of PS should prompt a diligent search for associated congenital abnormalities, the most frequent association being the tetralogy of Fallot (ventricular septal defect, RV hypertrophy, and overriding aorta).

Pulmonic Insufficiency

Gabriel Adelmann, M.D., and Neil J. Weissman, M.D.

201. What are the most frequent causes of pulmonic insufficiency (PI)?
PI can be functional, resulting from RV dilation or pulmonary hypertension, or structural, resulting from rheumatic disease, carcinoid, endocarditis, or other masses. Echocardiography is ideally suited for showing these causes.

202. How is the severity of PI graded by Doppler echocardiography?
There is no good standardization for grading the severity of PI. Most use the jet area and grade PI as trace, mild, moderate, or severe. Jet width (at the origin of the PI) should be a better marker for the grade of PI than jet length. Occasionally, pulmonary flow reversal is detected in the pulmonary artery in patients with severe TR. This sign is similar to the flow reversal in the aorta in patients with severe AI (Fig. 25).

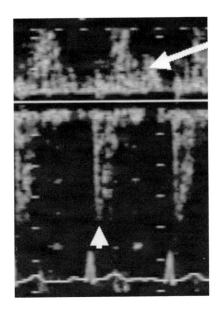

FIGURE 25. Diastolic flow reversal (*large arrow*) and normal forward systolic blood flow (*arrowhead*) in the pulmonary artery, in a patient with severe PI. Appreciate the importance of ECG for timing these events. An identical picture is seen in the aorta in the case of severe AI. (See also Color Plates, Figure 17.)

Prosthetic Valves

Steven A. Goldstein, M.D., Neil J. Weissman, M.D., and Gabriel Adelmann, M.D.

203. What are the main types of prosthetic heart valves?
Prosthetic heart valves can be of two types: mechanical or bioprosthetic (Fig. 26).

MECHANICAL VALVES	BIOPROSTHETIC VALVES
Ball-cage (Starr-Edwards)	Heterografts (animal, such as porcine or bovine). Heterografts may be stented or stentless
Disk	
Floating disk	
Tilting disk (single disk) (Medtronic-Hall, Omniscience)	Homografts (human)
Bileaflet (two disks) (St. Jude, Carbomedics)	Autologous (as in the Ross procedure, when the patient's own pulmonary valve is transferred to the aortic position)

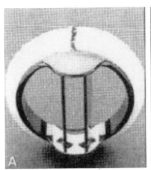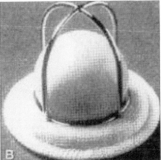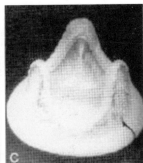

FIGURE 26. The main types of prosthetic valves. Three popular types of prosthesis *A,* Bileaflet St. Jude prosthesis in fully opened position (there are two lateral major flow orifices and a minor central orifice). *B,* Starr-Edwards prosthesis (model 6120). *C,* Porcine heterograft (frame-mounted- glutaraldehyde-preserved). (From Schaff HV: Prosthetic valves. In Giuliani ER, Gersh BJ, McGoon MD, et al (eds): Mayo Clinic Practice of Cardiology, 3rd ed. St. Louis, Mosby, 1996, pp 1484–1496, with permission.)

204. What causes prosthetic valves to open and to close?

In bioprosthetic and mechanical valves, the opening and closing depends on changes in blood flow and pressure gradients.

205. What are the main components of a prosthetic mechanical valve?

1. The **occluder,** which represents the mobile component of the prosthesis, usually is constructed of plastic, coated with a layer of carbon for strength and durability and to inhibit thrombosis. Occluders may be **ball-shaped** (older types of prosthetic valves, no longer made) or **diskoid** (the currently used type, with one or two disks).

2. The **restraining system** restricts the motion of the occluder. Depending on the shape of the occluder, the restraining system may consist of a **cage** (for ball-shaped occluders) or **projections** ("struts") attached to the sewing ring (for disk-shaped occluders).

3. The **sewing ring** attaches the valvular prosthesis to the vessel.

206. Describe the fluid dynamics of mechanical prosthetic valves.

A wide variety of mechanical valves are available, and the flow profiles across each of these vary substantially. Few are similar to flow across a normal native valve. With **ball-cage valves,** blood flows around the ball occluder on all sides. **Tilting disk valves** have two orifices in the open position, one larger and one smaller (major and minor openings), resulting in an asymmetric flow profile. Variations depend on the shape of the disk (convex vs. concave) and on the sewing ring design. **Bileaflet mechanical valves** have complex fluid dynamics. With the leaflets open, there are two large lateral orifices and a small central orifice. The flow velocity profile shows three peaks corresponding to these orifices. There is more acceleration of flow across the narrow central orifice, resulting in localized high-pressure gradients in this region of the valve. These local gradients may be substantially higher than the overall gradient across the valve, especially for small size (e.g., sizes 19 and 21 mm) aortic prosthetic valves.

207. Define physiologic regurgitation through a prosthetic valve.

The concept of *physiologic regurgitation* mainly refers to prosthetic valve designs that result in a mild degree of regurgitation when the valve is closed. The orientation of the regurgitant jet depends on the structural characteristics of the valve (Fig. 27).

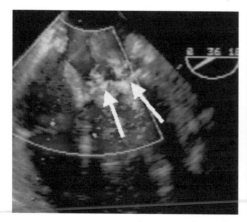 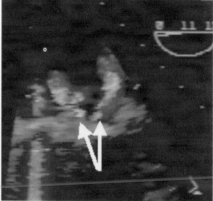

FIGURE 27. Physiologic valve regurgitation (*arrows*) through a St. Jude prosthetic valve in the mitral position. The characteristic jets may appear as convergent or divergent, depending on the transducer angulation (TEE). (See also Color Plates, Figure 18.)

208. What is the echocardiographic importance of physiologic regurgitation through a prosthetic valve?

The type of prosthetic valve should be known in advance to be able to differentiate normal from abnormal prosthetic valve regurgitation.

209. How can physiologic regurgitation of a prosthetic valve be distinguished from pathologic regurgitation?

Physiologic valve regurgitation has several features that help to differentiate it from pathologic regurgitation (Fig. 28):

1. The flow is contained within the sewing ring (i.e., central versus periprosthetic pathologic jets). Periprosthetic regurgitation is *always* abnormal.

2. The flow is usually laminar (i.e., not turbulent).

3. The regurgitation jet usually extends for no more than 2–3 cm into the receiving chamber.

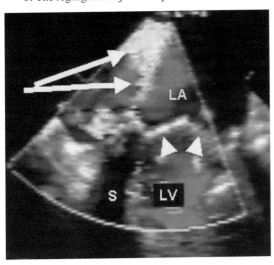

FIGURE 28. Pathologic prosthetic valve regurgitation through St. Jude valve (*large arrows*); the St. Jude valve is in the mitral position (*small arrow heads*). LA = left atrium, LV = left ventricle. Note the periprosthetic origin of the regurgitant jet. Additionally, note the shadowing artifact produced by the prosthetic valve (S). This artifact often makes prosthetic mitral valve assessment by TTE difficult or impossible (this figure is from a TEE study). (See also Color Plates, Figure 19.)

210. What are the main components of a bioprosthetic valve?

The bioprosthetic valves have the same main components as the mechanical valves:

- The mobile part is constructed of tissue (e.g., semilunar valves from pigs or humans or pericardium from cows)
- A metallic sewing ring
- A metallic restraining system (stents or struts) that supports the tissue. Newer generations of prosthetic valves (especially in the aortic position) have small or absent stents (stentless valves), a structural characteristic meant to improve the hemodynamic profile of these valves, increasing durability and decreasing the risk of thrombotic complications.

211. Describe the fluid dynamics of bioprosthetic valves.

Most bioprosthetic valves are trileaflet in shape and have the following characteristics:

1. The opening is circular in systole, resulting in a flow pattern similar to that of native valves (i.e., central and laminar).

2. The antegrade velocity is increased compared with that through a normal native valve because the opening is narrowed by the sewing ring and stents or struts. The older generation of bioprosthetic valves have an intrinsic degree of mild or moderate stenosis, the exact degree of stenosis depending on the type, size, and insertion specifics. This limitation is largely avoided with the newer stentless valves, which have dynamics more closely approximating normal valve function.

212. Should *all* patients with prosthetic valves have a baseline postoperative Doppler echocardiography evaluation?

Yes. One of the main aspects of management after valve replacement is patient follow-up, aimed at detection of prosthetic malfunction (pathologic regurgitation or obstruction). It is occasionally difficult to establish whether regurgitation or increased velocities detected through a prosthetic valve are a pathologic process or are normal for that patient. (Nearly all prosthetic valves have an intrinsic degree of stenosis and regurgitation). Follow-up studies of prosthetic valves imply a comparison with a specific baseline situation, which must be known in advance (review of previous studies). The baseline assessment can be performed before patient discharge or at the time of the first postoperative visit (usually 2–3 weeks after discharge).

213. What is prosthetic valve dysfunction?
- Obstruction by thrombus, vegetation, or tissue ingrowth (pannus)
- Dehiscence of the valve ring caused by infection or improper suturing at the time of surgery (see Figure 28)
- Structural damage to the occluder (mechanical valves) or to the leaflets (bioprosthetic valves)

Prosthetic valve dysfunction is identified and its severity is quantified by echocardiography (two-dimensional and Doppler).

214. Frequently used measurements for assessment of aortic prosthetic valve function include aortic valve area and the dimensionless index. Why?

The dimensionless index (the ratio between the blood velocity through the aortic valve and through the LVOT) and the aortic valve area have several advantages. The gradients through a prosthetic valve tend to vary widely depending on the valve type and the cardiac output. The dimensionless index and aortic valve area, generally independent of cardiac output, are useful in this setting. Calculation of the dimensionless index does not require an outflow tract diameter measurement, which can be particularly difficult in patients with prosthetic aortic valves owing to intense shadowing and reverberations. The normal dimensionless index in a prosthetic valve usually ranges between 0.30 and 0.50.

215. List the possible explanations of high Doppler gradient (blood flow velocity > 2.5–3.0 m/sec) in a patient with a prosthetic aortic valve.
- True prosthetic dysfunction (obstruction)
- Increased cardiac output (hyperdynamic syndromes, AI)
- Subaortic (dynamic) obstruction with normal prosthetic valve function
- Discrepancy between peak-to-peak (catheterization) and peak instantaneous (Doppler) gradients

216. Transvalvular aortic gradients measured by Doppler are systematically higher than gradients assessed in the catheterization laboratory. What is the relevance of this statement for patient follow-up after aortic valve replacement?

Echocardiography is the procedure of choice for patient follow-up after aortic valve replacement, and it is possible to compare inadvertently the follow-up echocardiographic gradient with a baseline catheter-determined gradient. In these patients, the discrepancy usually results from the difference between the two methods, rather than from true prosthetic valvular dysfunction.

217. What is the pressure recovery phenomenon?

Pressure recovery is a phenomenon affecting the invasive measurement of pressure gradients (in the catheterization laboratory) and is partly responsible for the discrepancy between the invasively and noninvasively measured pressure gradients. Pressure recovery results in a lower measured gradient by the invasive method because the lowest pressure is just beyond the prosthetic valve, then the pressure "recovers" and increases further downstream in the aorta. See the Cardiac Catheterization section for a detailed discussion of the pressure recovery phenomenon.

218. In which situations is the phenomenon of pressure recovery of practical importance?

It is especially important with small-diameter aortic mechanical prostheses (sizes 19 and 21 mm).

219. What is pannus?

Pannus (tissue ingrowth) is excessive endothelial proliferation at the site of a prosthetic valve. Pannus can invade and obstruct the prosthetic valve orifice. The main differential diagnosis of pannus is **prosthetic valve thrombosis,** an especially important distinction because pannus is not amenable to anticoagulation or thrombolytic therapy and requires surgical removal whenever it causes significant obstruction.

220. Can valvular thrombus be distinguished from tissue ingrowth (pannus) by echocardiography?

Echocardiography has a sensitivity of only 50–70% for the detection of pannus. Features suggesting thrombus are:
- Size (thrombi tend to be larger than pannus and often extend beyond the sewing ring)
- Texture (thrombus tends to be "softer" (less echo-dense) than pannus)
- A suggestive clinical context (i.e., suboptimal anticoagulation suggests the presence of thrombus)

Pannus and thrombus can coexist in the same patient.

221. What are the echocardiographic characteristics of prosthetic valve dehiscence?
Mechanical valve dehiscence
- An exaggerated mobility of the valvular ring ("rocking" motion of the valve)
- Structural damage of the occluder or restraining system
- The presence of pathologic regurgitant jets (see questions 207–209)

Bioprosthetic valve dehiscence
- Different degrees of valvular degeneration and destruction
- Eccentric regurgitant jets with a complex three-dimensional morphology and generally moderate or severe in intensity

222. What is the role of TTE in the evaluation of prosthetic valves?

TTE is the **cornerstone** of prosthetic valve evaluation. This is due to the good alignment between the TTE Doppler beam and the transvalvular blood flow, especially in the case of an aortic valve prosthesis. Artifacts (mainly reverberation and acoustic shadowing), which can mask regurgitation, represent the major limitation of TTE. If suspected regurgitation is not seen by TTE (especially in patients with a prosthetic mitral valve), a confirmatory TEE must be performed.

223. When should TEE be performed for the assessment of prosthetic valves?
- Patients with nondiagnostic TTE
- Patients in whom the TTE findings are not concordant with the clinical picture
- Patients with problems related to mitral (as opposed to aortic) valve prosthesis. TEE is especially suited for assessment of MR (pathologic jets through a mitral prosthesis are often eccentric and require a substantial number of transducer angulations for optimal visualization) and for assessment of the posterior sewing ring of a prosthetic mitral valve (overshadowed by the anterior portion of the sewing ring on TTE)
- Patients with known or suspected endocarditis, in whom persistent fever and positive blood cultures despite appropriate antibiotic therapy raise the suspicion of a cardiac abscess
- Patients with suspected prosthetic valve thrombosis, including patients after stroke (as discussed in Chapter 8, intracardiac clots are fine, non–echo-dense structures, best detected by TEE)

224. Summarize the most frequent complications of prosthetic heart valves.

COMPLICATION	CAUSE
Valve obstruction	Thrombosis (Fig. 29A)
	Fibrous tissue ingrowth (pannus)
Valve regurgitation	Dehiscence
	Degeneration (bioprostheses) (Fig. 29B)
Structural problems that can result in either	Infection (prosthetic valve endocarditis)
obstruction or regurgitation	Structural deterioration (mechanical
	prostheses)
	Suboptimal hemodynamics/hydraulics

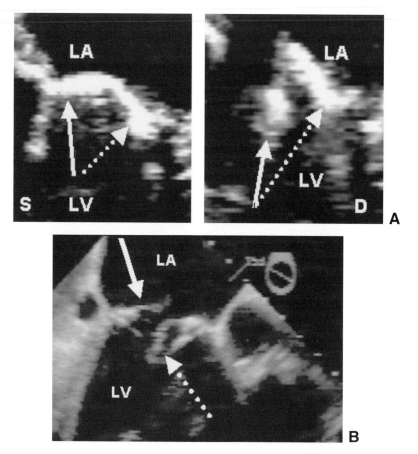

FIGURE 29. *A,* Partly thrombosed St. Jude valve in the mitral position. Note the almost vertical position of the mobile leaflet (*solid arrow*) in diastole as opposed to the virtually unchanged position of the thrombosed leaflet (*dotted arrow*). D = diastole, S = systole, LA = left atrium, LV = left ventricle. *B,* Degenerated bioprosthetic valve in the mitral position. Note the abnormal shape of both leaflets (*arrows*) with a flail motion of the posterior leaflet (*solid arrow*). The tunnel-like space between the leaflets is the origin of a severe, eccentric MR jet. LA = left atrium, LV = left ventricle.

225. What are prosthetic valve "strands"?

Filamentous structures representing fibrin deposition on the surface of a prosthetic valve (Fig. 30). They are a frequent finding and generally are not associated with embolic complications. Their main importance consists in the necessity to differentiate them from thrombi.

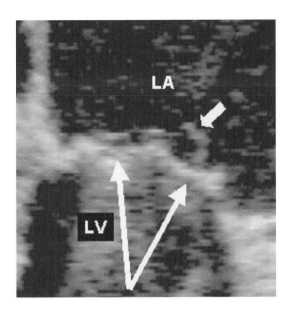

FIGURE 30. Fibrinous strand (*short arrow*) attached to a mitral St. Jude prosthetic valve (*long arrows*). LA = left atrium, LV = left ventricle.

MAGNETIC RESONANCE IMAGING

Anthon R. Fuisz, M.D., and Gabriel Adelmann, M.D.

226. What is the current practical role of magnetic resonance imaging (MRI) in the diagnosis of valvular heart disease?

As is the case with echocardiography, MRI can show valvular stenosis or regurgitation based on the turbulent transvalvular blood flow. Paradoxically the introduction of new MRI technology has made this assessment more difficult because the rapid acquisition sequences of the newer equipment minimize and sometimes eliminate the turbulence-related artifact. MRI remains valuable for assessment of ventricular function and volumes, but this assessment is significantly more complex and time-consuming than Doppler echocardiography.

227. How can valvular heart disease be assessed by MRI?

- Visualization of a regurgitant jet by the "white blood technique" (Fig. 31A)
- Assessing the **signal void** (depicted in black) produced by turbulent transvalvular blood flow (Fig. 31B)
- Application of Bernoulli's equation to MRI-measured transvalvular flow velocities
- Flow quantitation by echo-planar imaging
- Assessment of **valve morphology**
- Direct assessment of **valvular motion**

228. Is the signal void produced by stenotic lesions different from that corresponding to regurgitant lesions?

No. Stenotic and regurgitant lesions are characterized by turbulent blood flow depicted as a "signal void" (black area). The direction, timing (systole versus diastole), and geometric characteristics of this signal void (width, length) are used to distinguish valvular regurgitation from stenosis.

229. What is velocity-encoded MRI?

This method generates a velocity map of blood flow through a heart valve, based on the interplay between the electromagnetic properties of flowing blood and the speed and direction of blood flow. Transvalvular gradients can be measured, by applying Bernoulli's equation to the measured peak blood velocity. By integrating the measured flow over a given three-dimensional volume, actual blood flow volumes can be calculated.

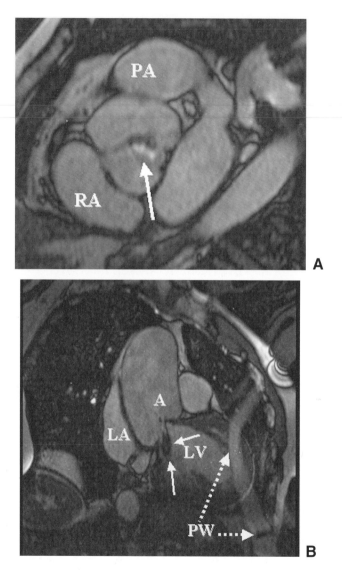

FIGURE 31. AI (*arrow*) demonstrated by the white blood technique (gradient-echo MRI) (*A*) and by the black blood technique (signal void) (*arrows*) (*B*). Also note the phenomenon of "phase wrap" (PW, *dotted arrows*), here depicted by one of the patient's limbs appearing on the opposite side of its actual anatomic location. This problem is seen in large patients.

230. What are the main pitfalls of velocity-encoded MRI?

(1) Potential malalignment between the direction of flow and the direction of flow encoding (processing of the MRI signal emitted by flowing blood) and (2) flow aliasing.

231. What is echo-planar imaging?

This method of rapid image acquisition and phase velocity mapping sequences allows quantitation of blood flow and direct observation of valvular motion.

232. What are the principles of regurgitant flow quantitation by MRI?

MRI quantitation of a regurgitant valvular flow can be achieved by:

1. Phase velocity imaging to produce direct measurements of blood flow across different planes.

2. Assessment of the length, width, and area of the corresponding signal void, similar to corresponding measurements performed in the echocardiography laboratory on regurgitant jets visualized by color Doppler. The results of this method are influenced substantially by patient-dependent factors (regurgitant orifice size and geometry, loading conditions) and by machine-dependent factors.

3. The PISA method: This method has been applied successfully in the quantitative assessment of aortic regurgitation.

4. Calculation of the RV and LV stroke volume (and the difference in the RV and LV stroke volume) in patients with single, isolated regurgitant lesions. The main shortcoming of this method is that its accuracy substantially decreases in patients with more than one regurgitant valvular lesion.

233. On which principles is MRI quantitation of valvular stenosis based?

- Calculation of transvalvular gradients using Bernoulli's equation
- Calculation of valvular area by means of the continuity equation

234. Is it possible to assess mechanical prosthetic valves by MRI?

With the exception of the ball-in-cage Starr-Edwards valve, MRI is safe in this setting. The exact role of MRI in the diagnosis of prosthetic valve dysfunction remains to be defined. Figure 32 demonstrates a prosthesis in the mitral position.

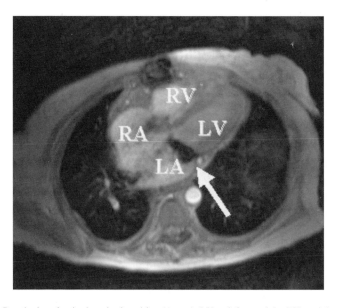

FIGURE 32. Prosthetic valve in the mitral position (*arrow*). LV = left ventricle, RV = right ventricle, LA = left atrium, RA = right atrium.

NUCLEAR MEDICINE

Manuel D. Cerqueira, M.D., Jonathan G. Tall, CNMT, and Gabriel Adelmann, M.D.

235. What information is provided by nuclear imaging in patients with valvular heart disease?
- LV and RV ejection fraction
- LV and RV volume
- Magnitude of regurgitation (regurgitant fraction)
- Presence, extent, and severity of concomitant coronary artery disease

236. What is the major indication for nuclear imaging in patients with valvular disease?
The only class I indication for nuclear imaging is the serial evaluation of LV ejection fraction at rest and after exercise-induced stress. In the absence of significant concomitant coronary artery disease, a decrease in LV ejection fraction implies a greater severity or progression of the underlying valvular disease and the necessity to consider surgical intervention (valvular repair or replacement) before the onset of irreversible myocardial damage.

237. Explain the importance of stress myocardial perfusion imaging in the preoperative evaluation of patients scheduled for valvular surgery.
Although valvular surgery is occasionally necessary in young, otherwise healthy patients, most patients present with either multiple risk factors or already established coronary artery disease. Detection and quantification of inducible ischemia are important. The presence and extent of underlying coronary artery disease should be documented by coronary arteriography at the time of definitive measurement of the extent of the valvular disease. In patients with borderline coronary artery stenosis, perfusion imaging may be useful to identify the hemodynamic significance of the observed lesions to decide whether the patient will require revascularization.

238. How can the severity of valvular regurgitation be assessed by nuclear imaging?
In patients with MR or aortic regurgitation or both, the difference in cardiac output (radioactive counts) between the two ventricles provides an index of the severity of LV volume overload. This method is not often used, owing to several shortcomings:
- Difficulty of separating total counts or volume between the enlarged ventricles and atria—a prerequisite step for accurate measurements
- Limitation in patients with multivalvular regurgitation—a common scenario in this setting of valvular heart disease

Echocardiography is the procedure of choice for the assessment of valvular disease.

239. What is the LV transit time?
The LV transit time, assessed by first-pass radionuclide angiography, represents the time elapsed between the first appearance of the radiotracers in the LV cavity and the moment when no radioactive signal is detected any longer.

240. State the importance of the LV transit time in the diagnosis of valvular heart disease.
The LV transit time is prolonged in patients with valvular regurgitation, owing to the recirculation of contrast material between the aorta, LA, and LV.

CHEST X-RAY

*Rina Sternlieb, M.D., Gabriel Adelmann, M.D., Matthew Brewer, M.D.,
and Curtis E. Green, M.D.*

241. Describe the findings of valvular disease on chest radiography.
- Structural or functional changes of the **valves themselves** (valvular calcification, prosthetic valve "rocking" or obstruction)

- The effect of valvular disease on the **heart chambers** (enlargement of the atria or the ventricles or both)
- The effect of valvular disease on the **pulmonary circulation** (pulmonary congestion or oligemia)
- The effect of valvular disease on the **great arteries** (poststenotic aneurysmal dilation)

242. Discuss the importance of valvular calcification in the diagnosis of valvular heart disease.

Valvular calcifications are seen on chest x-rays as radiopacities (bright, white spots) in the projection areas of the mitral and aortic valves. Occasionally, calcification involves the entire perimeter of the mitral or aortic valve annulus. The greatest diagnostic importance of valvular calcification refers to the radiographic identification of degenerative AS. Valvular calcification has high specificity but low sensitivity for the diagnosis of valvular disease. Care must be exercised to avoid misinterpretation of myocardial, pericardial, or coronary artery calcification for calcification of the valves.

243. What are the radiographic findings in prosthetic valve dysfunction?

Fluoroscopy is a simple and effective method for diagnosing prosthetic valve dysfunction. The findings may include:

- Excessive valvular motion (rocking), in case of valvular dehiscence
- Restricted motion of the prosthetic valvular occluder device (leaflets, ball) (Fig. 33)

244. What are the mechanisms of ventricular dysfunction secondary to valvular heart disease, and what are the associated radiologic findings?

Pressure overload—an increased resistance to ventricular emptying (AS, PS, systemic or pulmonary hypertension). The radiographic finding associated with pressure overload is ventricular hypertrophy. As noted earlier, isolated ventricular hypertrophy is not detected by chest x-ray. In the late stages of the disease, pressure overload may be associated with significant ventricular dilation.

Volume overload—an increased volume of blood filling the ventricles in diastole (owing to MR, TR, left-to-right shunt, or an increased blood volume). The radiographic finding of volume overload is ventricular dilation, which can be detected radiographically.

245. Is it possible to distinguish radiographically between ventricular dilation caused by volume overload and that associated with advanced pressure overload lesions?

Although this distinction generally is not possible based on chest x-ray alone, volume overload lesions are generally responsible for greater degrees of ventricular dilation than pressure overload lesions. The presence of gross ventricular dilation should suggest volume overload physiology.

246. What is *cor bovinum*?

This is the Latin term for "cow's heart." This term designates the extreme LV dilation seen in severe AI. This is the greatest degree of LV dilation seen in any disease.

247. How is the LV affected by MR?

MR is often associated with LV dilation and failure. There are two possible explanations for this association:

1. LV disease caused by the chronic volume overload of MR. This is a feature of advanced chronic MR and may be irreversible. Early detection of LV dysfunction secondary to MR is achieved by echocardiography. The treatment of choice in these patients is mitral valve repair or replacement.

2. Idiopathic or secondary LV dilation causing annular dilation and significant MR. The management of these patients involves an aggressive search for reversible causes of LV dysfunction (e.g., reversible myocardial ischemia).

The distinction between these two pathophysiologic mechanisms is of great practical importance but cannot be achieved based on chest x-ray alone.

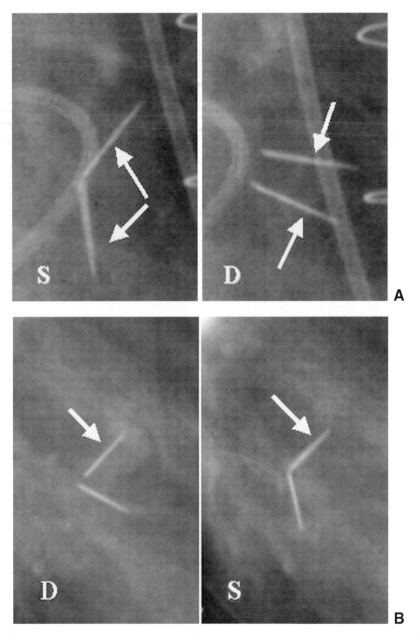

FIGURE 33. *A,* Normal prosthetic valve function by fluoroscopy. Normal St. Jude valve in the mitral position: the two leaflets have a similar range of motion (*arrows*). S = systole, D = diastole. *B,* Prosthetic valve dysfunction by fluoroscopy. Thrombosed St. Jude valve in the mitral position: one of the leaflets has a severely restricted range of motion (*arrows*). S = systole, D = diastole.

248. What are the radiographic findings of the RV in patients with valvular disease?

The most frequent finding involving the RV is dilation, best diagnosed on a lateral film (RV-sternal contact extending cranially beyond the lower third of the distance between the sternal angle and the diaphragm). RV dilation can be secondary to:

- Aortic or mitral disease (either stenosis or insufficiency) with a retrograde transmission of the elevated LA pressure to the pulmonary vasculature and ultimately to the RV
- Right-sided volume overload, as seen in severe TR or left-to-right shunt
- Severe chronic right-sided pressure overload, when RV dilation superimposes on the pre-existing RV hypertrophy.

249. How does valvular disease affect the atria?

The atrial response to valvular disease (stenosis and regurgitation) is usually chamber dilation.

250. State the main causes of atrial dilation.

1. Increases in ventricular diastolic pressure (ventricular failure); this may be due to either pressure overload valve diseases (AS or PS) or to volume overload lesions (AI or PI).

2. Obstructed blood flow from the atrium to the ventricle in diastole (MS or TS).

3. Increased diastolic volume of blood in the atrium (MR or TR, left-to-right shunt).

251. Can LA dilation be diagnosed by chest radiography?

Yes. The type of cardiac chamber enlargement most easily detected by chest x-ray is LA enlargement. There is a good concordance between the radiographic and echocardiographic diagnosis of LA dilation.

252. What are the radiographic signs of LA enlargement?

The LA is assessed best from the lateral view, where it forms the posterior border of the heart. The frontal chest x-ray plays a lesser role in the diagnosis of LA dilation because the only part of that chamber visualized on frontal films is the LA appendage (which forms the lower portion of the middle arch of the left cardiac border).

Early signs
- Bulging of the posterior border of the heart on a lateral film
- Encroachment of the esophagus by the dilated LA, on a barium swallow (lateral film) (see Figure 35B)
- Bronchial splaying > 105° on a frontal chest x-ray

Late stages
- *Double contour* along the right inferior border of the heart on a frontal chest x-ray film. The outer contour belongs to the RA, whereas the inner contour represents the dilated LA.
- *Giant LA,* a sign similar to the double contour but the right border of the heart is represented by the LA, whereas the inner contour reflects the RA. This sign is seen almost exclusively in chronic severe MR. Radiographic criteria for distinguishing a giant LA from lesser LA dilation (double contour) have been described, but in current practice this distinction usually is accomplished by echocardiography.

253. Is the double contour sign seen in MS or MR?

Both because both can be responsible for LA enlargement.

254. List the most frequent radiographic findings associated with LA dilation.

- LV dilation
- Mitral valve calcification, in patients with MS
- RV dilation
- Pulmonary venous hypertension (pulmonary congestion)
- Pulmonary arterial hypertension

255. Can RA dilation be diagnosed by chest x-ray?
Yes. RA dilation is the most difficult heart chamber dilation to diagnose by chest x-ray, however.

256. What are the radiographic signs of RA dilatation?
A bulge in the lower arch of the right cardiac border on a posteroanterior film (see Figure 38). RA dilation is associated most often with RV dilation.

257. List the radiographic findings in patients with MS.
- LA dilation
- Mitral valvular calcification
- Different degrees of pulmonary congestion
- Secondary RA and RV dilation
- Enlargement of the pulmonary trunk (Fig. 34)

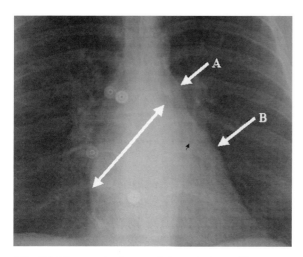

FIGURE 34. Mitral stenosis. PA chest x-ray film in a patient with mitral stenosis. A = convex pulmonary artery trunk; B = prominent LA appendage; double-headed arrow = LA.

258. Which nonvalvular condition mimics MS?
An LA myxoma causing obstruction of LV filling. The only patients in whom chest radiography can make this diagnosis are patients with tumor calcification. The imaging procedures of choice for atrial myxomas are echocardiography and cardiac MRI.

259. Which of the findings listed in question 256 is most specific for MS?
Enlargement of the pulmonary trunk is generally not present in patients with isolated MR or LV failure and helps distinguish MS from these conditions.

260. List the typical radiographic findings in patients with MR.
- LA dilation
- LV dilation
- Different degrees of pulmonary congestion
- Secondary RA and RV dilation and pulmonary trunk dilation (Fig. 35)

261. Does the presence of pulmonary congestion in a patient with MR have the same significance as in a patient with MS?
No. Pulmonary congestion is the result of an increased LA pressure, which has a different pathogenesis and significance in each of these two valvular disorders:
In patients with MS, the increased LA pressure results from the nature of the valvular dis-

ease itself. Pulmonary congestion in these patients indicates the presence of increased pressure gradients across the mitral valve, either as a result of severe anatomic MS or as a result of increased blood flow through the mitral valve (e.g., tachycardia).

In patients with MR, the increased LA pressure is associated with an increase of LV end-diastolic pressure, which generally indicates severe, irreversible myocardial damage as a result of the chronic pressure overload. In these patients, mitral valve replacement or repair usually is indicated.

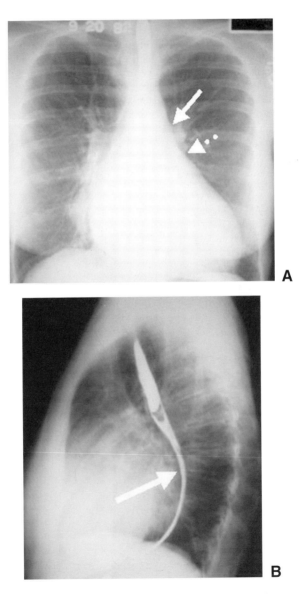

FIGURE 35. *A,* Mitral regurgitation (PA view). In this patient with MR, the frontal chest x-ray film demonstrates pulmonary artery trunk dilation (*continuous arrow*) as well as LA appendage dilation (*dotted arrow*). The normal concavity of the middle arch of the left cardiac border is lost. *B,* Mitral regurgitation (lateral view). A lateral view in the same patient shows a markedly dilated LA (*arrow*), which compresses the esophagus (barium swallow).

262. Is it possible to distinguish between acute and chronic MR by chest radiography?

The hallmark of **acute** MR is the presence of severe pulmonary congestion (pulmonary edema), in the absence of LV or LA enlargement. The chest x-ray must always be interpreted in light of the clinical information; in patients with a radiographic suspicion of acute MR, a clinical course suggestive of MI or bacterial endocarditis corroborates the diagnosis.

Chronic MR is generally associated with lesser degrees of pulmonary congestion, compensatory dilation of the LA (an adaptive mechanism for maintaining a relatively low atrial pressure in the face of severe LA volume overload), and different degrees of LV dilation.

263. Is it possible to establish the etiologic diagnosis of MR based on chest radiography?

Although chest radiography is usually unable to establish an etiologic diagnosis in patients with MR, it may offer indirect clues:

- Enlargement of the LA appendage in rheumatic heart disease
- Skeletal anomalies (e.g., pectus excavatum) in patients with mitral valve prolapse
- Enlargement of the ascending aorta in patients with Marfan's syndrome
- LV aneurysm or myocardial calcification or both in patients with a history of MI
- The *absence* of LV and LA dilation in a patient with pulmonary edema may suggest acute MR, caused by valvular disruption owing to MI or endocarditis

264. What is the diagnostic significance of aortic valvular calcification?

The **presence** of AS—the radiographic diagnosis of AS relies on this sign because isolated LV hypertrophy cannot be diagnosed (Fig. 36)

The **cause** of AS—valvular calcification is characteristic of degenerative AS.

The **severity** of AS—extensive valvular calcification is characteristic of severe AS.

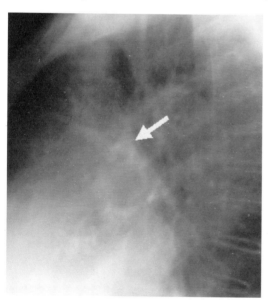

FIGURE 36. Aortic stenosis. Lateral chest x-ray. Note the aortic valvular calcification (*arrow*).

265. What cases of AS typically are missed by chest x-ray?

The radiographic diagnosis of AS is based on the identification of valvular calcification. Consequently the diagnosis is missed in patients who do not show this finding. These include:

- Patients with mild degrees of AS
- Patients with rheumatic AS
- Patients with AS secondary to bicuspid aortic valve

As previously noted, aortic valvular calcification suggests of severe, degenerative AS.

266. Name the typical radiographic findings in patients with AI.
- Tortuosity of the ascending aorta (Fig. 37)
- LV dilation; in its extreme forms, this is termed *cor bovinum*

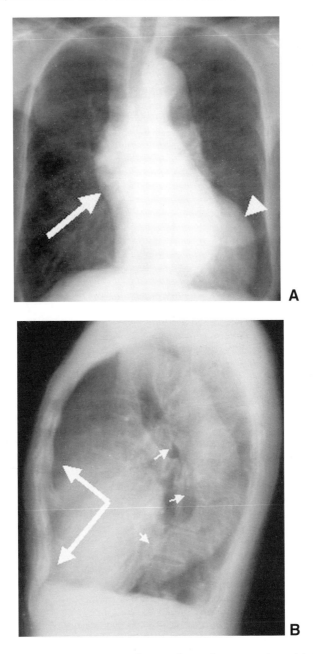

FIGURE 37. *A,* Aortic regurgitation (PA view). The ascending aortic aneurysm (*arrow*) is the underlying cause for AI in this patient. The significantly dilated LV (*arrowhead*) almost touches the left lateral wall of the thorax. *B,* Aortic regurgitation (lateral view). Dilated RV (*long arrows*) and tortuous aorta (*small arrows*) in a patient with aortic regurgitation.

267. Is it possible to establish an etiologic diagnosis of AI based on chest radiography?

In the absence of associated AS and of systemic hypertension, the presence of an enlarged, calcified ascending aorta suggests an aortic root problem as the cause of regurgitation (see Figure 37A). A normal ascending aorta suggests a valvular cause for the AI.

268. Name the radiographic findings in patients with TS.

The typical finding is RA dilation. Rheumatic TS often is associated with involvement of the mitral valve.

269. What are the radiographic findings in TR?

1. **Isolated TR** presents as RV enlargement.

2. In patients with **secondary TR,** chest x-ray detects the findings corresponding to the underlying disorder (MS, LV dilation) (Fig. 38)

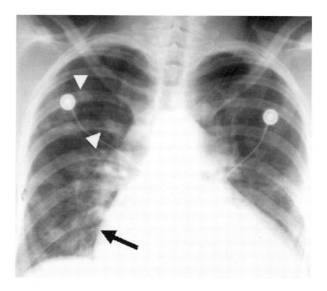

FIGURE 38. Tricuspid regurgitation in an intravenous drug abuser. Note the dilated right atrium (*arrow*) and the multiple septic pulmonary infarcts (*arrowheads*).

270. What are the radiographic findings of PS?

The sole radiologic finding is poststenotic aneurysmal dilation of the pulmonary trunk or the left pulmonary artery (or both) (Fig. 39).

271. Is it possible to differentiate between PS and pulmonic atresia by chest radiography?

Yes. The difference is a normal pulmonary vasculature in most patients with PS.

272. Is it possible to distinguish between idiopathic dilation of the pulmonary artery (IDPA) and poststenotic dilation in a patient with PS?

There are no definitive radiographic criteria to distinguish between these two entities, but:

1. PS is more common then IDPA.

2. Both conditions may be associated with dilation of the pulmonary trunk and of the left pulmonary artery; however, the left pulmonary artery is involved more often in patients with PS, whereas isolated pulmonary trunk involvement suggests IDPA.

273. List the causes of clinically significant PI.
- Secondary to MS (most cases) (Fig. 40)
- Idiopathic (IDPA)

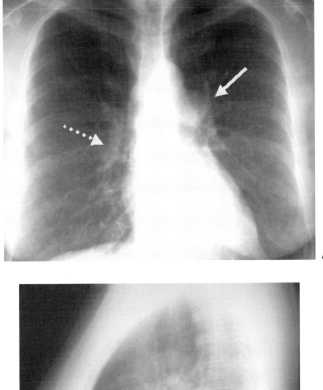

A

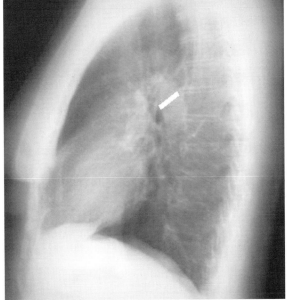

B

FIGURE 39. *A*, Pulmonic stenosis (PA view). Frontal chest x-ray in a patient with pulmonic stenosis. Continuous arrow = dilated pulmonary artery trunk and left main pulmonary artery; dotted arrow = normal right main pulmonary artery. *B*, A lateral view in the same patient confirms the left pulmonary artery dilatation (*white line*).

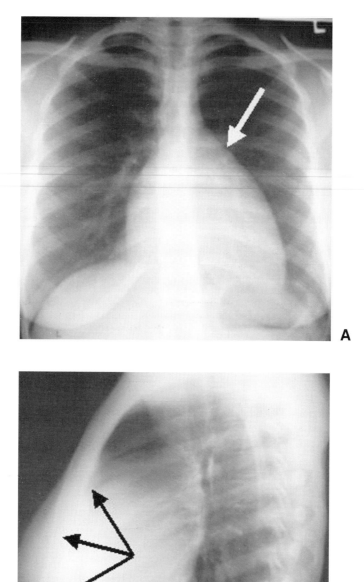

FIGURE 40. *A,* Pulmonic insufficiency (PA view). Note the dilated pulmonary trunk (*arrow*). *B,* Pulmonic insufficiency (lateral view). Note the extensive contact between the right ventricle and the interior wall of the thorax, characteristic of RV dilatation (*arrows*).

274. How can IDPA be distinguished from secondary PI by chest radiography?

The only radiographic findings in **IDPA** are pulmonary trunk and RV dilation. In patients with **secondary PI,** chest x-ray shows pulmonary hypertension and signs pertaining to the underlying condition (e.g., MS).

275. How is the pulmonary circulation affected by valvular heart disease?

The pulmonary vascular markings may be **normal, increased** (pulmonary venous hypertension, also called *pulmonary congestion*) in mitral or aortic disease, or **decreased.** Decreased pulmonary vascular markings may indicate:

- Pulmonary hypertension, the most frequent cause of decreased pulmonary vasculature in adults (this is manifest as peripheral oligemia, also called *vascular pruning*)
- Significant right-to-left shunt (Eisenmenger's syndrome)
- PS, pulmonic atresia, or tricuspid atresia; these conditions are seen most often in the children and may be isolated or part of a complex congenital cardiac syndrome.

276. How are the great arteries affected by the presence of valvular disease?

Radiographic findings include:

- Poststenotic aneurysmal dilation, in case of severe AS or PS
- The presence of a small-caliber pulmonary artery trunk and branches, in the case of pulmonic atresia or significant right-to-left shunt

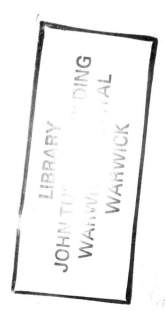

7. PERICARDIAL DISEASE

CARDIAC CATHETERIZATION

Gabriel Adelmann, M.D., and Benjamin Kleiber, M.D.

1. What information is obtained in the catheterization laboratory regarding patients with pericardial disease?

The main information pertains to pericardial constriction or tamponade.

1. **Fluoroscopy,** often performed in the catheterization laboratory (cath lab), may reveal pericardial calcification in patients with constrictive pericarditis.

2. **Assessment of intrapericardial pressures,** rarely performed routinely in clinical practice, may show increased pericardial pressure in patients with massive or rapidly accumulating pericardial effusion.

3. **Catheterization of the heart chambers** may reveal increased intracardiac pressures and different degrees of decrease in the right ventricle (RV) and left ventricle (LV) ejection fraction; additionally, specific patterns of pressure variation may be shown.

2. How is the assessment of pericardial pathology in the cath lab different from that of other cardiac structures (coronary, ventricular, and valvular function)?

The characteristic feature of pericardial assessment resides in its indirect nature. As mentioned in question 1, intrapericardial pressures are only rarely measured; the main value of cardiac catheterization in these patients is in the assessment of the hemodynamic consequences of pericardial effusion or fibrosis (constriction).

3. What is the hallmark of cardiac tamponade on cardiac catheterization?

Pulsus paradoxus, consisting of a decrease of systolic blood pressure > 10 mmHg on inspiration (Fig. 1). The mechanism is as follows: In normal subjects, the decreased intrathoracic pressures generated by inspiration result in increased venous return to the right atrium (RA) and to the RV. The RV accommodates this increase in blood flow by increasing its volume by an outward motion of the RV free wall. In patients with a pericardial effusion, however, the RV is compressed by the intrapericardial fluid and can expand only by distention of the interventricular septum. This moves the septum toward the LV. The LV cavity decreases in inspiration, resulting in a decreased LV stroke volume and a consequent decrease in systolic blood pressure.

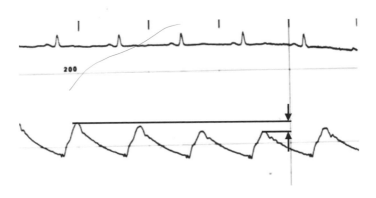

FIGURE 1. Pulsus paradoxus. Peak systolic pressure drop > 10 mmHg in inspiration, in a patient with pericardial tamponade.

4. How is pulsus paradoxus observed in the intensive care unit?

Many patients admitted to the intensive care unit, especially patients with hemodynamic instability, have an arterial catheter installed, which offers on-line invasive measurement of the systemic blood pressure. By observation of either the pressure curves or the actual blood pressure values, a decrease in systolic blood pressure > 10 mmHg in inspiration can be noted.

5. Is pulsus paradoxus specific for cardiac tamponade?

No. The pathophysiologic mechanism of pulsus paradoxus also occurs in patients with constrictive pericarditis or severe chronic obstructive pulmonary disease. The association of pulsus paradoxus and pericardial effusion (especially if large or rapidly accumulating) is highly suggestive for cardiac tamponade.

6. What is the basic pathophysiologic mechanism of hemodynamic disturbances in patients with constrictive pericarditis?

The heart is encased in a rigid "shell" (the calcified pericardium). The normal ventricular diastolic volume increase is severely restricted, leading to a rapid equalization of the atrial and ventricular pressure in diastole. The major part of the ventricular diastolic filling is accomplished at the beginning of diastole, with an almost absent transtricuspid and transmitral flow beyond that point.

7. Describe the catheterization findings in a patient with constrictive pericarditis.

Fluoroscopy, often performed before the invasive assessment of the heart cavities and arteries, may reveal pericardial calcification in patients with constrictive pericarditis. Pericardial calcification is neither sensitive nor specific for this condition.

Hemodynamic measurements reveal:

- An equalization of the diastolic pressures in the four heart chambers
- Increased diastolic pressures in the heart cavities
- Decreased cardiac output
- A particular pattern of LV pressure variation in diastole

The pattern consists of an initial decrease in pressure (owing to the rapid distention of the LV in the initial phase of diastole, corresponding to an increased rate of filling from the LA), followed by a rapid increase in LV pressure, which "plateaus" by the end of early diastole and subsequently remains unchanged until the onset of the next systole. This pattern is termed *dip-and-plateau* (Fig. 2) or, because of its particular graphic aspect, the *square root* sign. (In normal subjects, there is a gradual increase in LV chamber pressure throughout diastole, and the LV end-diastolic pressure is only slightly greater than 0).

8. What is the echocardiography parallel of the dip-and-plateau sign?

Although a particular motion pattern of the LV free wall reproducing the dip-and-plateau sign may be observed on an M-mode tracing, the most important echocardiography parallel to the invasive findings is a tall E wave and an almost absent A wave, reflecting the fact that the near-totality of LV filling is completed in early diastole.

9. What is the Kussmaul sign, and when is it seen?

In normal subjects, inspiration produces a decrease in the intrathoracic pressure, with a consequent decrease in the central venous pressure. The normal RV is able to distend sufficiently to accommodate this increased blood flow, resulting in a decrease in central venous pressure in inspiration. In patients with constrictive pericarditis, the *restrained* RV is unable to handle the increased venous return, a fact resulting in an accentuation in the neck vein congestion in these patients. The Kussmaul sign, an increased jugular venous distention with respiration, is relatively specific to constrictive pericarditis (Fig. 3).

10. State the finding on the right heart chamber pressure tracing when there is a Kussmaul sign.

The expression of the Kussmaul sign on a Swan-Ganz catheter tracing consists of an increase in RA pressure during inspiration.

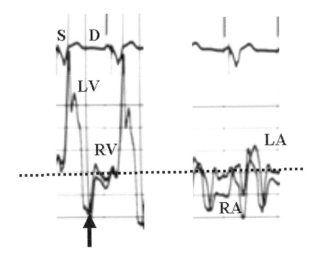

FIGURE 2. Constrictive pericarditis: "dip-and-plateau." In patients with constrictive pericarditis, the early diastolic LV distention (LV pressure decrease) stops abruptly, and there is virtually no ventricular filling in mid- and late diastole. This results in a classical "dip-and-plateau" configuration (*arrow*). There is diastolic pressure equalization in the four heart chambers (*horizontal line*). S = systole, D = diastole.

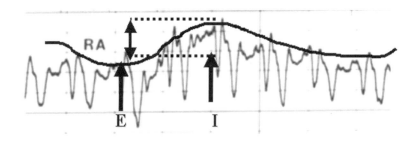

FIGURE 3. Constrictive pericarditis: Kussmaul's sign. In constrictive pericarditis, peak right atrial (RA) pressure rises with inspiration (*double-headed arrow*). This is observed clinically as an inspiratory rise in jugular venous pressure. E = expiration, I = inspiration.

11. Define the fluid challenge test in the diagnosis of constrictive pericarditis.

The hallmark hemodynamic findings of constrictive pericarditis (an equalization of the elevated pressures in the four heart chambers) can be absent in dehydrated patients. The rapid infusion of 100–200 mL of saline elicits these typical findings, helping to differentiate constrictive pericarditis from restrictive cardiomyopathy (in the latter setting, even after fluid challenge, the LA pressure is greater by at least 5 mmHg than the RA pressure).

12. Besides the fluid challenge test, how can right heart catheterization help with the differentiation of constrictive pericarditis from restrictive cardiomyopathy?

In patients in whom neither echocardiography nor invasive pressure measurement is able to differentiate between constrictive pericarditis and restrictive cardiomyopathy, the demonstration of histologic findings typical of sarcoidosis, amyloidosis, or other infiltrative diseases by myocardial biopsy of the RV may establish the diagnosis. Myocardial biopsy is carried out by right heart catheterization.

ECHOCARDIOGRAPHY

Gabriel Adelmann, M.D., Steven A. Goldstein, M.D., and Neil J. Weissman, M.D.

13. Name the two layers of the pericardium.
The **visceral pericardium,** which is continuous with the epicardium, and the **parietal pericardium.**

14. What is the *transverse sinus*?
The parietal and visceral layers of the pericardium extend a short distance superiorly along the great vessels (aorta and pulmonary artery) and meet to close the "ends of the pericardial sac." This small pocket of pericardium is termed the *transverse sinus.* This structure can harbor small effusions, which occasionally are fibrinous and can masquerade as a periaortic abscess or as a thrombosed left main coronary artery (Fig. 4).

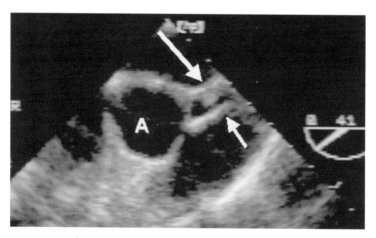

FIGURE 4. Transverse sinus (*small arrow*) with a thrombus within (*large arrow*) at the level of LMCA (TEE). The transverse sinus is distinguished from LMCA by its larger diameter. A = aorta.

15. What is the normal amount of pericardial fluid?
The space between the two layers of pericardium is filled with pericardial fluid that lubricates the surface of the heart so that motion can occur without friction or damage to the epicardial surface. Normally the pericardial sac contains 20–50 mL of clear serous fluid. Usually this small amount of fluid either is not detectable by two-dimensional echocardiography or is seen as a thin posterior echo-free space present only in systole. There are no established criteria for distinguishing normal pericardial fluid from a small pericardial effusion.

16. Name the echocardiography signs of pericarditis.
The echocardiography hallmark of pericarditis is **pericardial effusion,** seen as an echo-free space that first accumulates behind the LV posterior wall (as a result of gravity) and, in later stages, surrounds the heart.

17. Does the absence of a pericardial effusion on two-dimensional echocardiography exclude the diagnosis of pericarditis?
No. Patients with pericarditis may have no effusion, effusion of any size (small, moderate, or large), or just pericardial thickening (a finding difficult to diagnose by echocardiography). Peri-

carditis is a clinical diagnosis that cannot be made independently by echocardiography. The presence of pericardial effusion has a limited sensitivity for the diagnosis of pericarditis.

18. Does the presence of pericardial effusion imply the presence of pericarditis?

No. Pericardial effusion may be present as a result of a systemic disease (e.g., hypoalbuminemia, lymphatic blockage caused by malignancy, lupus), in the absence of pericardial inflammation. The presence of pericardial effusion has a limited specificity for the diagnosis of pericarditis.

19. What is the echocardiographic grading of the severity of pericarditis?

Small pericardial effusion—posterior only (i.e., behind the LV free wall), usually ≤ 1 cm in width

Moderate pericardial effusion—anterior and posterior (i.e., surrounding the heart), usually ≤ 2 cm in width

Large pericardial effusion—anterior and posterior, ≥ 2 cm in width (Fig. 5)

The size and location of a pericardial effusion are important for assessing the risk of cardiac tamponade and planning the therapeutic strategy; large, anterior effusions are readily accessible to pericardiocentesis.

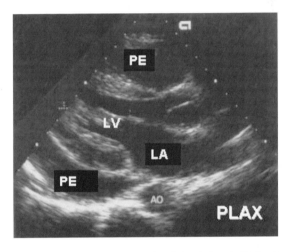

FIGURE 5. Echocardiographic distinction between pericardial and pleural effusion. Large pericardial effusion (PE) both anterior and posterior to the left ventricle (LV). LA = left atrium, Ao = aorta.

20. Can echocardiography establish the cause of pericardial effusion?

No. The character of a pericardial effusion (i.e., serous, serosanguineous, hemorrhagic, chylous, or purulent) cannot be diagnosed reliably by the echocardiography appearance. Certain characteristics of the fluid, interpreted in light of the patient's historical and clinical data, may offer clues as to the nature of the fluid (e.g., the presence of clot in the pericardial effusion in a hypotensive patient after percutaneous transluminal coronary angioplasty suggests coronary perforation and bloody pericardial effusion).

21. List some conditions that may simulate pericardial effusion echocardiographically.

- Epicardial fat (the most common condition mimicking pericardial effusion)
- Anterior mediastinal tumors
- Ascites
- Pleural effusions

22. What is the main echocardiography criterion to differentiate anterior epicardial fat from anterior pericardial effusion?

Both conditions present as an anterior echo-free space. The main *difference* is that pericardial effusion first accumulates posteriorly, owing to gravity. Pericardial fat often has some subtle echos within it because of fibrous material within the fat.

An isolated anterior echo-free space usually represents epicardial fat, and an isolated posterior echo-free space is usually a pericardial effusion. A combined anterior and posterior echo-free space is usually a pericardial effusion with or without associated epicardial fat. Nothing in medicine is absolute, however, and a loculated anterior pericardial effusion may not have an associate posterior effusion. Also, rarely, posterior epicardial fat deposition can occur either in isolation or associated with anterior fat.

23. Is the location of an echo-free space the only echocardiography criterion for differentiation of epicardial fat from pericardial effusion?

No. Fat is slightly more echogenic or "granular" than fluid and usually has some echoes within it, whereas fluid is usually black. (This distinction is not absolute because occasionally fibrinous pericardial effusion also may have a speckled appearance.)

24. What is the definitive imaging modality for differentiation of epicardial fat from pericardial effusion?

Magnetic resonance imaging (MRI).

25. Which echocardiography findings differentiate a pericardial effusion from an anterior mediastinal tumor?

Anterior mediastinal tumors are usually more echo-dense than either free fluid or fat. Occasionally, they may appear relatively echo-free because of necrotic centers.

26. How can pericardial effusion be distinguished from pleural effusion echocardiographically?

The relation between the echo-free space and the descending thoracic aorta is helpful for distinguishing pericardial versus left pleural effusion. Pericardial effusion lies anterior to the descending thoracic aorta (see Figure 5). This is noted best in a parasternal long-axis view at the level of the LA and LV. Pleural effusion lies posterior, lateral, or posterolateral to the descending aorta.

Another view that is occasionally helpful is the apical four-chamber view. When fluid is seen adjacent to the RA in this view but not seen in any other imaging plane, the fluid is most likely pleural.

27. Name the echocardiography criteria for differentiation of pericardial effusion from ascites.

Ascites may appear as an echo-free space anterior to the heart in a subcostal view and can be mistaken for a loculated pericardial effusion. Ascites can be differentiated from pericardial effusion by its contour (deviates away from the heart) and by its relation to the liver. Ascites is not seen "around" the heart from the parasternal images (high up on the chest wall).

28. What is cardiac tamponade?

The elevation of pericardium fluid pressure to values sufficient to restrict cardiac filling.

29. What is the spectrum of severity of cardiac tamponade?

Cardiac tamponade can range from early, asymptomatic hemodynamic effects to severe cardiac compression and severely decreased cardiac output (circulatory collapse).

30. Discuss the pathophysiology of low cardiac output in patients with cardiac tamponade.

Abnormal ventricular filling results in a low cardiac output despite a (generally) normal LV contractility. Abnormal filling is caused by accumulation of fluid in the pericardium and increased intrapericardial pressure; the pericardial fluid not only interferes with diastolic expansion of the ventricles, but also compresses both atria and the RV (the thick LV generally is not directly affected). The LV and RV free walls are limited in their excursion by the pericardial effusion so that any change in volume of one ventricle forcibly affects the other ventricle by deviating the septum. During inspiration, blood rushes into the RV, causing RV expansion and deviation of the septum toward the LV and a decrease of LV volume. This results in "respiratory variation" of mitral and tricuspid flow in tamponade and respiratory changes in systemic blood pressure (pulsus paradoxus).

31. List the factors that determine whether a pericardial effusion will cause tamponade.

1. Amount of fluid (the greater the amount of fluid, the higher the pressure and the higher the chance of tamponade).

2. Rate of fluid accumulation. Significant increases in intrapericardial pressure may occur with rapid accumulation of a relatively small amount of fluid (e.g., in the catheterization laboratory, after laceration of an artery).

3. Pericardial distensibility (the greater the capacity of the pericardium to accommodate the effusion, the lower the chance that the effusion significantly will compress the heart).

32. List the most important echocardiography signs suggesting cardiac tamponade.

1. Two-dimensional
   RA invagination
   RV diastolic invagination
   Decreased collapsibility of the inferior vena cava (IVC)
2. Doppler
   Increased respiratory variation of the mitral and tricuspid diastolic blood flow
3. M-mode
   Evidence of RA and RV compression in diastole
   Evidence of decreased IVC collapsibility

33. Is RA invagination a good criterion to use for the diagnosis of cardiac tamponade?

RA compression is a fairly sensitive (but nonspecific) echocardiography sign of cardiac tamponade. This is one of the first signs because the RA is usually the lowest pressure chamber in the heart and it is the easiest to be compressed.

34. Is RA compression a specific sign for cardiac tamponade?

No. Invagination ("compression") of the RA wall is indirect evidence of elevated intrapericardial pressure and a transient reversal of the normal gradient between the RA and the intrapericardial space. Although this situation does occur with cardiac tamponade, it has a low specificity, and slight RA invagination is seen occasionally with hemodynamically insignificant effusions (e.g., with dehydration and a low RA pressure of almost 0). An additional diagnostic element is the duration of RA invagination: The longer this duration relative to the cardiac cycle length, the more likely the diagnosis. Atrial compression for longer than one third of the cardiac cycle has a high specificity for tamponade. Careful frame-by-frame analysis is needed for this evaluation.

35. What is the value of RV diastolic invagination in the echocardiographic diagnosis of cardiac tamponade?

RV diastolic invagination ("collapse") occurs when intrapericardial pressure exceeds RV diastolic pressure. This sign is less sensitive but more specific than RA compression for the diagnosis of tamponade (Fig. 6).

36. What is the value of IVC collapsibility assessment in the echocardiography diagnosis of tamponade?

Normally the IVC diameter decreases by approximately 50% with inspiration. Absence of IVC collapsibility indicates elevated RA pressure, nearly always present with tamponade. Increased RA pressure is not specific for tamponade, however, and may be present in a variety of conditions.

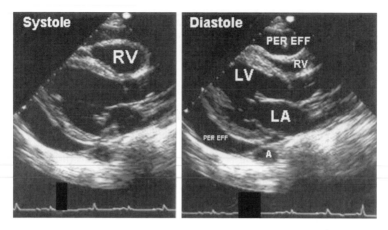

FIGURE 6. Cardiac tamponade. Diastolic collapse of the right ventricular free wall (RV). RA = right atrium; LV = left ventricle; LA = left atrium; A = aorta; PER EF = pericardial effusion.

37. Does the presence of normal IVC collapsibility rule out the diagnosis of tamponade?

No. "Low-pressure" tamponade in a volume-depleted patient can be associated with normal IVC diameter decrease with inspiration. If volume depletion is not a possibility, the presence of normal IVC collapsibility virtually rules out the diagnosis of tamponade.

38. What is respiratory variation of mitral and tricuspid blood flow?

With significant respiratory variation, there is a >25% increase in the mitral E-wave velocity with expiration and a > 40% increase in the tricuspid E wave velocity with inspiration.

39. One of the electrocardiography signs in patients with large pericardial effusions is electrical alternans, consisting of a cyclic increase and decrease in the height of the R wave. What is the corresponding echocardiographic sign?

In these patients, the heart has a "swinging motion" (i.e., has different positions in the fluid-filled pericardial sac at different points in time, such as at the end of two consecutive systoles). The swinging motion of the heart results in a different distance between the heart and the electrocardiogram electrodes, with consequent differences in the recorded amplitudes of the R waves.

40. What is echocardiography-guided pericardiocentesis?

Echocardiography can be used to determine the optimal site and direction of pericardiocentesis needle. The information provided by echocardiography in this setting includes:

- The location where pericardial effusion is the largest and the closest to the transducer
- Confirmation of the intrapericardial location of the needle by instillation of agitated saline, which can be identified by echocardiography (Fig. 7)

41. Describe the pathophysiologic changes in patients with constrictive pericarditis.

The heart is encased in a rigid pericardium, and as a result LV filling occurs almost exclusively at the beginning of diastole. At the end of this rapid filling period, the LV is limited in its excursion by the rigid pericardium so that there is virtually no ventricular filling beyond the first part of diastole. The main resultant hemodynamic disturbances are:

- Rapid increase in LV pressure at the beginning of diastole
- Rapid posterior movement of the LV free wall in early diastole, followed by the virtual absence of further ventricular expansion beyond that point
- Rapid, characteristic anterior motion of the interventricular septum in early diastole
- High diastolic pressure, which is virtually equal in all four heart chambers

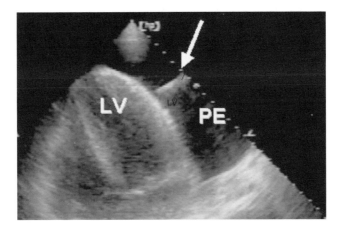

FIGURE 7. Echo-guided pericardiocentesis. Pericardiocentesis needle (*arrow*). PE = pericardial effusion; LV = left ventricle.

42. Summarize the main echocardiography findings in constrictive pericarditis.
Two-dimensional findings (which often can be observed on the M-mode study):
- Pericardial thickening
- Abnormal motion of the interventricular septum
- Diastolic flattening of LV posterior wall
- Dilated IVC, which lacks normal inspiratory collapse

The Doppler findings include respiratory variation of the mitral and tricuspid blood flow, similar to that seen in pericardial tamponade.

43. Can echocardiography of pericardial thickening reliably establish or rule out constrictive pericarditis?
No. This is due to several factors:

1. Echocardiography cannot reliably quantitate pericardial thickness: Echocardiography gain adjustments can erroneously overestimate- or underestimate pericardial thickness.

2. Pericardial thickening may involve different regions around the heart, some of them isolated and not readily accessible to echocardiography.

3. Pericardial thickening and constriction are not always directly related. Constriction can occur with only mild thickening of the pericardium.

44. Name the imaging methods of choice for the diagnosis of pericardial thickening.
MRI or computed tomography (CT).

45. How do the echocardiography signs of constrictive pericarditis and cardiac tamponade compare?
The **similarity** consists of an abnormal ventricular filling caused by extrinsic compression of the heart. The **difference** is that tamponade usually impairs diastolic filling throughout diastole, whereas constriction allows early diastolic filling with abrupt termination of filling in mid diastole. The abrupt posterior motion of the LV posterior wall in early diastole with subsequent leveling off, represents the *dip-and-plateau* or the *square root* sign of constrictive pericarditis. This sign is absent in patients with tamponade.

46. What is the "septal bounce" of constrictive pericarditis?
This is one of several echocardiography signs corresponding to the typical abnormal filling pattern of constrictive pericarditis. In these patients, there is rapid early filling of the LV, owing

to the high LA pressure. The expansion of the LV is stopped abruptly when the limits of the rigid pericardium are reached, however, and a "septal bounce" is seen at that point (Fig. 8).

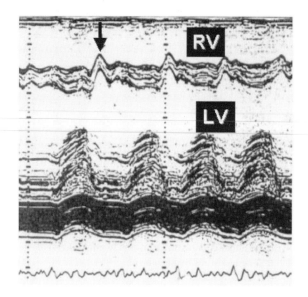

FIGURE 8. M mode echo demonstrating septal "bounce" (*arrow*) in constrictive pericarditis. LV = left ventricle, RV = right ventricle.

47. What is the significance of a dilated, noncollapsible IVC in a patient with constrictive pericarditis?

This sign reflects an increase pressured in the right heart chambers and is similar to what is seen in cardiac tamponade.

48. What should always be listed in the differential diagnosis when considering constrictive pericarditis?

Constrictive pericarditis must be distinguished from restrictive cardiomyopathy. This differential diagnosis is discussed in Chapter 3. Constrictive pericarditis usually has respiratory variation in Doppler patterns, and cardiomyopathy does not. Occasionally, it is impossible to distinguish between the two conditions by imaging methods (echocardiography, MRI, cardiac catheterization), and myocardial biopsy is indicated.

49. Name the common echocardiography signs of constrictive pericarditis and cardiac tamponade.

1. Respiratory variation of the mitral and tricuspid blood flow
2. Dilated, noncollapsible IVC

These findings reflect the similar pathogenesis of the two conditions, which involves limitation of the diastolic ventricular expansion owing to pericardial pathology.

50. What are intrapericardial strands?

Fibrinous and hemorrhagic pericarditis may produce intrapericardial strands extending from the visceral to the parietal pericardium. These typically appear as a series of linear echoes of varying thickness that divide the pericardial space into a series of compartments (Fig. 9). Sometimes, these strands do not cross the pericardial space completely,and their free ends undulate with cardiac motion. The significance of intrapericardial strands is that they often loculate the pericardial fluid. In such instances, pericardiocentesis may fail to drain an effusion completely, and surgery may be required.

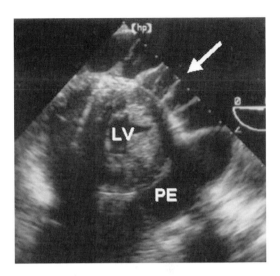

FIGURE 9. Intrapericardial "strands" (*arrow*). PE = pericardial effusion; LV = left ventricle.

51. Which tumors most commonly metastasize to the heart and pericardium?

Lung, breast, lymphoma, leukemia, melanoma, and sarcoma. Lung and breast are the most common but that is because these are common cancers. Lymphoma, leukemia, and melanoma have the greatest propensity to migrate to the pericardium. Nevertheless, all malignant neoplasms have the potential to metastasize to the heart and pericardium.

52. What is the echocardiography hallmark of metastatic involvement of the pericardium?

Pericardial effusion. Occasionally an intrapericardial mass may be visualized on two-dimensional echocardiography.

53. How do metastatic tumors cause pericardial effusion?

Most metastatic (secondary) tumors of the heart invade the visceral pericardium. Direct invasion of the pericardium with subsequent exudation of fluid is the most common mechanism. Less common mechanisms include lymphatic obstruction and malnutrition leading to hypoalbuminemia.

MAGNETIC RESONANCE IMAGING

Gabriel Adelmann, M.D., and Anthon R. Fuisz, M.D.

54. How can the pericardium be visualized by MRI?

The normal pericardium is identified as the space between the epicardial and the pericardial fat. The thickness of this space is usually 1–2 mm and 4 mm in some normal subjects.

55. Name an imaging technique other than MRI in which demonstration of the pericardial space is based on visualizing the epicardial and pericardial fat.

A classic x-ray sign of pericardial effusion is the so-called **Oreo cookie sign** (see Figure 12), which visualizes the pericardial space based on visualization of epicardial and pericardial fat. The Oreo cookie sign, however:

- Shows pericardial **effusion,** not the normal pericardium
- Visualizes the pericardial effusion as a **white space between two black layers,** whereas MRI visualizes the normal pericardium as a black space between two white layers (on the usual T1-weighted images)

56. Can MRI visualize pericardial effusion?

MRI is a sensitive technique for detection of pericardial effusion and of its hemodynamic complications (cardiac tamponade). The pericardial fluid appears as either black or white, depending on the MRI technique being used (Fig. 10).

57. How does MRI compare with echocardiography in the diagnosis of pericardial effusion?

MRI can offer elements of information not readily available by echocardiography:

* Easy visualization of loculated pericardial effusion
* Differentiation of pericardial exudates and hemorrhage from pericardial transudates, based on the specific MRI properties of proteinaceous material
* Differentiation of pericardial effusion from epicardial fat

58. List the MRI characteristics of pericardial involvement in a malignant process.

* Pericardial mass
* Pericardial thickening
* Local nodular pericardial lesions
* Hemorrhagic pericardial effusion

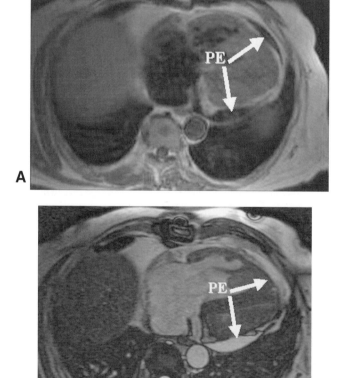

FIGURE 10. Pericardial effusion can be visualized in either black (*A*) or white (*B*), depending on the technique being used. The possibility to display the pericardial material in different colors by different techniques indicates that one is dealing with pericardial effusion, as opposed to pericardial thickening.

59. What is the role of MRI in the diagnosis of pericardial effusion?

Although echocardiography is the imaging modality of choice because if its portability and cost, MRI is indicated for the diagnosis of complex pericardial effusion (especially if loculated) and for the differentiation of pericardial effusion from epicardial fat.

60. What are the MRI signs of constrictive pericarditis?

The great value of MRI in the diagnosis of constrictive pericarditis is the accurate assessment of pericardial thickness. Pericardial thickness > 4 mm (Fig. 11) is strong circumstantial evidence in favor of the diagnosis of constrictive pericarditis over that of restrictive cardiomyopathy. Radiofrequency tagging can show areas of adhesion between the pericardium and epicardium. Newer MRI techniques allow complex hemodynamic evaluation of patients with suspected constrictive pericarditis.

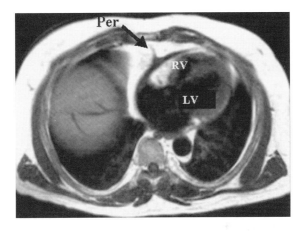

FIGURE 11. Constrictive pericarditis. Thick pericardium (*arrow*). Other MR images in the same patient demonstrated adhesion of the pericardium to the RV myocardium and abnormal interventricular septal motion. The diagnosis was confirmed at surgery.

61. Is pericardial thickening mostly diffuse or localized?

Pericardial thickening most often is localized over the area of the RV. In other patients, it can be localized to a discrete area of the cardiac surface (i.e., the atrioventricular groove).

62. Does the absence of pericardial thickening rule out constrictive pericarditis?

No. Pericardial thickening may be discrete or localized over a small area, in which case it may be missed by MRI. The absence of demonstrable pericardial thickening, even by high-resolution imaging such as cardiac MRI, does not rule out constrictive pericarditis but makes it much less likely.

63. Does the presence of pericardium thickening imply the presence of constrictive pericarditis?

No. Pericardial thickening is a nonspecific finding, sometimes (although infrequently) seen in patients with prior cardiac surgery who do not have clinical evidence of constriction. Hemodynamic assessment is an essential component of the diagnosis of constrictive pericarditis. The hemodynamic changes themselves are not diagnostic, and consequently the diagnosis is based on a combination of anatomic and hemodynamic findings.

64. Name one important feature of constrictive pericarditis easily diagnosed by x-ray methods (radiography, CT) but typically not visualized by MRI.

Pericardial calcification.

65. How does MRI compare with CT in the diagnosis of constrictive pericarditis?

The advantage of MRI over CT is the ability to obtain images in multiple planes (versus the typical vertical slices of a CT study) and of simultaneously assessing LV function. Newer CT techniques (external-beam CT) may provide accurate three-dimensional visualization of the cardiac structures. MRI may be better than CT for measuring the thickness of a noncalcified pericardium.

The advantage of CT over MRI is the ability to visualize pericardial calcification, a common finding with constrictive pericarditis.

66. Describe the anatomic characteristics of congenital absence of the pericardium.

Congenital absence of the pericardium may be complete or partial. Partial left-sided absence of the pericardium is the most frequent variant and usually benign. Patients with partial absence of the left side of the pericardium are, however, at risk for herniation of the atria or the ventricles (or both) through the pericardial defect, a potentially lethal complication.

67. Is congenital absence of the pericardium associated with other cardiac anomalies?

In 3% of patients, partial congenital pericardial defect is associated with atrial septal defect, patent ductus arteriosus, or mitral valve abnormalities.

68. What is the role of MRI in the diagnosis of congenital absence of the pericardium?

MRI is ideally suited for:
- Direct identification of the anomaly
- Identification of leftward protrusion of the LA appendage or of the main pulmonary artery
- Demonstration of lung tissue between the aorta and the pulmonary artery and between the base of the heart and the left hemidiaphragm.
- Identification of any associated cardiac anomalies
- Identification of cardiac herniation through the pericardial defect

69. What are pericardial cysts?

Benign lesions resulting from islands of pericardial tissue left behind ("pinched off") during the different phases of embryogenesis.

70. List the MRI characteristics of pericardial cysts.
- Have well-defined borders
- Have water-density contents unless they are hemorrhagic (with blood-density contents)
- Are located in the right cardiophrenic angle, contiguous to the normal pericardium.
- Are round or ovoid-shaped

71. What is the role of cardiac MRI in the diagnosis of pericardial cysts?

MRI and cardiac CT are the imaging procedures of choice for the diagnosis of pericardial cysts.

CHEST X-RAY

Gabriel Adelmann, M.D., Rina Sternlieb, M.D., Matthew R. Brewer, M.D., and Curtis E. Green, M.D.

72. List the main pericardial conditions that can be diagnosed by chest radiography.
- Pericardial effusion
- Pericardial cysts
- Pericardial calcification
- Congenital pericardial defects

73. What is the most frequent pericardial condition shown by chest x-ray?

Pericardial effusion, a common cause of cardiomegaly.

74. What is the role of chest radiography in the diagnosis of pericardial effusion?

Chest radiography has a low sensitivity and specificity for this diagnosis, and more sophisticated imaging procedures, such as echocardiography or MRI, are the diagnostic procedures of choice.

75. How can pericardial effusion be differentiated from LV enlargement as the cause of cardiomegaly?

Typical findings associated with pericardial effusion include:

1. **Cardiomegaly in the absence of pulmonary venous congestion:** This finding must be differentiated from congestive heart failure treated with diuretics, when pulmonary congestion has resolved. The clinical setting is important for making this distinction (patients with a history of chest trauma, recent cardiac surgery, chronic renal failure on dialysis, collagen-vascular disease, and cancer as well as patients after radiation therapy are prone to pericardial effusion).

2. The **Oreo cookie sign:** In patients with pericardial effusion, the radioopaque pericardial fluid is bordered on either side by echo-dense pericardial fat (Fig. 12).

3. A **posterior bulge** of the cardiac silhouette on a lateral film forms an obtuse angle with the left hemidiaphragm.

4. The **double density sign** consists of a second, much weaker cardiac contour seen beyond the heart shadow and represents the pericardial effusion (in the absence of significant amounts of blood, the effusion fluid has a significantly lower radioopacity than the heart itself).

5. The **water bottle** sign is a globular shape of the heart visible on upright films, with a blunted left heart border.

6. **Enlarged azygos vein.**

7. **Enlarged venae cavae.**

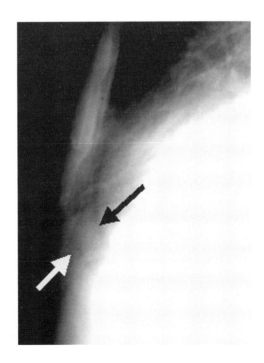

FIGURE 12. The "Oreo cookie" sign in a patient with pericardial effusion. Note the dark-light-dark appearance, representing pericardial fluid bordered on either side by epicardial fat.

76. Can chest radiography provide an etiologic diagnosis of pericardial effusion?

Chest radiography is generally unable to provide significant information regarding the underlying cause of pericardial effusion. Examination of the lung fields may offer occasional diagnostic clues. The presence of pulmonary tumor or infection may point to a malignant or infectious cause of the pericardial effusion. Similarly the presence of ectopic calcification may suggest chronic renal failure as the underlying disorder.

77. What is the role of chest radiography in the diagnosis of cardiac tamponade?

Chest radiography is one of the least sensitive methods for diagnosing cardiac tamponade. Massive pericardial effusion is more prone to lead to tamponade, but most massive effusions are not associated with tamponade physiology. Cardiac tamponade can be caused by small amounts of pericardial fluid, if it accumulates rapidly.

78. Name the radiographic finding with malignant infiltration into the pericardium.

Pericardial effusion.

79. What is the radiographic finding with a pericardial cyst?

Pericardial cysts are usually seen as space-occupying lesions in the cardiophrenic angles. Their radiodensity is intermediate between that of the heart and the surrounding lung tissue. Their main importance lies in the necessity to distinguish them from mediastinal tumor. The imaging procedures of choice are CT and MRI.

80. How can pericardial and myocardial calcification be differentiated by chest radiography?

Pericardial calcification:

- Has a typical crescentic shape, usually following the contour of the heart over several centimeters (as opposed to myocardial calcification, which usually consists of pinpoint speckling) (Fig. 13)
- Is often associated with constrictive pericarditis; radiographic signs of potential predisposing conditions (sternotomy or clips after coronary artery bypass graft surgery, pulmonary tuberculosis) may help with the differentiation from myocardial calcification
- Is often seen in the area of the right heart chambers, a finding practically never present with myocardial calcification

81. My patient has unexplained right heart failure. On reviewing her chest x-ray, I am concerned about the possible presence of pericardial calcification. Do I need to clarify this issue further?

Yes. The concern about finding pericardial calcification is its possible association with constrictive pericarditis; this may be the occult cause of the patient's symptoms. CT scan is the procedure of choice to diagnose pericardial calcification. Echocardiography would be indicated for further assessment of the RV size and function and common causes of RV failure, such as LV dysfunction.

82. What are the chest x-ray findings in patients with pericardial defects?

Pericardial defects can be either left-sided or right-sided and partial or complete.

Partial left-sided pericardial defect is the typical form and characteristically causes an isolated prominence of the LA appendage and pulmonary trunk (Fig. 14). It is important to be alert to the possibility of this malformation to avoid a false diagnosis of pulmonary hypertension (which otherwise might be suggested by the bulge in the middle arch of the left cardiac border).

Complete defects cause a shift of the heart shadow to be affected side.

The diagnostic procedure of choice in the case of pericardial defects is MRI.

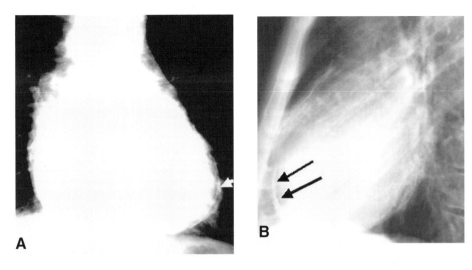

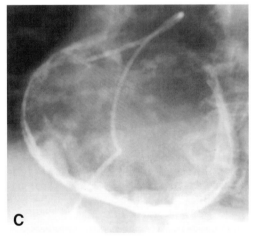

FIGURE 13. Pericardial calcification. *A,* PA view (*arrow*). *B,* Lateral view. Crescent-shaped linear pericardial calcification (*arrow*). *C,* Constrictive pericarditis. Extensive pericardial calcification, enclosing the heart in a rigid "shell."

FIGURE 14. Congenital pericardial defect. Prominent pulmonary artery trunk (*continuous arrow*) and left atrial appendage (*dotted arrow*) in a patient with congenital pericardial defect.

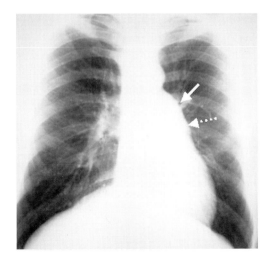

8. CARDIAC MASSES

CARDIAC CATHETERIZATION

Benjamin Kleiber, M.D., and Gabriel Adelmann, M.D.

1. What information can be obtained by cardiac catheterization concerning intracardiac masses?
- The **presence** of a tumor in the heart chambers
- The **vascular or nonvascular nature** of the tumor
- The **coronary anatomy** in surgical candidates

2. How can the presence of a cardiac tumor be identified in the catheterization laboratory?
- By **fluoroscopy** (calcified tumors)
- By **injection of contrast material** into the left and right **cardiac chambers,** which helps identify a space-occupying lesion (Fig. 1)
- By **coronary angiography,** in the case of vascular tumors, which are supplied with blood by the epicardial coronary arteries; in these patients, an unexpected capillary territory corresponding to the tumor (*tumor blush*) can be identified by intracoronary injection of contrast material

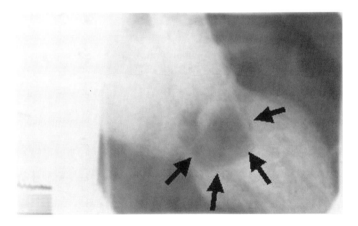

FIGURE 1. Intracardiac tumor, manifesting as a "filling defect,"—i.e., a nonopacified area surrounded by contrast (*arrows*).

3. Explain the practical importance of identifying tumor blush.

This finding indicates the vascular (versus cystic or thrombotic) nature of a cardiac space-occupying lesion. In certain cases, the coronary branch supplying the tumor may be coiled, severing the vascular supply, which results in partial or total tumor necrosis. Coiling therapy may lead to significant shrinkage of a previously inoperable tumor and make it amenable to surgical excision.

4. Is it possible to distinguish between a benign and a malignant cardiac tumor, based on cardiac catheterization?

Although it is occasionally possible to determine the malignant nature of a tumor based on its invasive character and irregular borders, cardiac catheterization is neither sensitive nor specific for identification or histologic characterization of cardiac tumors.

5. How important is coronary catheterization in the diagnosis and management of cardiac tumors?

In occasional patients, a cardiac tumor is identified first on cardiac catheterization. The role of catheterization in patients with cardiac tumor is generally limited, however, to assessment of the vascular or nonvascular nature of the tumor and assessment of the coronary anatomy.

6. Discuss the importance of cardiac catheterization in the diagnosis of cardiac thrombus.

Although intraventricular thrombus occasionally may be identified by left ventriculography as an avascular mass, the presence of a known cardiac thrombus is an absolute contraindication for insertion of catheters into the left ventricle (LV) because of the high embolic risk. Left ventriculography also may suggest a higher risk for thrombus formation, by identification of LV aneurysm.

ECHOCARDIOGRAPHY

Steven A. Goldstein, M.D., Neil J. Weissman, M.D., and Gabriel Adelmann, M.D.

7. List the diagnostic possibilities when a cardiac mass is visualized by echocardiography.
- Thrombus
- Vegetation
- Tumor
- Man-made devices
- Normal variants

8. What is the role of echocardiography in evaluating intracardiac masses?

Echocardiography detects intracardiac masses and helps characterize the following:
1. Size and shape
2. Number of masses (single versus multiple)
3. Texture (solid versus cystic) and margins (smooth versus irregular)
4. Location and the form of attachment to the heart structures (e.g., pedunculated versus sessile, infiltration of the neighboring tissues)
5. Associated abnormalities (e.g., a regional wall motion abnormality)

Thrombus

9. Where does cardiac thrombus form?

Thrombus can form in the left atrium (LA), can form in the LV, or pass through the heart (atrial septal defect, patent foramen ovale [PFO]) from the venous circulation.

10. List risk factors for intracardiac clot formation and embolization.
- Nonvalvular atrial fibrillation (45%)
- Acute myocardial infarction (MI) with mural thrombus (15%)
- LV aneurysm (10%)
- Rheumatic mitral stenosis (10%)
- Prosthetic heart valves (10%)
- Other sources (10%), including infective endocarditis, intracardiac tumors, aortic atherosclerotic debris, paradoxical embolism via PFO, atrial septal aneurysm, spontaneous echo contrast, (SEC), nonspecific valve "strands," and calcification of the mitral annulus

11. What are the general echocardiographic characteristics of an LV thrombus?

LV thrombus generally appears as a space-occupying lesion adjacent to an area of abnormality (akinetic or aneurysmal region of the LV). The size, shape, and mobility of an LV thrombus are variable. The echodensity also can vary widely but is generally lower than that of the surrounding myocardium if the thrombus is relatively new.

Figure 2 shows LV thrombi of different sizes, shapes, and locations.

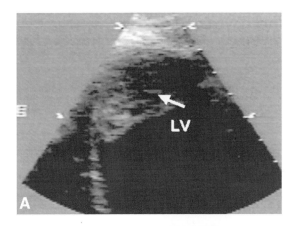

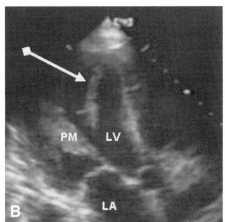

FIGURE 2. *A,* Large clot in the LV apex *(arrow)* 1 week after myocardial infarction. *B,* Apical thrombus *(arrow)* in a patient with dilated cardiomyopathy. Note the substantial dilatation of the left ventricle (LV). LA = left atrium; PM = papillary muscle. *C,* Large spherical thrombus *(arrow)* in the LV. *(continued)*

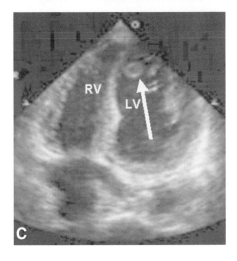

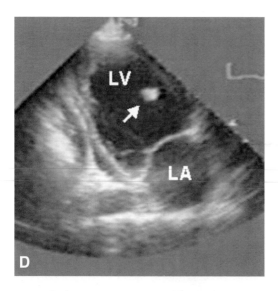

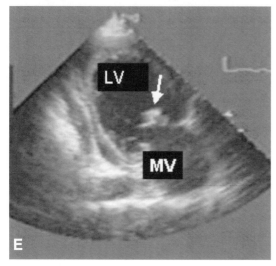

FIGURE 2. (*continued*) *D,* Free thrombus in the LV (*arrow*). *E,* Free thrombus in LV cavity adjacent to the mitral valve. LV = left ventrilce, MV = mitral valve; arrow = thrombus.

12. Name the most frequent location of an LV thrombus.
The apex.

13. What are the risk factors for LV thrombus formation?
LV thrombi are most likely to occur whenever there is intracavitary stasis of blood, as occurs in the case of:
- Recent anterior MI
- Dilated cardiomyopathy (especially when ejection fraction < 30–35%)
- LV aneurysm

14. How quickly after an anterior MI do thrombi form?
LV thrombi start forming within hours after acute MI. Most LV thrombi are detected by echocardiography 3–7 days after the event.

15. Does the absence of an LV thrombus on echocardiography reliably rule out this disorder?

No. There are at least four clinical settings in which echocardiography can fail to detect LV thrombi:

1. Early after MI ($<$ 3 days) when the thrombus may still be small

2. If the thrombus already has embolized

3. If the thrombus is layered (mural thrombus) against the LV wall, which makes it difficult to detect

4. If the echo is technically limited

One of the main goals of echocardiography in these patients is to detect structural changes of the LV known to be associated with a high rate of thrombosis (LV aneurysm) (Fig. 3).

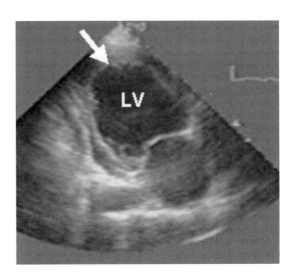

FIGURE 3. LV cavity after thrombus embolization. An important role of echo in the context of suspected LV thrombus is detection of predisposing factors, such as LV aneurysm (*arrow*).

16. Does the presence of a thrombus detected by two-dimensional echocardiography after an acute MI predict the likelihood of stroke?

Yes. Cerebral embolism occurs in approximately 20% of patients after acute MI who have thrombi detected by echocardiography, if untreated. Inversely, embolization occurs in $<$ 1% of patients in whom no thrombus is detected.

17. List the echocardiographic features of LV thrombi that are predictive of embolization.

• Large size
• Protruding into the LV cavity (as opposed to layered thrombi)
• Mobile
• Sonolucent at the center ("fresh")

18. What are the pitfalls of the echocardiographic diagnosis of LV thrombus?

False-positive or false-negative diagnosis of LV thrombus may be due to:

1. Machine-dependent artifacts (e.g., near-field "noise" artifact)

2. Normal LV structures that may be mistaken for thrombi (prominent LV muscle trabeculations, papillary muscles, false tendons)

3. The failure to distinguish layered thrombi from the underlying myocardium (which is often "thinned out" so that the thrombus lining this segment is mistaken for the endocardial aspect of the myocardium)

4. Failure to diagnose fresh thrombi that may be less echogenic than older clots (Fig. 4)

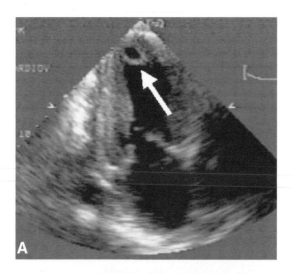

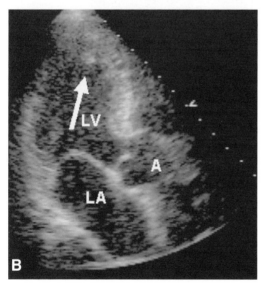

FIGURE 4. *A,* Pseudo-LV thrombus: LV false tendon *(arrow),* mimicking apical thrombus. *B,* Pseudo-LV thrombus. Foreshortened section through the LV, mimicking apical thrombus *(arrow).*

19. Is transesophageal echocardiography (TEE) superior to transthoracic echocardiography (TTE) for detecting LV thrombus?

No. This is due to frequent suboptimal imaging of the apex by TEE because:

1. The LV apex is an anterior structure and is in the far field relative to the posterior TEE probe.

2. It is often difficult to obtain a true longitudinal section through the LV by TEE.

20. List the clinical conditions most commonly associated with thrombi in the LA and LA appendage (LAA).

- Mitral stenosis
- Atrial fibrillation or flutter
- Prosthetic mitral valve
- LV systolic or diastolic dysfunction

Patients with mitral stenosis are at highest risk for atrial thrombosis, but mitral stenosis is not prevalent in Western nations; atrial fibrillation is the most common cause of LA thrombus in the United States.

21. What is the most common site of atrial thrombi?

Atrial clots are found most frequently in the LAA. This is most likely due to the LAA being shaped as a long, narrow chamber (*cul-de-sac*), fostering slow blood flow, and an increased internal surface area because of the presence of pectinate muscles on the inner surface of the LAA (Fig. 5).

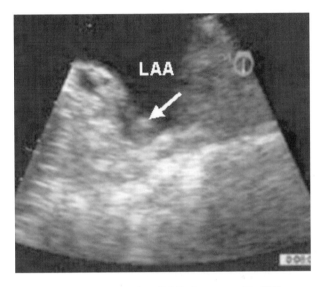

FIGURE 5. Thrombus in the left atrial appendage (LAA), demonstrated by TEE.

22. In addition to the *morphologic* characteristics outlined in the previous question, is there any echocardiography method for assessing the contractility (*function*) of the LAA?

LAA function can be assessed echocardiographically by measuring the change in LAA area from atrial diastole to systole and the velocity of blood entering and leaving the LAA.

23. What is the prognostic importance of these functional assessments?

There is a correlation between decreased LAA flow velocity and:
- Systemic thromboembolism
- The success of cardioversion from atrial fibrillation to sinus rhythm and maintenance of sinus rhythm (the higher the flow velocities, the higher the chances)

24. What is the most commonly employed method of LAA functional assessment?

Flow velocity assessment is used most frequently for this indication. This assessment is best performed by TEE, placing the pulse wave Doppler sample volume in the LAA and recording the peak filling and emptying velocities. It is appropriate to sample at the site of maximal flow velocities, while avoiding wall motion artifacts. The preferred sampling side is the proximal third of the LAA. Peak emptying velocities > 40 cm/sec generally are considered to be normal, whereas velocities < 20 cm/sec are abnormal.

25. List the most frequent causes of LAA dysfunction.

- Atrial fibrillation and flutter
- Rheumatic heart disease

- Amyloid heart disease
- Dilated cardiomyopathy

26. What are the technical limitations of LAA imaging on TTE?

Because of its relatively small size, complex anatomy (most LAAs are bilobed or multilobed), and posterior location, the LAA is rarely visualized by TTE (only seen in approximately one third of subjects).

27. Name the preferred views for LAA imaging by TTE.

The parasternal short-axis view of the base of the heart and the apical two-chamber and four-chamber views.

28. What is the role of TEE in the assessment of the LAA?

Because of the significant technical problems of TTE imaging of the LAA, TEE is mandatory to visualize the LAA reliably. Despite the superior quality, even TEE may give a **false-positive diagnosis** (owing to prominent pectinate muscles and separation ridges between lobes) or a **false-negative diagnosis** (small thrombi in multilobed appendages) (Fig. 6).

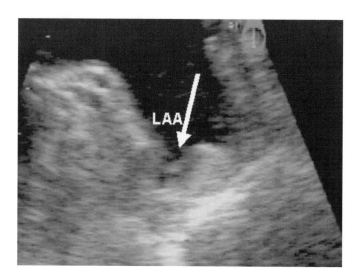

FIGURE 6. Pectinate muscle (*arrow*) in the left atrial appendage (LAA) mimicking a thrombus.

29. What is "smoke"?

Spontaneous echo contrast (SEC), known as "smoke," consists of dynamic, smokelike echoes with a characteristic swirling motion. SEC is the result of slow flow and is seen most often in the LA, but occasionally may be seen in the other heart chambers or in the great vessels (Fig. 7).

30. Explain the pathogenesis of SEC.

SEC is a manifestation of increased red blood cell aggregation seen in slow-flow states. The increased amplitude of backscattered ultrasonic signals causes the typical smoke appearance.

31. What clinical conditions are associated with SEC in the LA?

The risk factors for SEC generally coincide with those for LA thrombus and include any clinical setting resulting in slow intracardiac blood flow.

32. State the clinical significance of SEC.

SEC is associated with an increased incidence of LA thrombosis and systemic thromboembolism (SEC is a marker for previous and future embolic events).

33. What is the relationship between LA thrombosis and SEC?

Almost all LA thrombi are accompanied by LA SEC. In respect to LA thrombosis, SEC can be:
- The cause (smoke as a prethrombotic condition).
- The consequence (slow and erratic intracavitary flow resulting from the presence of an LA thrombus). In this case, SEC can be seen as a marker of LA thrombus.

34. What is the clinical importance of right atrium (RA) thrombosis?

RA thrombus places the patient at higher risk for pulmonary embolism (Fig. 8).

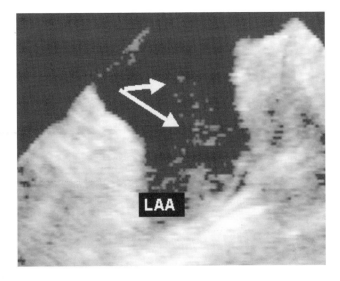

FIGURE 7. Spontaneous echo contrast ("smoke"; *arrows*) in the left atrial appendage (LAA) (TEE).

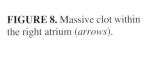

FIGURE 8. Massive clot within the right atrium (*arrows*).

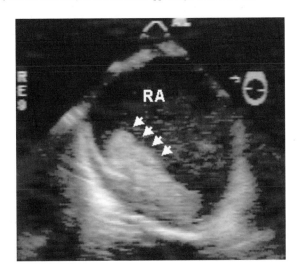

35. Can the origin of RA thrombus be established by echocardiography?

RA thrombus may be formed in situ, secondary to blood stasis, or at a distal site, such as a lower limb vein (deep venous thrombosis). Although echocardiography cannot establish definitely the origin of an RA thrombus, a long, mobile blood clot usually originates in a leg vein and represents a "cast" of the blood vessel in which it has formed.

Normal Cardiac Structures Appearing as Masses

36. What is an atrial septal aneurysm (ASA)?

A prominent bulging (usually mobile) of the fossa ovalis or the entire interatrial septum, which frequently oscillates back and forth between the two atria. An ASA protrudes at least 1.5 cm from the plane of the interatrial septum (Fig. 9).

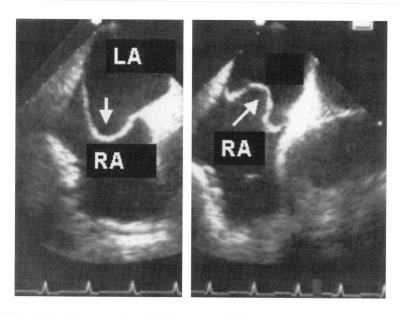

FIGURE 9. Atrial septal aneurysm "to-and-fro" movement of the interatrial septum (*arrows*) in a patient with atrial septal aneurysm.

37. Explain the clinical significance of an ASA.

Most ASAs (≥ 75%) are associated with either a secundum atrial defect or a PFO. There may be an association between ASA and cardioembolic stroke, although this association is controversial.

38. How might an ASA cause a stroke?

The postulated mechanisms include:
- Development of thrombus within the aneurysm
- Paradoxical embolism by PFO or atrial septal defect
- Association with atrial arrhythmias (e.g., atrial fibrillation)

39. What is the moderator band?

A prominent muscular trabeculation found in the right ventricle (RV) and present in most people. Echocardiographically the moderator band is imaged best in the apical four-chamber view; it appears as a thick, echo-dense band extending from the lower ventricular septum, across the RV cavity, to the base of the anterior papillary muscle. It can be confused with a thrombus in the RV.

40. State the clinical importance of the moderator band.

It identifies the "true" anatomic RV in patients with congenital heart disease (this is particularly important in transposition of the great vessels).

It may be mistaken for a pathologic structure (tumor or thrombus).

41. What is a PFO?

The foramen ovale is an opening in the midportion of the fetal atrial septum at the junction of the septum primum and the septum secundum. Before birth, it is kept open by flow from the RA to the LA. After birth, the normal pulmonary circulation increases LA pressure and closes the opening. In some instances, the septum primum and septum secundum do not fuse, and the PFO remains open; in other instances, a previously closed PFO is "stretched open" by an increase in the LA or RA pressure.

42. What is the clinical relevance of a PFO?

PFOs can cause:

1. Hypoxemia and cyanosis in patients with elevated RA pressure and right-to-left shunt; in these patients, hypoxemia is often unexplained until a PFO is identified.

2. Paradoxical systemic embolism by a thrombus passing through the PFO from the RA to the LA.

43. What is the prevalence of PFO in the general population?

PFO has been shown in 20–35% of all individuals by autopsy and contrast echocardiography (TTE or TEE).

44. How can a PFO be detected echocardiographically?

- Two-dimensional echocardiography without contrast enhancement (direct visualization, which is rare)
- Two-dimensional echocardiography contrast echocardiography using agitated saline or other contrast agents (passage of contrast material across the PFO is the most common method to diagnose a PFO)
- Color Doppler (right-to-left, left-to-right, or bidirectional shunting) (Fig. 10)

45. In a patient with hypoxemia or paradoxical systemic embolism and a PFO shown by echocardiography, what is the likelihood of a causal relationship?

Unknown. In most cases, the causal role of a PFO is presumptive. The likelihood may be increased if:

1. The PFO is large with a high degree of right-to-left shunting.

2. There are other associated clinical circumstances (deep vein thrombosis and elevated RA pressure).

46. What is negative contrast through a PFO?

In patients with left-to-right shunt through the PFO, blood passing through the PFO from the LA is free of contrast material. As this blood enters the RA, which is filled with contast material, a black "indentation" of contrast-free blood on the white background of contrast material is formed. This pattern is called *negative contrast*. It is important not to confuse a pattern of **negative contrast** with a diagnositic result of a **negative contrast study.**

Vegetation

47. Define vegetation?

Pathologically a vegetation is an amorphous mass of fibrin and platelets containing large colonies of microorganisms and variable numbers of inflammatory cells.

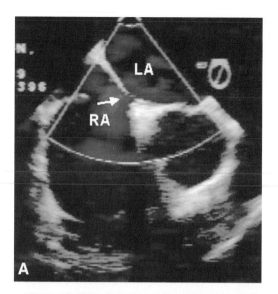

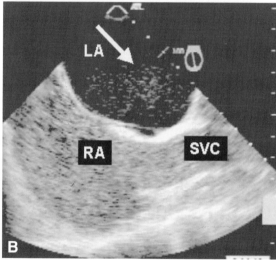

FIGURE 10. *A*, Color Doppler demonstration of left-to-right flow (*arrow*) through a patent foramen ovale (PFO). LA = left atrium; RA = right atrium. (See also Color Plates, Figure 20.) *B*, Demonstration of right-to-left PFO flow (*arrow*) by contrast (agitated saline). LA = left atrium; RA = right atrium; SVC = superior vena cava.

48. Describe the echocardiographic characteristics of vegetations.

Echocardiographically, vegetations are localized echodensities or masses that are usually irregularly shaped, may be sessile or pedunculated, rarely impair valve motion, and often flutter or vibrate in concert with valvular motion (Fig. 11).

49. Where do vegetations typically occur?

Vegetations almost always occur on valves, usually where the endocardium has been damaged by a pathologic jet (e.g., valvular regurgitation) or a valve that is congenitally abnormal. Vegetations usually form on the:

- Atrial aspect of the mitral or tricuspid valve
- Ventricular aspect of the aortic or pulmonic valve
- RV aspect of a ventricular septal defect.

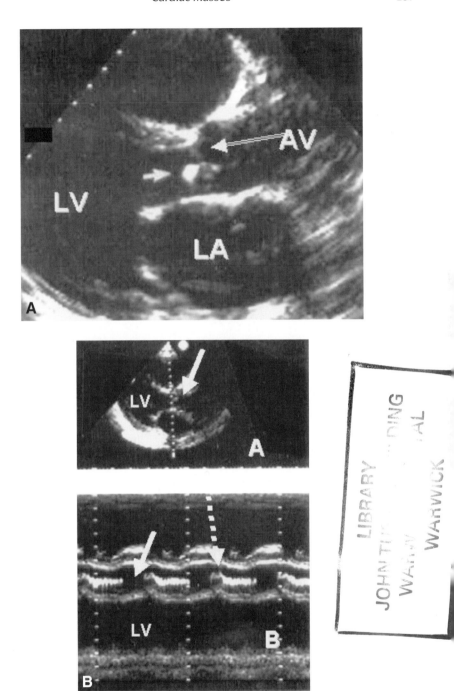

FIGURE 11. *A,* Two-dimensional study from the parasternal long axis in a patient with endocarditis. Vegetation (*short arrow*) on the left atrial side (LA) of the aortic valve (AV; *long arrow*). LV = left ventricle. *B,* M mode of the aortic valve. Note the fine undulations of the aortic valve, due to vegetation (*dashed arrow*). Solid arrow = aorta; LV = left ventricle. (Panel A shows the two-dimensional view used as a guide for the M mode study.)

50. Do vegetations ever occur on sites other than valves?

Yes. Some unusual sites of vegetation include:

- Native structures, including mural endocardium, chordae tendinae, eustachian valves, and Chiari network (Fig. 12)
- Acquired lesions, such as mural thrombus
- Man-made devices, such as pacemaker wires

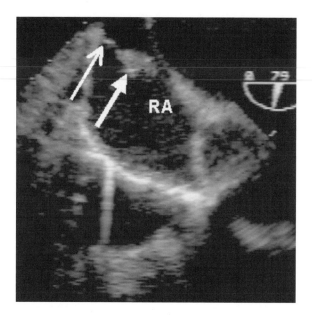

FIGURE 12. Thrombus vs. vegetation (*thick arrow*) on the Eustachian valve (*thin arrow*). RA = right atrium.

51. Can new and old ("healed") vegetations be distinguished by echocardiography?

The echocardiographic distinction between new and old vegetation is not reliable. New vegetations (which are usually soft and friable) may be less echogenic (less bright) than a "healed" vegetation (which underwent fibrosis, endothelialization, and calcification).

52. How do the Duke criteria for infective endocarditis incorporate the echocardiography findings?

Although the clinical and bacteriologic findings are essential in the diagnosis of infective endocarditis, echocardiography is an important diagnostic tool. In 1994, investigators from Duke University proposed new criteria for the diagnosis of infective endocarditis that incorporate echocardiographic findings.

Major Criteria

1. Positive echocardiogram for infective endocarditis
   a. Oscillating intracardiac mass on valve or supporting structures *or* in the path of regurgitant jets, *or* on implanted material, in the absence of an alternative anatomic explanation, *or*
   b. Abscess, *or*
   c. New partial dehiscence of prosthetic valve, *or*
2. New valvular regurgitation (increase or change in preexisting murmur not sufficient)

Minor Criteria

Echocardiogram consistent with infective endocarditis but not meeting a major criterion.

53. What is the mitral-aortic intervalvular fibrosa (MAIVF) region, and how can it be affected by endocarditis?

The MAIVF is the interannular junction between the anterior mitral leaflet and the aortic valve. This region in particularly susceptible to complications of infective endocarditis, including abscess, aneurysm, and perforation into the LA. Figure 13 shows an aneurysm of the MAIVF.

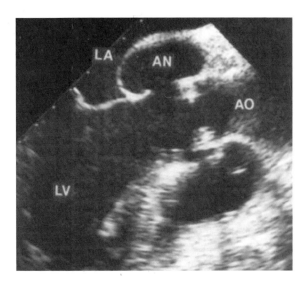

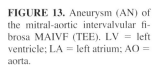
FIGURE 13. Aneurysm (AN) of the mitral-aortic intervalvular fibrosa MAIVF (TEE). LV = left ventricle; LA = left atrium; AO = aorta.

54. What is the differential diagnosis of an echocardiographic vegetation?

Several native, acquired, or man-made structures may be mistaken for vegetation, including:
- Ruptured chordae tendinae
- Myxomatous degeneration, thickening, or calcification of heart valves
- Retained mitral leaflets and chordae after mitral valve replacement
- Lambl's excrescences
- Thrombi
- Tumors
- Sutures, pledgets, and other prosthetic material for prosthetic valves

55. What are the main reasons for false-negative TTE studies in patients with infective endocarditis?

Vegetations can be missed by TTE in patients with:
- Poor acoustic windows, leading to suboptimal or incomplete visualization of the heart valves
- Small (diameter < 3 mm), sessile vegetations
- Vegetations on thickened or calcified valves
- Vegetations on or around prosthetic valves

56. What is the echocardiographic procedure of choice for the diagnosis of valvular vegetation?

Because of the high image resolution, TEE is ideally suited for the diagnosis of vegetation. TEE often is performed after TTE already has made the diagnosis to evaluated more fully the extent of infection (e.g., TTE may visualize an aortic valve vegetation accurately but fail to show a coexisting periaortic abscess).

57. Should TEE be performed on *all* patients with known or suspected endocarditis?

Performing a TEE in all patients with known or suspected endocarditis is controversial. Some recommend this approach, whereas others advocate TEE for select high-risk patients. Reasonable indications for TEE include:

- Strong clinical suspicion for endocarditis and negative or nondiagnostic TTE
- Persistent bacteremia (abscess suspected)
- Suspected prosthetic valve endocarditis
- Hemodynamic instability
- Clinical embolic event

If surgery is being considered:

- Staphylococcal aortic valve endocarditis
- TTE is technically inadequate
- TTE reveals vegetation, but size, mobility, and extent are unclear

Conversely, TEE is probably not required in patients in whom:

- TTE clearly reveals a small focal vegetation, and the patient is responding appropriately to treatment
- There is a low index of suspicion for endocarditis (e.g., fever in a patient with another source identified)
- The only abnormality is one isolated blood culture

The indications for TEE are discussed in more detail in the American College of Cardiology/American Heart Association "Guidelines for the Clinical Applications for Echocardiography."

58. What are the prognostically important echocardiography characteristics of vegetation?

The presence (as opposed to absence) of a vegetation on TTE has an adverse prognosis (higher incidence of death, emboli, heart failure, and need for surgery). Additional risk factors of complications include:

- Size (diameter > 1 cm)
- Mobility
- Abscess
- Otherwise unexplained pericardial effusion
- Extensive valve destruction with regurgitation

59. List the main complications of endocarditis that are shown by echocardiography.

- Valvular perforation, resulting in severe regurgitation
- Rupture of the mitral or tricuspid subvalvular apparatus, resulting in flail leaflets and severe regurgitation
- Cardiac abscess and fistula
- Purulent pericarditis

60. What are the echocardiographic features of cardiac abscess?

A cardiac abscess usually appears as a walled-off, echo-free space (Fig. 14). Less common findings include:

- Focal thickening of the aortic wall
- The presence of an echodensity in the ventricular septum
- "Rocking" of a prosthetic valve (suggesting dehiscence)

61. Describe the echocardiographic characteristics of a cardiac fistula.

A fistula is an abnormal communication between two cavities. Intracardiac fistulas can be a complication of aortic valve endocarditis forming an abnormal communication between the aorta and the LA or the aorta and the LV.

Tumor

62. Are most primary intracardiac tumors benign or malignant?

Benign (75%).

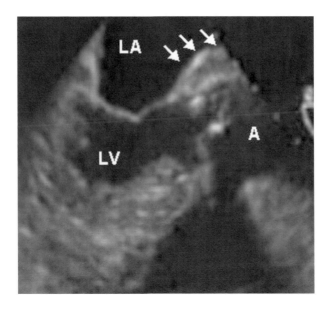

FIGURE 14. An abscess usually appearing on echo as a walled-off echo-free space (*arrow*). LV = left ventricle; LA = left atrium; A = aorta (TEE).

63. How do intracardiac tumors present clinically?

Most are asymptomatic and are detected incidentally at autopsy or by imaging such as echocardiography. The rest may cause:

- Obstruction (e.g., LA myxoma may cause obstruction of the mitral valve orifice)
- Embolization
- Constitutional manifestations (e.g., fever, anemia, malaise, arthralgias, hypergammaglobulinemia)
- Syncope

64. Are there any echocardiographic features that are helpful in differentiating benign versus malignant tumors?

The only reliable echocardiographic feature that can distinguish a malignant tumor is the presence of **invasion** into surrounding structures.

65. Summarize the importance of cardiac tumor invasion into the surrounding structures.

Diagnostic—It suggests a malignant nature of the tumor.

Prognostic—Extensive invasion has a poor prognosis.

Therapeutic—The degree and site of invasion greatly influence the feasibility and technique of surgery.

66. Is TEE superior to TTE for detecting left-sided intracardiac tumors?

TTE is generally excellent for detecting myxomas, the most common intracardiac tumor, and other left-sided intracardiac tumors. TEE is sometimes useful for further evaluation of these intracardiac masses. TEE can provide additional important information about the sites of attachment, acoustic characteristics, and extension into or impingement on adjacent structures.

67. Name the most frequent benign cardiac tumors.

Myxomas, lipomas, and fibroelastomas.

68. What are the echocardiographic characteristics of cardiac myxomas?

Cardiac myxomas:

1. Usually have regular borders and do not invade the neighboring tissues.

2. Most frequently are located in the LA, although they may be encountered in any heart chamber and even on the heart valves.

3. Are attached to the interatrial septum by a stalk.

4. Are single (in 95% of cases).

5. Are of variable dimension.

69. Describe the echocardiographic characteristics of papillary fibroelastomas.

Papillary fibroelastomas typically appear as small, round structures attached to the heart valves. The aortic valve most frequently is involved. Papillary fibroelastomas usually are located on the atrial aspect of the atrioventricular valve and on the ventricular aspect of the aortic valve.

70. Name the main complication of papillary fibroelastomas.

Papillary fibroelastomas may produce embolic events.

71. List some intracardiac structures that can be confused with tumors.

LOCATION	ENTITY
RA	Catheters, pacemakers
	Eustachian valve
	Chiari network
	Lipomatous hypertrophy of atrial septum
	Fat in tricuspid annulus
	Crista terminalis
LA	Ridge between left upper pulmonary vein and LAA
	Calcified mitral annulus
	Compression of LA wall by tortuous descending aorta
RV	Thrombus
	Moderator band
LV	Thrombus
	Papillary muscle
	Anomalous muscle band
	False tendon

72. Which tumors invade the RA via the inferior vena cava?

The most common tumor is renal cell carcinoma (Fig. 15). Other tumors, far less common, include uterine leiomyoma and leiomyosarcoma, rhabdomyosarcoma, adrenal carcinoma, and hepatocellular carcinoma.

73. What man-made object in the hearts can be distinguished by echocardiography?

- **Therapeutic devices,** such as catheters (Swan-Ganz, pacing, dialysis, parenteral nutrition catheters), the presence of which is usually known. Typically, they appear as elongated, thin, linear echodensities coursing through the superior vena cava, inferior vena cava, RA, RV, or RV outflow tract. Catheters often create multiple linear reverberations, occasionally detected in other chambers (e.g., LA or LV) (Fig. 16A).
- **Other objects,** such as bullets, nails, or needles (Fig. 16B)

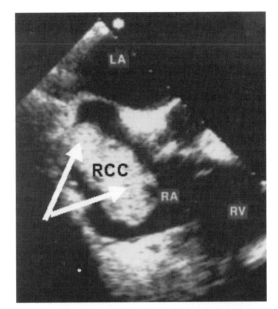

FIGURE 15. Metastatic renal cell carcinoma (RCC; *arrows*) in the right atrium (RA).

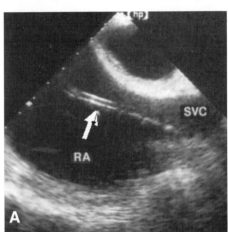

FIGURE 16. *A,* Catheter (*arrow*) in the RA. SVC = superior vena cava. *B,* Foreign body (bullet) in the right ventricle (RV) (*large arrow*). The exact size of the metallic fragment is difficult to assess, due to intense reverberation (*small arrows*).

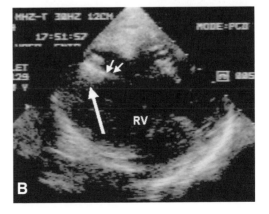

74. What is the echocardiographic appearance of a LV assist device?

Usually, echocardiography visualizes the LV apical cannula of the device and its aortic site of implantation (Fig. 17). It is possible to suspect a malfunction or thrombosis of the device by showing an increased blood flow velocity through the cannula and, rarely, by visualizing the thrombus itself.

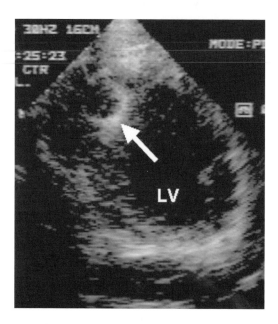

FIGURE 17. Left ventricular assist device (LVAD) cannula in left ventricular (LV) apex (*arrow*).

75. How can surgical sutures be differentiated from thrombi and vegetations?

Surgical sutures often are seen around the sewing ring of prosthetic valves or at the margins of prosthetic patch material (Fig. 18). Important differences include:

Shape—sutures are regular, vegetations often elongated or bulbous.

Spacing—sutures are regularly spaced.

Echodensity—sutures are often brighter than vegetations.

Mobility—sutures are consonant with cardiac motion, whereas vegetations generally have independent mobility.

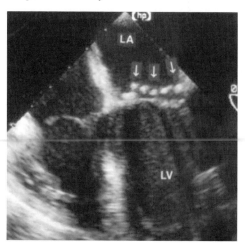

FIGURE 18. Sutures of a mitral valve prosthesis (*arrows*). LA = left atrium.

76. What is the structure shown in Figure 19?

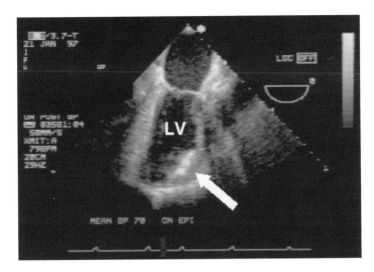

FIGURE 19. Air in the LV (*arrow*), immediately after cardiac surgery. This echocardiogram was obtained in the operating room, at the end of the surgical procedure but before extracorporeal circulation was discontinued. Identification of air in the LV is one of the most important tasks of intraoperative TEE and prompts the performance of certain surgical maneuvers for removing it before the extracorporeal circulation is discontinued.

MAGNETIC RESONANCE IMAGING

Anthon R. Fuisz, M.D., and Gabriel Adelmann, M.D.

77. Describe the magnetic resonance imaging (MRI) appearance of cardiac thrombi.

Thrombi are avascular structures and do not enhance after contrast administration. The MRI appearance of cardiac thrombi depends on their age. Relatively fresh thrombi can produce high signal intensity, and older thrombi typically produce low signal intensity.

78. What is the role of MRI in the diagnosis of cardiac thrombi?

Although MRI is not usually the first test of choice, it can be used to assess for an LV thrombus. Its role in assessing small LA thrombus has not yet been established.

79. Regardless of the imaging modality, significant motion abnormality of the LV apex in a stroke patient has important implications; what are they?

1. Normal systolic function of the apex is associated with an extremely low probability of thrombus.

2. Severe apical contraction abnormalities generally indicate the necessity for long-term anticoagulation in eligible patients, even in the absence of a clearly visualized thrombus.

80. What elements of information regarding cardiac tumors may be obtained by MRI?

- The presence of the tumor
- The dimensions of the tumor
- The site of a primary malignancy, such as pulmonary carcinoma invading the heart directly or through the pulmonary veins
- The composition of the tumor, based on relatively characteristic MRI signal intensities corresponding to muscle, fat, and myxomatous tissue

81. Name the most frequent benign tumors of the heart.
Myxomas and lipomas.

82. Summarize MRI findings that suggest cardiac myxoma.
- Location in the LA, most frequently attached to the interatrial septum at the fossa ovalis
Myxomas are located most frequently in the LA, and the most frequent tumor type in the LA is myxoma. Cardiac myxomas can involve any of the cardiac chambers or valves, however.
- Pedunculated tumors
- Contrast enhancement after intravenous administration of gadolinium

83. List MRI findings that suggest the diagnosis of cardiac lipomas.
1. Location in the RA (although lipomas can be located in any heart chamber)
2. Sessile, polypoid, or infiltrative tumors
3. MRI density similar to that of fat

84. List the findings that suggest the diagnosis of malignant cardiac tumor.
1. Origin from, or extension into, neighboring tissues or organs (Fig. 20)
2. A broad implantation base
3. Characteristic behavior on T1-weighted and T2-weighted images

85. Can MRI provide accurate histologic characterization of cardiac tumors?
Although certain MRI characteristics may suggest the nature of the tumor, MRI does *not* provide a histologic diagnosis.

86. What is the most frequent cardiac tumor in children, and what are the specific problems of its identification by cardiac MRI?
Rhabdomyomas. Because they have the same MRI characteristics as the surrounding myocardium, rhabdomyomas occasionally may be missed. Special attention to any myocardial wall distortion and a high index of suspicion are essential in this setting.

87. Discuss the role of cardiac MRI in the evaluation of cardiac tumors.
Although echocardiography is the first-line imaging procedure in most patients with cardiac disease (including suspected cardiac tumor), MRI has an important place in the definition of tu-

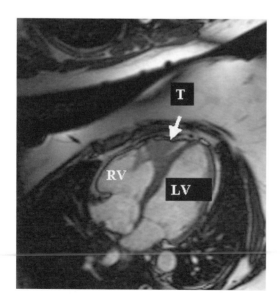

FIGURE 20. LV mass (*arrow*) not seen by standard transthoracic echocardiography.

mor extension and in identifying a primary malignancy, in the case of metastatic cardiac malignancy. The advantages of MRI over computed tomography (CT) include the ability of MRI to image the heart from different planes, providing information important for planning surgical intervention in eligible patients. (Latest generation CT systems also are able to provide complex three-dimensional reconstruction of the heart.) In addition, MRI avoids the x-ray exposure and considerable doses of contrast agents necessary with CT techniques.

CHEST X-RAY

Curtis E. Green, M.D., Gabriel Adelmann, M.D., and Matthew Brewer, M.D.

88. What is the role of chest radiography in the diagnosis of cardiac masses?

As mentioned in Chapter 1, chest radiography is generally of low utility when it is necessary to separate a low-density structure from surrounding higher density tissues. Generally, cardiac tumors have a low density and are not diagnosed by chest x-ray. "Classic" radiology may be useful, however, for the diagnosis of **calcified tumors** and **intracardiac or intra-aortic man-made devices.**

89. List the main man-made devices that can be visualized by chest radiography.

- Venous catheters
- Pacemakers
- Intra-aortic counterpulsation devices

90. What is the role of radiography in the management of these patients?

Radiography is a cheap and readily available diagnostic modality for assessing the proper placement of these catheters. This is extremely important because catheters can be malpositioned (leading to inaccurate pressure tracing) or can perforate the cardiac or vascular walls.

91. Describe the radiographic characteristics of a correctly positioned central venous catheter.

The **course** of the catheter should be parallel to that of the superior vena cava; catheter coiling or angulation may indicate perforation of the vessel wall.

The **tip** of the catheter should be superior to the upper border of the RA (i.e., cranial to the lower half of the posterior cardiac border, on a lateral film); catheters in the RA or the RV may produce arrhythmia or cardiac perforation or both.

92. Describe the radiographic characteristics of a correctly positioned Swan-Ganz catheter.

The tip of the Swan-Ganz catheter should be located in the right or left main pulmonary artery or in one of their major lobar branches:

If the tip of the catheter is located too proximally (i.e., in the pulmonary artery or in the RV), the pressure tracing will not reflect the pulmonary capillary wedge pressure.

If the tip of the catheter is located too distally, there is an increased risk for pulmonary infarction or pulmonary artery branch rupture on inflation of the balloon.

92. Describe the radiographic characteristics of a correctly positioned cardiac pacemaker.

The following elements should be assessed on a chest x-ray in a patient with a cardiac pacemaker:

- The pacemaker **generator:** The presence of excessive wire looping around the pacemaker "box" may indicate that the patient has excessively rotated the generator in its subcutaneous "pocket," a fact that may lead to pacemaker dysfunction.
- The **course of the pacemaker wires:** Wire rupture is noticeable as a lack of wire continuity.

- The **tip of the pacemaker wires:** The tip of the pacemaker lead should project within the area of the RV; in patients with a DDD pacemaker, the tip of the atrial lead should project within the area of the RA. Projection of the tip of the pacemaker lead >3 mm beyond the cardiac contour should raise the possibility of cardiac perforation.

94. Describe the radiographic characteristics of a correctly positioned intra-aortic balloon.

The radiopaque tip of the counterpulsation intra-aortic balloon should be positioned at the junction between the aortic arch and the descending aorta (more precisely, the position should be immediately distal to the origin of the left subclavian artery, but it is not possible to assess this by chest x-ray alone). A more proximal position of the device tip may occlude the left subclavian or the left carotid artery or both and lead to limb or brain hypoperfusion, whereas a more distal position diminishes the efficacy of the intra-aortic balloon (inadequate coronary circulation).

9. CONGENITAL HEART DISEASE

CARDIAC CATHETERIZATION

Abraham Rothman, M.D., Luis Gruberg, M.D., and Gabriel Adelmann, M.D.

1. What information can be obtained in the catheterization laboratory regarding congenital heart disease?

- The **structure** of the heart chambers and of the great vessels
- The **connections** between the heart chambers and the great vessels
- The presence of **associated coronary artery anomalies**
- The presence of **associated atherosclerotic coronary disease,** in the occasional adult with risk factors scheduled for corrective surgery of congenital heart disease
- The presence of **collateral vessels** (e.g., in patients with aortic coarctation)
- The presence of intracardiac or extracardiac pathologic connections (**shunt**)
- The functional impact of the cardiac anomaly on the function of ventricles (**systolic dysfunction**)
- The presence or absence of **pulmonary hypertension**
- The structure and function of surgically implanted corrective **devices** (conduits, baffles)

2. Discuss the role of cardiac catheterization in the diagnosis of congenital heart disease.

For many decades, cardiac catheterization was the gold standard imaging modality for diagnosis. With the advent of newer, noninvasive imaging technologies (transesophageal echocardiography [TEE], magnetic resonance imaging [MRI], spiral computed tomography [CT]), the use of cardiac catheterization has decreased dramatically. This diagnostic modality remains useful, however, in the following settings:

1. Assessment of associated coronary artery anomalies (the procedure of choice for this indication is cardiac MRI; however, this imaging modality is not yet widely available)

2. Assessment of congenital heart disease in centers that may not have access to newer technology (mainly in developing nations)

3. Invasive assessment of the pulmonary artery pressures, in patients in whom echo Doppler does not provide conclusive results or in patients with a branch stenosis of the pulmonary artery in whom Doppler measurement of the transtenotic gradients is difficult or impossible

3. What is the role of cardiac catheterization in the treatment of congenital heart disease?

Initially considered as an exclusively diagnostic procedure, cardiac catheterization has become increasingly involved in treatment. A detailed discussion of the different indications for percutaneous therapy of congenital cardiac lesions is beyond the scope of this text, but some of the most frequent indications include:

- Balloon occlusion of **atrial septal defect (ASD)** and **patent foramen ovale (PFO)**
- Coil occlusion in patients with **patent ductus arteriosus (PDA)**
- Coil occlusion in patients with **pulmonary arteriovenous malformations**
- Coil occlusion of **pulmonary artery branches,** in certain syndromes associated with an increased pulmonary blood flow

4. Describe the role of cardiac catheterization in the follow-up of patients after corrective surgery for congenital heart disease.

Because of its invasive nature, cardiac catheterization rarely is indicated solely for follow-up in these patients, especially if noninvasive tests do not reveal a problem and the patient is asymptomatic. In cases in which additional surgery is contemplated, cardiac catheterization may be useful for structural and functional assessment, as outlined in questions 1 and 2.

5. What is the hallmark angiographic sign of ASD?

The finding of a communication at the level of the interatrial septum, through which contrast material injected into the right atrium (RA) can progress freely into the left atrium (LA) (Fig. 1).

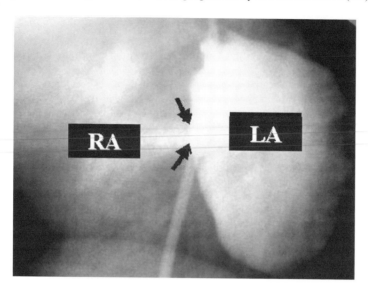

FIGURE 1. Atrial septal defect. Contrast can be seen progressing from RA to the LA through a secundum atrial septal defect (*arrows*).

6. List the indications for ASD closure.

- A left-to-right shunt > 1.8:1, in the absence of significant irreversible pulmonary hypertension
- Clinical symptoms such as paradoxical embolism or atrial rhythm disturbances, even in the presence of a minimal shunt

7. Which patients are candidates for percutaneous ASD closure?

The indications for percutaneous occlusion of ASD are rapidly evolving and depend on the type of occluder that is being used. Candidacy for percutaneous closure is assessed based on the following characteristics of the ASD (generally shown by echocardiography):

1. The **type** of ASD: most currently used devices require that the ASD be of the secundum type, which ensures a sufficient "tissue rim" around the interatrial communication for proper tethering of the occluder device.

2. The **"stretched diameter"** of the ASD, which represents the size of the communication when a balloon is inflated across it; generally, a diameter < 34 mm is compatible with percutaneous closure.

3. A **distance > 5 mm from the margins** of the defect to the coronary sinus, atrioventricular valves, and right upper pulmonary vein.

4. The **absence of associated congenital cardiac** anomalies, which would require cardiac surgery anyway (e.g., ventricular septal defect [VSD], PDA).

5. **Associated anomalous pulmonary vein drainage** (the presence of this anomaly is a contraindication to percutaneous closure).

6. The presence of a **single** (as opposed to multiple) **ASD** that can be covered adequately by a single device.

8. Which patients with PFO are candidates for percutaneous shunt closure?

PFO is a frequent and generally innocuous anomaly, found in 25–30% of adults in autopsy series and in 20% of adults using contrast echocardiography. There has been an increasing awareness of the potential role of PFO in patients with cryptogenic stroke (i.e., stroke in the absence of any detectable cause; this entity accounts for 40% of strokes). In these patients, small blood clots in the RA, which usually would not cause any detectable pulmonary embolic complications, might cross the interatrial communication (PFO) and embolize to the cerebral circulation. It has been suggested that PFO closure in these patients may prevent further cerebral embolic events, a hypothesis tested in an ongoing study. Pending the results of the study, percutaneous PFO closure remains controversial.

9. What are the main challenges of surgical PDA ligation, which may be overcome by the use of percutaneously delivered occluder devices (coils)?

Surgical ligation is problematic in patients with:
- Calcified PDA, which may be too rigid to be compressed by the surgical suture
- Short window-type PDA, in which it is difficult to find an optimal site for suture placement
In these patients, percutaneously delivered coils may be the optimal solution.

10. Summarize the contraindications of percutaneous PDA occlusion.

In addition to irreversible pulmonary hypertension (pulmonary vascular resistance), which is a general contraindication for interventional PDA closure by any method, specific contraindications for percutaneous PDA occlusion include:
- Low body weight (a potential problem in infants)
- Presence of associated congenital cardiac anomalies, which would require cardiac surgery anyway, such as a VSD, aortic coarctation, and ASD.

11. Can percutaneous closure be applied to VSD?

Yes. Percutaneous VSD closure can be carried out in patients with acceptable body weight (this problem generally concerns the pediatric population). The inclusion criteria refer to:

1. The **nature** of the VSD; muscular-type VSD is an indication, whereas membranous VSD and VSD associated with tetralogy of Fallot (TOF) are contraindications to percutaneous closure.

2. The **location** of the VSD; a distance of ≥ 3 mm between the muscular communication and the ventricular apex is necessary for percutaneous closure.

3. The absence of **associated cardiac anomalies,** which would require surgical intervention anyway.

4. **Residual VSD** after previous surgical closure.

12. What are the angiographic findings in patients with TOF?

All the typical components of TOF: VSD, overriding aorta, right ventricle (RV) hypertrophy, pulmonic stenosis (Fig. 2).

13. What is the role of cardiac catheterization in patients with pulmonary arteriovenous malformations?

Pulmonary arteriovenous malformations are congenital pathologic communications between the pulmonary arteries and veins. The hemodynamic importance depends on the magnitude of blood flow (shunt). In patients with high shunt flows, RV volume overload and high-output cardiac failure may ensue. Cardiac catheterization is the mainstay of management in these patients and has a double role, as follows:
- **Diagnostic:** Cardiac catheterization is the procedure of choice for assessing the presence and number of malformations and the magnitude of flow through the pulmonary anomalous communication.
- **Therapeutic:** Coiling provides definitive therapy for arteriovenous malformations.

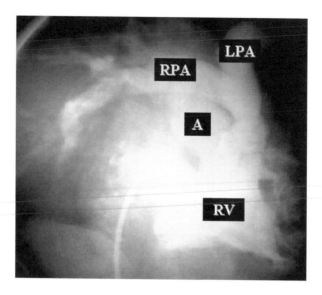

FIGURE 2. Tetralogy of Fallot. Ventricular septal defect and overriding aorta (A) in a patient with tetralogy of Fallot. LPA = left pulmonary artery, RPA = right pulmonary artery.

14. Summarize the findings on ventriculography in a patient with valvular pulmonic stenosis.

- Thickened, rigid pulmonic valve leaflets, with frequent association of pulmonic regurgitation (Fig. 3)
- Poststenotic dilation of the pulmonary artery, sometimes aneurysmal
- RV hypertrophy

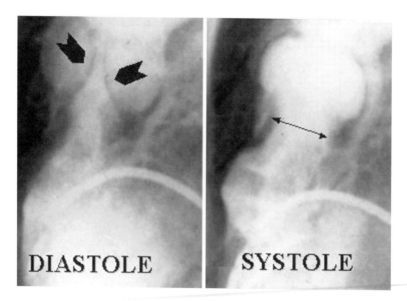

FIGURE 3. Valvular pulmonary stenosis. Note thickened pulmonic valve leaflets with incomplete valve opening in systole and leaflet malcoaptation in diastole and poststenotic dilatation of the pulmonary artery root (*double-headed arrow*).

15. Discuss the role of cardiac catheterization in follow-up of patients after corrective surgery for congenital heart disease.

Cardiac catheterization gradually is being replaced by newer techniques, such as MRI/magnetic resonance angiography (MRA). Cardiac catheterization still may be useful, however, when these modalities are not available. Information regarding calcification of conduits connecting different heart chambers can be obtained easily by fluoroscopy, which is performed immediately before the catheterization procedure itself. Figure 4 show different examples of catheterization findings in patients who underwent previous corrective surgery for congenital heart disease.

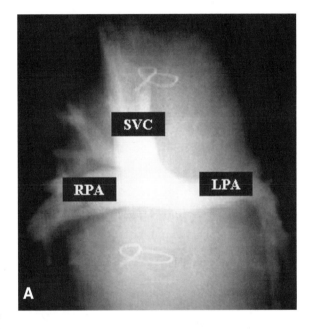

FIGURE 4. *A*, The Fontan operation. The Fontan operation is used in patients with a single functional ventricle and consists of connecting the systemic venous return directly to the pulmonary arteries. In this patient, the SVC is connected to the pulmonary arteries (*arrows*). *B*, Calcified Rastelli conduit. The Rastelli repair usually utilizes a valved homograft from the right ventricle to the pulmonary artery in patients with different congenital carded malformations, especially transposition of the great arteries with associated VSD and pulmonic stenosis. Homografts frequently calcify or become too small as patients grow, making replacement necessary. (*continued*)

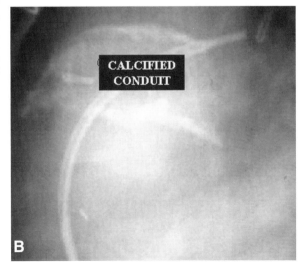

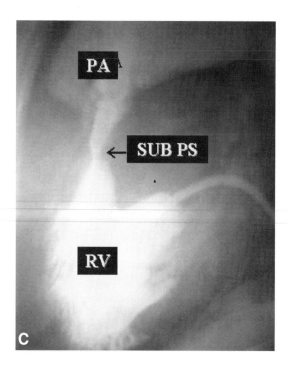

FIGURE 4. (*continued*) *C,* Dynamic subvalvular infundibular obstruction after relief of pulmonary valve stenosis. Long-standing pulmonary valve stenosis causes RV hypertrophy, typically involving the infundibular (subvalvular) region. Immediately after balloon dilation, relief of obstruction at the level of the valve often causes dynamic subvalvar infundibular obstruction (SUB PS, *arrow*). This infundibular obstruction may be severe enough to compromise forward pulmonary flow and, consequently, cardiac output. PA = pulmonary artery.

16. Which patients with congenital heart disease need cardiac catheterization?

According to the American Heart Association guidelines, there are two important indications for cardiac catheterization in these patients, both referring to the coronary anatomy: assessment for associated coronary anomalies and assessment for atherosclerotic coronary artery disease in patients with risk factors.

Target catheterization also can be used for anatomic assessment of the congenital malformation itself, but, in this regard, MRI or MRA, if available, is the procedure of choice

ECHOCARDIOGRAPHY

Gabriel Adelmann, M.D., and Neil J. Weissman, M.D.

17. What is the main difference between echocardiography in a patient with congenital heart disease and echocardiography performed for any other cardiac indication?

In noncongenital cases, the sonographer has a mental picture of what the heart should look like (see Chapter 2) and is looking for any deviation from the rule that may exist in a specific patient (similar to a person exploring an unknown house with a clear idea of which room is the living room, the bedroom, and the kitchen, despite the different decoration schemes he or she will discover).

In congenital disease, the sonographer must piece together mentally the different segments of the heart (chambers, valves, great arteries) into a coherent picture, which is sometimes substantially different **in organization** from normal.

18. What is the difference between the following terms: *morphologic RV* and *functional RV*?

In some patients, the connection between the different components of the heart (atria, ventricles, great arteries) is abnormal (e.g., the aorta connecting to the RV). In this case, a chamber may exhibit morphologic characteristics associated (in **normal** subjects) with a given chamber (e.g., RV), while fullfilling the **function** normally accomplished by a different chamber (e.g., a morphologic RV connected to the aorta functions as a "systemic" ventricle, functioning as a left ventricle [LV]).

19. Explain the segmental approach to the echocardiographic diagnosis of congenital heart disease.

This approach individually identifies all the cardiac components ("pieces of the puzzle") without relying on their association with other structures (e.g., the left atrium [LA] sometimes may be connected to the RV rather than the LV; a ventricular chamber connected to that LA that drains the pulmonary veins is not necessarily the LV; the true identity of this chamber must be assessed based on its own, intrinsic, characteristics, rather than on identification of the atrium to which it connects).

20. Describe the main characteristics of the morphologic RV.

The features that identify a ventricle as being the morphologic RV regardless of its atrial and arterial connections are:
- A triangular external shape
- An internal surface rich in thick muscle bundles (trabeculations)
- Attachment of the papillary muscles to the surface of the interventricular septum
- The presence of a moderator band that separates the RV outflow tract (the part of the RV that immediately leads to the great artery to which this chamber is connected) from the rest of the ventricle

21. Identify the characteristics of the morphologic LV.

A conical shape and a smooth internal surface, with the exception of fine apical trabeculations.

22. Identify the characteristics of the morphologic RA.

1. It is the atrium that drains the coronary sinus, the inferior vena cava, and the superior vena cava.
2. It has a larger appendage than the LA.
3. It also could drain some or all of the pulmonary veins (anomalous pulmonary vein drainage).

23. Describe the characteristics of the morphologic LA.
- It does not drain any of the systemic veins (except for a rare congenital malformation).
- It normally drains all of the pulmonary veins, although some or all of these veins occasionally may drain into the RA (partial or total anomalous pulmonary vein drainage).

24. The diagnosis of congenital heart disease most often is based on morphologic identification of the different heart chambers, rather than on the relationship between them. There are two anatomic relationships, however, that can serve as "stable milestones" for the mental reconstruction of the cardiac anatomy. Name these relationships.

1. The visceroatrial situs
2. The relationship between the ventricles and the atrioventricular valves

25. What is the visceroatrial situs?

The pattern of arrangement of the atria in the thorax, which can serve as a "point of departure" for the step-by-step process of mental reconstruction of the heart anatomy. Regardless of the complexity of congenital heart syndromes, the relationship between the atria and the abdominal organs is preserved:

The morphologic LA is on the same side as the gastric bubble.
The morphologic RA is on the same side as the liver.

26. What is the relationship between the ventricles and atrioventricular valves?

The mitral valve is always attached to the LV, and the tricuspid valve is always attached to the RV. With the exception of patients with atrioventricular canal malformation (discussed later), the tricuspid valve is apically displaced from the mitral valve. This displacement provides additional information to determine which ventricle is the anatomic RV.

27. Describe the different positions of the heart in the chest cavity.

Levocardia: The cardiac apex points leftward, and the heart is located predominantly in the left chest.

Dextrocardia: The cardiac apex points rightward, and the heart is located predominantly in the right chest .

Mesocardia: The heart is positioned in the midline, and the apex points inferiorly.

Dextroposition: The apex points leftward, but the heart is located predominantly in the right chest.

28. Which of the patterns outlined in question 27 is normal, and what is the importance of identifying the abnormal patterns?

The normal position of the heart in the chest is levocardia. It is important to identify dextrocardia, mesocardia, and dextroposition because they often are associated with congenital cardiac anomalies (and may be the first factor to raise the suspicion of these associated conditions). These abnormal patterns of cardiac position within the thorax may confuse the interpretation of the electrocardiogram (EKG), angiography, and echocardiography.

29. What is the atrioventricular alignment?

This term describes which atrium opens into which ventricle. There are two possibilities:

1. **Atrioventricular concordance**—the RA opens into the RV, and the LA opens into the LV (normal pattern).

2. **Atrioventricular discordance**—the RA opens in to the LV, through the mitral valve, and the LA opens into the RV, through the tricuspid valve.

30. What is the ventriculoarterial alignment?

This term describes which ventricle opens into which great artery. There are several possibilities:

1. **Ventriculoarterial concordance**—the RV opens into the pulmonary artery, and the LV opens into the aorta.

2. **Ventriculoarterial discordance (transposition)**—the RV opens into the aorta, and the LV opens into the pulmonary artery.

3. **Double-outlet RV**—both great arteries originate from the RV.

4. **Double-outlet LV**—both great arteries originate from the LV.

5. **Truncus arteriosus**—a single great artery leaves the heart, supplying blood to the systemic and the pulmonary circulation.

31. Practically, how do I go about piecing together the anatomy of a heart with congenital malformations?

Echocardiography in congenital heart disease is probably one of the most technically demanding fields of medicine. Substantial experience is required for "solving the puzzle" of these hearts. There are no set recipes, but here are some useful hints:

1. Identify the position of the heart in the thorax (situs solitus, situs inversus, situs ambiguous, dextrocardia).

2. Identify the morphologic ventricles and atria.

3. Identify the great vessels.

4. Identify the relationship between the atria, the ventricles, and the great arteries (atrioventricular and ventriculoarterial alignment).

32. List the most common cardiac malformatioxns.
- PFO (30% of the population)
- Mitral valve prolapse (3–8% of the population)
- Bicuspid aortic valve (1–2% of the population)

33. What are the echocardiographic findings in patients with PFO?
Echocardiographic visualization of PFO is done best from the subcostal view, where all four heart chambers are seen and the direction of the ultrasound is perpendicular to that of the interatrial septum.

On two-dimensional echocardiography:
Direct visualization of a gap in the interatrial septum, at the level of the foramen ovale, is rarely possible
Intravenously injected contrast material (agitated saline) is visualized traversing from the RA into the LA across the PFO

On Doppler echocardiography:
Visualization of color flow between the two atria, across the interatrial septum, is also rare.

34. Does a positive PFO contrast study (i.e., progression of an intravenously injected contrast agent from the RA to the LA) indicate pathologically increased pressures in the right heart chambers?
No. There are physiologic variations in the pressure relationship between the two atria that enable echocardiographic contrast material to cross the PFO from the RA into the LA, even in normal patients. Nonetheless, during a contrast study to assess for PFO, if the initial attempt is negative, a patient is asked to perform the Valsalva maneuver, transiently increasing the RA pressure over the LA pressure; this maneuver occasionally helps to reveal a PFO.

35. What are the contrast substances used for visualization of PFO?
The contrast agent of choice is **agitated saline solution.** Agitated saline contains small air bubbles, which reflect ultrasound and can be followed from the RA to LA. More expensive, commercially available contrast agents designed to persist across the pulmonary circulation to provide LV opacification are not optimal for this situation. If contrast material is seen in the LA, the operator may not be able to tell if this is due to passage through the PFO or through the lungs. The echogenic air in agitated saline diffuses through the alveolar/capillary interface in the lungs and generally does not reach the left heart chambers. Visualization of contrast material within the LA is usually diagnostic of a PFO.

36. What is the clinical importance of a PFO if 30% of the population has one?
A PFO may have clinical significance in the following settings:
1. Systemic embolism (most frequently stroke) of unknown origin. A venous thrombus may progress from the RA into the LA and go into the systemic circulation (**paradoxic embolus**).
2. Patients with significantly increased PA pressure may have a significant right-to-left shunt through the PFO, which may cause oxygen desaturation of the systemic blood. This is seen most often in intensive care unit patients on a ventilator, in whom the positive pressures generated by the breathing machine may lead to an increased pressure in the right heart chambers.

37. How can congenital heart defects be classified based on the degree of cyanosis that they produce?
Acyanotic does not cause cyanosis.
Cyanotic causes cyanosis and implies the existence of a right-to-left shunt.

38. List the most frequent acyanotic congenital heart defects in the adult.

VSD	Subvalvular aortic stenosis
ASD	Aortic coarctation

PDA   Ebstein's anomaly
Atrioventricular canal defect   Corrected transposition of the great arteries (TGA)
Pulmonary stenosis

39. Are all of the conditions listed in question 38 always acyanotic?
No. The designation *acyanotic defects* refers to the "usual case." In patients in whom pulmonary hypertension generates shunt reversal (i.e., left-to-right shunt becomes right-to-left shunt), cyanosis may complicate the course of these conditions. This is in opposition to *cyanotic* malformations, which always cause cyanosis in the affected patient.

40. Name the most frequent cyanotic congenital cardiac malformation in the adult.
TOF.

41. Name the types of VSD.
  • Membranous
  • Muscular
  • Canal
  • Supracristal
  • Malalignment

42. What are the echocardiographic signs common to all types of VSD?
VSDs are visualized by **two-dimensional echocardiography** as gaps in the interventricular septum and by **Doppler echocardiography** as a jet from the LV into the RV.

43. What is the role of contrast echocardiography in the visualization VSD?
Because these defects usually are seen by two-dimensional and Doppler echocardiography, contrast echocardiography has virtually no role in the diagnosis of VSD. Agitated saline bubbles cross from the RV into the LV only if the RV pressure is higher than the LV pressure. Commercial contrast agents cross the pulmonary circulation and opacify the RV before the LV. Blood flow across a VSD from the LV into the RV is not seen (the RV is already "white" from the contrast agent).

44. Which type of VSD is seen most frequently in adult patients?
Membranous VSD.

45. What are the echocardiographic characteristics of membranous VSD?
Membranous VSDs involve the upper part of the interventricular septum (Fig. 5). They are seen best from the parasternal short-axis view at the base of the heart, but also can be seen from the subcostal views and from apical views.

46. What are the echocardiographic characteristics of muscular VSD?
Muscular VSD is seen from the parasternal short-axis view and the apical views (Fig. 6). Muscular VSDs are often multiple, small-diameter openings in the interventricular septum and typically have a "Swiss cheese–like" appearance. It is easier to identify the opening of these VSDs on the LV side than on the RV side, owing to the smooth internal surface of the LV compared with the internal surface of the RV, which is typically rich in trabeculations. Doppler echocardiography is helpful in making the diagnosis because it identifies left-to-right jets of blood flow through the interventricular septum.

47. What are the echocardiographic characteristics of malalignment VSD?
Malalignment VSD is a feature of TOF and may be seen in the occasional adult presenting with this syndrome.

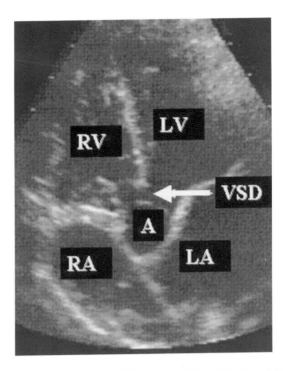

FIGURE 5. Membranous VSD (*arrow*). RV = right ventricle, RA = right atrium, LV = left ventricle, LA = left atrium, A = aortic valve.

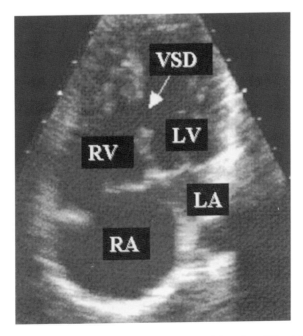

FIGURE 6. Muscular VSD (*arrow*). RV = right ventricle, RA = right atrium, LV = left ventricle, LA = left atrium, A = aortic valve.

48. What are the echocardiographic parameters that determine the severity of VSD?

The severity of a VSD ultimately depends on the magnitude of blood flow crossing the defect. This is determined primarily by the size of the defect: The larger the VSD, the greater the magnitude of the shunting and the smaller the chance for spontaneous closure. The relationship between the systemic arterial pressure and the pulmonary pressure determines the "drive" for left-to-right shunt through the VSD, but this is more a factor of shunt velocity and not shunt volume.

49. What are the main echocardiographic tips for correct measuring of the size of a VSD?

A VSD typically is elliptical in shape and, if possible, should be displayed in multiple views for accurate measuring.

50. In addition to the dimension of the VSD, what other important parameters regarding this lesion are delineated routinely by echocardiography?

Parameters that allow **evaluation of the hemodynamic significance of the VSD** include:
- The ratio of pulmonary blood flow to system blood flow (i.e., the shunt = Qp:Qs)
- Pulmonary hypertension
- The presence of LA and LV enlargement

Parameters that may be **important to the surgeon who performs the VSD repair** include:
- The margins of the VSD, which should be evaluated for chordae or papillary muscles straddling the defect (ignoring these structures may lead to valve dysfunction after the placement of the VSD patch)
- Prominent RV muscle bundles that may obscure the true dimensions of the VSD
- Associated malformations, such as subaortic membranes

51. How can pulmonary artery pressure be calculated in a patient with VSD?

By means of Bernoulli's equation, as follows:

1. If pulmonary artery pressure in systole = RV pressure in systole (this equation is true only in the absence of RV outflow tract obstruction or pulmonary stenosis), *then*

2. The RV pressure can be calculated by knowing the LV pressure (systemic blood pressure) and the gradient between the RV and LV, *and*

3. The LV-RV gradient = $4 v^2$, where v is the velocity of the VSD flow by Doppler.

52. How can the Qp:Qs be calculated by echocardiography, and what is its importance in the evaluation of the hemodynamic significance of VSD?

In normal subjects, the RV and the LV have the same cardiac output (e.g., the Swan-Ganz catheter measures the RV output as an indicator of the LV output; this is possible because in the absence of RV volume overload from a shunt, the RV and LV output are equal and can be substituted for one another). In patients with a shunt, the RV output is higher than the LV output by the amount of blood shunted from the LV to the RV. The ratio between the RV and LV output is a measure of shunt severity. The calculations are relatively easy (the LV output is calculated based on the diameter of the LV outflow tract and on the velocity of blood flow through the LV outflow tract; the RV output is assessed similarly in the pulmonary artery). At low Qp:Qs ratios, the echocardiographic determined ratio has a fair amount of variability, but still is clinically important for determining if the shunt is large or small.

53. List the main types of ASD.

Based on their embryologic formation and on their site within the interatrial septum, ASDs are classified as:
- Secundum ASD (the most frequently seen in adults)
- Primum ASD
- Sinus venosus ASD (the rarest form) (Fig. 7)

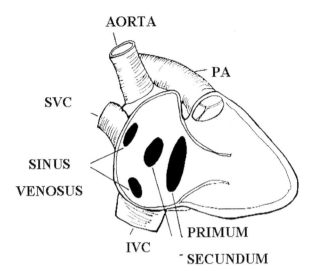

FIGURE 7. The different types of atrial septal defects.

54. How is echocardiography used to assess an ASD?
To assess:
- The type (location) of defect
- Its dimensions
- The presence of associated cardiac anomalies
- The presence and degree of RV dilation and failure secondary to the volume overload
- The presence and severity of associated pulmonary hypertension

55. What are common characteristics of the three types of ASD?
Regardless of its type, an ASD is visualized as a lack of continuity in the interatrial septum with associated blood flow shown by Doppler echocardiography or contrast enhancement. RV dilation and dysfunction may exist because of chronic volume overload.

56. What are the main echocardiographic tips for the correct measurement of ASD?
The size of an ASD should be measured at end-diastole (when the opening is largest), from at least two different orthogonal planes (because ASDs are often oval, with a long and a short axis).

57. Describe the most important echocardiographic views for visualization of ASD.
As in the case of PFO, the **subcostal view,** which presents the interatrial septum in an almost perpendicular orientation to the ultrasound beam, is the imaging projection of choice. The apical four-chamber view is also useful, but because the interatrial septum is approximately parallel to the ultrasound beam, there are two potential diagnostic problems:
1. Mistaking the commonly seen echo dropout in the middle portion of the interatrial septum for a secundum ASD (false-positive diagnosis)
2. Failure to visualize a true ASD because of the parallel orientation of the ultrasound beam relative to the interatrial septum (false-negative diagnosis).
Because of these problems with two-dimensional echocardiography detection of an ASD, the use of Doppler and contrast enhancement is important.

58. Identify the main characteristics of secundum ASD.
- It is located in the midportion of the atrial septum (Fig. 8).
- It is often an isolated defect (no associated cardiac anomalies).

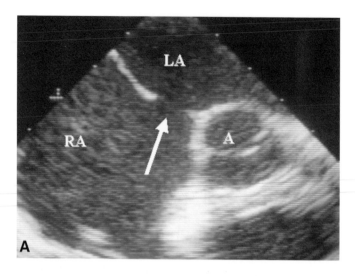

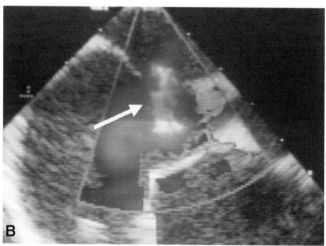

FIGURE 8. *A*, Secundum ASD (*arrow*) on two-dimensional TEE. LA = left atrium, RA = right atrium, A = aortic valve. *B*, Secundum ASD on color TEE (arrow). The flow through the ASD is depicted in lighter shades of blue than the "background" blood flow inside both atria; however, these shades of blue are not very bright, because the patient has a large ASD with decreased interatrial pressure gradient, and a consequent low-velocity left-to-right blood flow. (See also Color Plates, Figure 21.)

59. What additional echocardiographic information is especially important in a patient with an ASD?

The presence and width of tissue margins around the ASD opening is important in contemporary practice because patients with a sufficient rim of tissue around the communication may be candidates for percutaneous closure of the ASD. For further discussion of the use of occluder devices in ASD patients, see the section on cardiac catheterization.

60. List the echocardiographic characteristics of primum ASD.
- Located anterior and inferior to the fossa ovalis
- Crescent-shaped

- Frequently associated cleft anterior mitral valve leaflet
- May be part of a more complex congenital cardiac malformation, termed *atrioventricular canal defect*

61. Summarize the main characteristics of the atrioventricular canal defect.

This complex malformation frequently is associated with Down syndrome and includes:

- Primum ASD
- Membranous VSD
- Anomalies of the atrioventricular valves (in one of the extreme forms of this syndrome, the mitral and tricuspid valves are joined as a single atrioventricular valve straddling the VSD)
- A lack of normal apical displacement of the tricuspid valve relative to the mitral valve (in other words, the two valves are at the same level)

62. What are the echocardiographic characteristics of a sinus venosus ASD?

It is located posterior to the fossa ovalis.

It may be associated with partial anomalous drainage of the pulmonary veins, most frequently the right superior pulmonary vein.

63. Which type of ASD is the most difficult to diagnose by transthoracic echocardiography (TTE)?

Sinus venosus ASD. TTE has a sensitivity of only 44% for a sinus venosus defect compared with nearly 90% for primum defect and 89% for secundum defect.

64. What is the role of TEE in the diagnosis of ASD?

TEE is necessary in patients with suspected sinus venosus defect. There are two important elements of information that TEE is much better suited to provide than TTE:

1. The presence of the **anomaly**
2. The presence of **associated partial anomalous venous return**

65. What are the echocardiographic characteristics of PDA?

PDA connects the main pulmonary artery to the aorta. It is seen best from a parasternal short-axis view. PDA can be shown echocardiographically by:

- Direct visualization, which allows measurement of the diameter and length of the duct
- Doppler echocardiography, which visualizes flow between the aorta and the pulmonary artery

66. List associated abnormalities that should be sought in patients with PDA.

- Associated abnormalities of the aortic arch
- Pulmonary hypertension
- Dilation of the **left** heart chambers
- Diastolic flow reversal in the descending aorta caused by antegrade blood flow through the PDA into the pulmonary artery.

67. PDA and ASD result in a left-to-right shunt, but only an ASD causes dilation of the right heart chambers. What is the explanation?

As opposed to what is seen with ASD, the left-to-right shunt of PDA occurs beyond the right heart, so the RV does not have to cope with the excessive **volume** of blood. The LV has to cope with an increased pulmonary **venous** return, however, consisting of the physiologic return and the additional volume shunted directly to the pulmonary circulation. This LV volume overload may lead to LV dilation and failure.

68. List the echocardiographic characteristics of pulmonary valve stenosis.

- Thickened, fused valve leaflets
- Systolic doming of the valve leaflets

- Variable degrees of hypoplasia of the pulmonary annulus
- RV hypertrophy
- Poststenotic dilation of the pulmonary artery
- Possible association with other congenital anomalies, most frequently anomalies pertaining to the TOF

69. Name the main types of subvalvular aortic stenosis seen in adult patients.

Subaortic membrane and **dynamic subaortic obstruction** (in hypertrophic obstructive cardiomyopathy patients). For a discussion of these anomalies, see Chapters 3 and 6.

70. What is aortic coarctation?

A congenital narrowing of the thoracic aorta that can vary from a localized lesion to a diffuse hypoplasia of the aortic arch. Associated congenital anomalies include:

71. List congenital anomalies associated with aortic coarctation.

- Bicuspid aortic valve /valvular aortic stenosis
- Parachute mitral valve
- Subaortic stenosis

72. What is Ebstein's anomaly?

Ebstein's anomaly is characterized by the following findings (Fig. 9):

1. Apical displacement of the septal leaflet of the tricuspid valve. (Although the tricuspid valve normally is located more apically than the mitral valve, the distance between the insertion point of the two valves is normally ≤ 10 mm; in Ebstein's anomaly, the tricuspid valve is > 10 mm apically displaced compared with the level of the mitral valve.

2. The apical displacement of the tricuspid valve leads to "atrialization" of a portion of the RV (the portion of the RV situated above the tricuspid valve).

3. In addition to the abnormal insertion of the septal leaflet of the tricuspid valve, there may be other malformations, including presence of excessive valve tissue, tethering, or dysplasia (thickened valves, with "rolled-up" edges).

4. There is usually some associated tricuspid regurgitation or stenosis.

5. There may be an associated ASD.

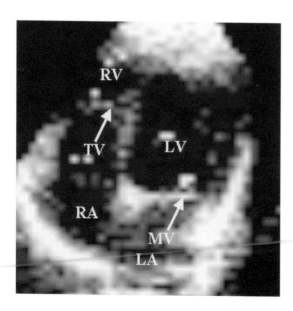

FIGURE 9. Ebstein's anomaly. Note the gross apical displacement of the tricuspid valve in this patient. RV = right ventricle, RA = right atrium, TV = tricuspid valve, LV = left ventricle, MV = mitral valve, LA = left atrium.

73. What is congenitally corrected TGA?

This malformation consists of:

Atrioventricular discordance: The RA opens into a right-sided morphologic LV through the mitral valve, whereas the LA opens into the left-sided morphologic RV through the tricuspid valve.

Ventriculoarterial discordance: The RV is connected to the aorta, and the LV is connected to the pulmonary artery.

74. Summarize the echocardiographic characteristics of congenitally corrected TGA.

- A morphologic LV situated to the right of the morphologic RV
- A left-sided atrioventricular (tricuspid) valve situated apically from the right-sided (mitral) atrioventricular valve
- A parallel course of the aorta and the pulmonary artery (in normal subjects, these two arteries are "wrapped" around each other)

75. What is uncorrected TGA?

A congenital cardiac anomaly usually seen in children, consisting of: **atrioventricular concordance** (the RA opens into the the the RV through the tricuspid valve; the LA opens into the LV through the mitral valve) and **ventriculoarterial discordance** (LV is connected to the aorta; RV is connected to the pulmonary artery).

In these patients, the pulmonary and systemic circulations essentially function in parallel and an intracardiac or extracardiac shunt is necessary for survival. Although this entity usually is seen in pediatric patients, children with this condition can live to adulthood if they have corrective surgery.

76. In patients with atrioventricular and ventriculoarterial discordance, the circulation is "congenitally corrected." Does this mean that these patients have a normal life expectancy?

No. Reasons for a decreased life expectancy in these patients include:

- Associated anomalies, such as VSD and anomalies of the ventricles and atrioventricular valves
- Progressive left atrioventricular (tricuspid) valve regurgitation
- Progressive systemic (morphologic right) ventricular failure, because of the inability of the relatively thin RV myocardium to cope with the demands of the systemic circulation over the long-term

77. What is TOF?

A complex congenital cardiac malformation including the following components:

- Pulmonary stenosis
- VSD
- Overriding aorta
- RV hypertrophy

78. What other congenital abnormality is associated with TOF?

In approximately 5% of patients with TOF, there is anomalous origin of the coronary arteries (left anterior descending artery originating from the right coronary artery, a single coronary artery, or a duplicated anterior descending coronary artery). Patients with this syndrome also may present with branch pulmonary artery stenosis.

79. What is an overriding aorta?

An aorta opening "above" the VSD. Rather than the aorta being continuous with the LV outflow tract, the aorta is continuous with the LV outflow tract and the RV portion adjacent to the VSD. Literally the aorta appears to "straddle" (override) the interventricular septum (Fig. 10).

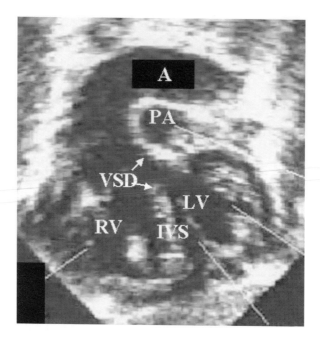

FIGURE 10. Tetralogy of Fallot from an inverted subcostal view. Note that the aorta "overrides" the interventricular septum—that is, it drains blood from both ventricles rather than just from the LV. RV = right to ventricle, LV = left ventricle, VSD = ventricular septal defect (*small arrows*), A = aorta.

80. What is the nature of the pulmonary stenosis with TOF?

In addition to valvular pulmonary stenosis, one also may encounter:
- Subvalvular stenosis, owing to the narrowing of the RV outflow tract
- Supravalvular stenosis, ranging from discrete branch pulmonary artery stenosis to diffuse hypoplasia of the pulmonary artery and its branches.

81. Identify the shortcoming of echocardiography in assessing TOF.

Echocardiography may fail to show distal branch pulmonary artery stenosis. In these patients, spiral CT or MRI may be necessary.

82. What is truncus arteriosus?

A congenital malformation with a single arterial trunk leaving the base of the heart. The pulmonary artery and the aorta are not separate, and the truncus must supply the pulmonary and the systemic circulation. Echocardiography typically shows a single great artery originating from the heart. This artery has a semilunar valve that overrides the interventricular septum.

83. What is a persistent left superior vena cava?

This is seen in 0.5% of normal subjects and 10% of patients with other congenital heart malformations. The hallmark of this syndrome is a dilated coronary sinus (best seen on parasternal long-axis view and on an apical four-chamber view), which results from the left superior vena cava drainage into the coronary sinus. The diagnosis of a left superior vena cava is made by injecting agitated saline into the left antecubital vein and visualizing the contrast material, which drains from the left arm into the persistent left superior vena cava then into the coronary sinus. As a result of this unique route, the contrast material opacifies the coronary sinus before it reaches the RA. (Injection of contrast material into a right arm vein, which drains into the "normal" [right] superior vena cava, opacifies the RA, but not the coronary sinus.)

84. List the main echocardiographic characteristics of Marfan's syndrome.
- Dilation of the aortic root, annulus, and sinuses of Valsalva
- Loss of a clearly defined sinotubular junction in the ascending aorta
- Redundant tissue in the anterior mitral valve leaflet (mitral valve prolapse)
- Increased risk of aortic regurgitation and aortic dissection

85. Describe the role of echocardiography in the follow-up of patients with Marfan's syndrome.

Echocardiography has an essential role in assessing the aortic root in this setting. It has been shown that when the aortic root diameter exceeds 50–55 mm, the risk of spontaneous rupture increases dramatically. Echocardiographic monitoring is a crucial component in the management of these patients.

86. What are the echocardiographic manifestations of sinus of Valsalva aneurysms?

A congenital aneurysm of the sinus of Valsalva appears as a narrow, "wind sock–like" projection extending from the aortic sinus into the adjacent cardiac structures. These aneurysms usually project into adjacent cardiac structures and may have an associated fistula, such as left coronary-to-LA fistula or right coronary-to-RV outflow tract fistula.

87. What are the echocardiographic manifestations of coronary arteriovenous fistula?

This is an uncommon anomaly usually consisting of a communication between a coronary artery and the coronary sinus or RA. These fistulas manifest as a murmur in a young adult and may be responsible for high-output cardiac failure or become involved in bacterial endocarditis.

88. Describe the echocardiographic findings of congenital pulmonary stenosis.

Similar to any other valvular stenosis, congenital stenosis of the pulmonary valve is characterized by an increased velocity of the systolic blood flow from the RV into the pulmonary artery (Fig. 11). Additional characteristics include:
- Thickening and doming of the pulmonary valve leaflets
- Fused or underdeveloped (hypoplastic) pulmonary valve leaflets
- Poststenotic dilation of the main pulmonary artery with true valvular stenosis
- Secondary RV hypertrophy

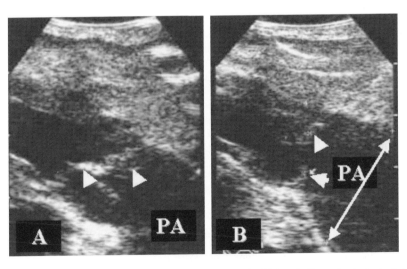

FIGURE 11. Congenital pulmonary stenosis. *A,* Diastole. Note the thickened, distorted valvular leaflets (*arrowheads*). *B,* Systole. Note the restricted opening of the valve leaflets (*arrowheads*). PA = pulmonary artery; double-headed arrow = poststenotic dilatation of the PA.

89. What are the important components of an echocardiogram in patients after corrective surgery for congenital heart disease?

Echocardiography in these patients is particularly challenging because of the complexity of the original disease and the surgical procedure, which further altered the patient's anatomy. Basically, the sonographer must show:

1. The original problem (congenital syndrome)
2. The surgical solution to the problem (surgically established corrective connections with or without implanted prosthetic material)
3. Complications of the surgical procedure
4. Remnant lesions from the original malformation

90. Summarize the concerns in patients after a VSD repair.

1. VSDs often are repaired by applying a synthetic or pericardial patch. This patch may be close to the His bundle and cause conduction defects.
2. Residual VSD should be meticulously looked for.
3. Follow-up assessment of the LV and RV function and of the pulmonary artery pressure is essential.

91. What is the concern after ASD repair?

Search for residual ASD and persistent pulmonary hypertension.

92. What is the concern after surgical correction for Ebstein's anomaly?

In addition to reassessing tricuspid flow (stenosis or regurgitation), it is important to assess LV function because LV dysfunction can progress in these patients despite successful treatment of the anomaly.

93. What are the concerns in the echocardiographic assessment of patients after surgical correction of TOF?

In addition to obvious issues related to the integrity of the VSD patch, it is essential serially to assess:

- RV function
- Degree of RV hypertrophy (this should regress after successful repair)
- Degree of RV dilation (related to residual or progressive pulmonary or tricuspid valve pathology of shunt)
- Degree of tricuspid regurgitation (occasionally, tricuspid regurgitation may progress despite successful repair if RV dilation complicates the late postoperative course)
- Degree of RA dilation
- Residual pulmonary stenosis or insufficiency
- Residual VSD
- Aneurysms of the RV outflow tract
- LV function (which may be decreased, especially in patients operated at an older age; the decrease in LV function is due mainly to the chronic volume overload resulting from long-standing VSD)

94. Summarize the possible causes of RV dysfunction after repair of TOF.

1. **Volume overload,** due to:
   a. Pulmonary valve regurgitation (in some patients the pulmonary valve is not replaced after it has been resected)
   b. Residual VSD
   c. Tricuspid regurgitation, secondary to RV dilation, which in turn is a late phase of ventricular response to RV outflow tract obstruction
2. **Pressure overload,** due to repeat RV outflow tract obstruction from:
   a. Failure of the outflow tract structures to grow with the overall body and heart growth (in children)

     b. RV outflow tract scarring
3. **Decreased RV inotropic function,** owing to:
     a. Sectioning of RV myocytes (ventriculotomy)
     b. The presence of a patch that cannot contract

Echocardiography is the procedure of choice for identification and severity assessment of all the above-mentioned elements.

95. What is the Fontan operation?

The Fontan procedure connects the RA to the pulmonary arteries through a synthetic conduit. Fontan and coworkers showed that blood flow to the lungs is not dependent on the presence of a functional RV. Blood can cross the lungs from the pulmonary artery into the pulmonary veins without having a "pump" to propel it through the circuit as long as there is a natural gradient between the RA and the LA.

MAGNETIC RESONANCE IMAGING

Anthon R. Fuisz, M.D., and Gabriel Adelmann, M.D.

96. Discuss the role of MRI in the evaluation of congenital heart disease.

The main challenge in the evaluation involves the three-dimensional complexity of some of these malformations. MRI is ideally suited to meet this challenge. In current practice, cardiac MRI is indicated whenever echocardiography is not able to supply all the necessary information. In view of the excellent imaging made possible by TEE and of the extensive experience accumulated in this field, echocardiography in the hands of experienced echocardiographers is sufficient in most patients with congenital heart disease. In cases in which the pulmonary arteries or the connections of extracardiac structures need to be well visualized, MRI may prove indispensable.

97. List the elements of information that can be provided by MRI in the diagnosis of aortic coarctation.

- Direct visualization of the coarctation
- Estimation of the pressure gradient across the coarctation
- Evaluation of the collateral blood flow
- Follow-up after surgery

98. List the elements of information that can be obtained by MRI for the diagnosis of ASD.

- Direct visualization of ASD (evident as a signal void) (Fig. 12)
- Visualization of any associated cardiac anomalies
- Assessment of the shunt through the ASD

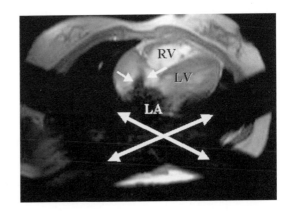

FIGURE 12. Atrial septal defect visualized by the " double slab technique," created by superimposing on the cardiac image two intersecting black rectangles, which create the necessary "background" contrast for visualization of the blood flow through the interatrial communication (*arrow*).

99. What is the main pitfall in the MRI diagnosis of ASD?
Although MRI generally is accurate for diagnosis of ASD, the diagnosis of secundum ASD must be made with special caution because the fossa ovalis occasionally may be mistaken for an abnormal interatrial communication. Specialized sequences that show left-to-right flow in the atria are often necessary to define the secundum ASD precisely.

100. Name the most common congenital abnormality missed by routine echocardiography and detected by subsequent MRI.
Sinus venosus ASD.

101. List the MRI characteristics of the anatomic RV that allow accurate identification of this chamber in patients with TGA.
1. The RV outflow tract separates the tricuspid from the pulmonary valve.
2. A muscular ring can be seen below the pulmonary valve.
3. The tricuspid valve is oriented more ventrally than the mitral valve.
4. A moderator band is present.
5. An irregular internal surface (trabeculations) is apparent.

102. List the elements of information provided by MRI in patients with TOF.
- Direct visualization of the different elements of the syndrome (pulmonary stenosis, VSD, overriding aorta, and RV hypertrophy)
- Assessment of flow through the VSD and through the stenotic pulmonary valve
- Assessment of peripheral pulmonary artery stenosis (a relatively common feature of this syndrome, which is difficult or impossible to diagnose by echocardiography)
- Assessment and follow-up of pulmonary insufficiency, which may complicate surgery in these patients
- Assessment and follow-up of RV mass, which may increase as a result of RV dilation secondary to severe pulmonary insufficiency

103. What are the advantages of cardiac MRI over echocardiography in the follow-up of patients after congenital heart disease repair?
MRI is superior to echocardiography for:
- Serial follow-up of extracardiac conduits (including direct visualization and blood flow assessment) (Fig. 13)
- Follow-up of the RV mass in patients with pulmonary insufficiency after surgical repair of the TOF (see question 102).

NUCLEAR MEDICINE

Manuel D. Cerqueira, M.D., Jonathan G. Tall, CNMT, and Gabriel Adelmann, M.D.

104. List the elements of information provided by nuclear imaging in adult patients with congenital heart disease.
- Ventricular function
- Presence, localization (intracardiac versus extracardiac), and direction (left-to-right versus right-to-left) of shunt
- Presence of concomitant myocardial ischemia

105. What is the role of nuclear cardiology in the diagnosis and management of adult patients with congenital heart disease?
The only class I indication for nuclear cardiology is the assessment of ventricular function. For all the other indications, echocardiography and cardiac MRI are the procedures of choice.

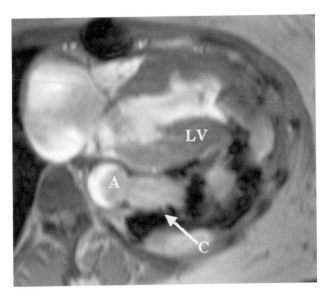

FIGURE 13. Follow-up MRI in a patient after repair of LVOT obstruction. A valve conduit (C) empties the apex of the left ventricle (LV) into the descending aorta (A).

106. What is the nuclear technique of choice for assessment of patients with cardiac shunt?

The detection and quantification of cardiac shunt necessitate a rapid acquisition of radioactivity as it passes through the heart; this can be best performed by first-pass radionuclide angiography.

107. Describe the nuclear findings in patients with cardiac shunts.

In patients with left-to-right shunt, first-pass radionuclide angiography shows persistent high levels of radioactivity in the lungs or RV or both, as a result of early recirculation (besides the "legitimate" [physiologic] blood flow, the lungs and RV receive an additional volume of radiolabeled blood because of the transit of radioactive tracer through the shunt).

In patients with right-to-left shunts, there is early visualization of the radioactive bolus in the left cardiac chambers, which it reaches prematurely, through the abnormal communication.

108. What is the pulmonary circulation time?

The delay between the moment when the radioactive tracer reaches the right heart chambers and the moment when it first appears in the left heart chambers.

109. State the importance of the pulmonary circulation time for the diagnosis of cardiac shunt.

Pulmonary circulation time is significantly shortened in patients with right-to-left shunt.

110. How can the site of blood shunting (intracardiac versus extracardiac) be established based on radionuclide angiography?

Time-activity curves may be derived from the acquired signals from both ventricles and can be used to establish the site of blood shunting.

CHEST X-RAY

Gabriel Adelmann, M.D., and Curtis E. Green, M.D.

111. What are the findings of congenital heart disease on chest radiography?

- Anatomic changes characteristic of the anomaly in question (e.g., the "3" sign in aortic coarctation) (Fig. 14)

- The effect of the cardiac anomaly on the heart chambers
- The effect of the cardiac anomaly on the pulmonary circulation

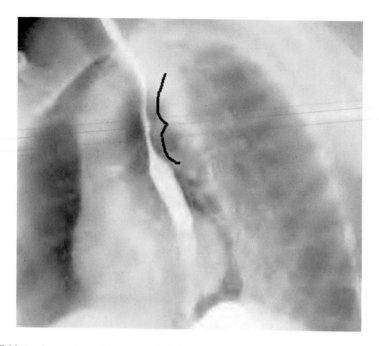

FIGURE 14. Aortic coarctation. The "inverted 3" sign represents the indentation produced by the local aortic narrowing on the barium-filled esophagus.

112. How important is radiography in the detection of cardiac anomalies?

Chest radiography provides a silhouette image of the heart (i.e., a superimposition on a single image with all the cardiac structures crossed by the x-rays). Chest radiography generally does not allow direct visualization of *intra*cardiac anomalies. Occasionally, *extra*cardiac anomalies can be seen directly (e.g., aortic coarctation or a calcified PDA).

113. What are the radiographic findings referring to the heart chambers in patients with congenital heart disease?

Congenital heart disease can cause either dilation or hypertrophy of the cardiac chambers. Chest x-ray can show atrial or ventricular dilation, whereas isolated hypertrophy of the ventricles cannot be diagnosed reliably by chest x-ray.

114. Summarize the impact of congenital heart disease on the pulmonary circulation.

Congenital heart disease may be responsible for:
- Pulmonary venous hypertension (cranial redistribution of the pulmonary circulation, prominent pulmonary trunk and main pulmonary arteries, Kerley B lines, pulmonary edema)
- Pulmonary arterial hypertension (enlarged central pulmonary arteries with peripheral "pruning")
- Pulmonary shunt physiology

115. Can left-to-right and right-to-left shunt be distinguished by chest radiograph?

1. **Isolated left-to-right shunt** (i.e., without associated right-to-left shunt) is characterized by:
   a. Dilated central pulmonary circulation (trunk, main pulmonary arteries) with gradual tapering toward the periphery
   b. RV and RA dilation

2. **Isolated right-to-left shunt** (i.e., without any remnant left-to-right shunt) is characterized by signs of pulmonary hypertension.

3. **Combined left-to-right and right-to-left shunt** is associated with features of both conditions.

116. List the main conditions associated with oligemia (decreased pulmonary circulation in the lung fields) on chest x-ray.

- TOF
- Ebstein's anomaly
- Tricuspid atresia

117. How can chest radiography distinguish between pulmonary hypertension and oligemia?

Both conditions cause a decrease in pulmonary vascularity. The **difference** is that:

- Pulmonary hypertension is associated with a dilated central pulmonary vasculature (pulmonary trunk, main pulmonary arteries).
- Oligemia is associated with a uniform decrease of pulmonary vascular markings over the entire area of both lungs.

118. What is Eisenmenger's syndrome?

The late complication of a chronic left-to-right shunt. In these patients, chronic volume overload generated by a left-to-right shunt causes irreversible changes in the pulmonary vasculature with secondary pulmonary hypertension. The pulmonary artery pressures attain values higher than those of the systemic pressure, resulting in shunt reversal (left-to-right becomes right-to-left shunt).

119. Identify the radiographic signs of Eisenmenger's syndrome.

Practically, the radiographic picture is that of pulmonary hypertension. (Fig. 15)

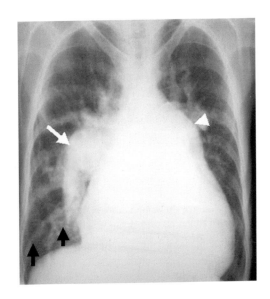

FIGURE 15. Eisenmenger's syndrome in a patient with ASD (PA film). Note the severely dilated right pulmonary artery (*white arrow*) and pulmonary trunk (*arrowhead*). The significant disproportion between the central circulation and the periphery of the lungs (*black arrows*) indicates pulmonary hypertension.

120. Explain the practical importance of the diagnosis of Eisenmenger's syndrome in a patient with cardiac shunt.

The presence of Eisenmenger's syndrome generally indicates that a surgical approach to the underlying shunt is contraindicated. In these patients, the right-to-left shunt is a compensatory mechanism by which the RV can meet that challenge of severely increased pulmonary artery pressures. Closure of the shunt would deprive the RV of this compensatory mechanism, resulting in acute RV failure.

121. What are the radiographic findings in patients with ASD?

The radiographic findings are due to left-to-right shunt causing a volume overload of the RV and pulmonary hypertension. A chest x-ray typically shows:

Signs of RA enlargement: posterior bulging of the lower half of the posterior cardiac border, on a lateral film

Signs of RV enlargement: a contact between the RV and the sternum extending cranially beyond the inferior one third of the distance between the sternal angle and the diaphragm, on a lateral film

Signs of pulmonary hypertension: increased diameter of the pulmonary trunk and main pulmonary arteries, with rapid tapering in diameter toward the lung periphery ("pruning") these findings occur later in the course of the disease and are due to irreversible pulmonary vasculature changes in the face of the chronic volume overload (see Figure 15)

122. What are the main radiographic findings in patients with VSD?

The radiographic signs typically show different degrees of:
- LV dilation: a cardiothoracic ratio > 0.5
- LV failure: pulmonary congestion

123. In the absence of Eisenmenger syndrome, ASD and VSD are associated with left-to-right shunt. The radiographic signs in the two conditions are different, however. For what reason?

The main difference between the two conditions is that ASD produces RV volume overload, whereas VSD does not.

124. List the main radiographic findings in patients with bicuspid aortic valve.

1. Aortic stenosis, causing LV hypertrophy; when isolated, this is not detected by chest radiography. LV dilation and LV failure in the late stages of severe aortic stenosis are associated signs that can be detected by chest x-ray.

2. Aortic insufficiency, responsible for LV dilation and failure.

3. Associated abnormalities, including aortic coarctation and aneurysmal dilation of the ascending aorta.

125. Name the main radiographic findings in patients with Ebstein's anomaly.

Ebstein's anomaly is characterized by apical displacement of the triscuspid valve, severe tricuspid regurgitation, and (often) the presence of an ASD. The radiographic findings include signs of **RA dilation, RV dilation,** and **pulmonary hypertension.**

126. Identify the main radiographic findings in patients with PDA.
- Signs of RV volume overload (RV dilation)
- Signs of RV pressure overload (pulmonary hypertension), when irreversible changes in pulmonary vasculature occur

127. What are the main radiographic findings in patients with aortic coarctation?
See Chapter 10.

128. List the main radiographic findings in patients with TOF.
- A characteristic shape of the LV, with the apex pointing superiorly (in normal subjects, the apex points downward, whereas in patients with RV hypertrophy, the apex is horizontal)
- Pulmonary oligemia, resulting from the associated pulmonary stenosis

10. THE AORTA AND THE GREAT VESSELS

CARDIAC CATHETERIZATION

Gabriel Adelmann, M.D.

1. What are the current indications for aortography?

Aortography is an easy and convenient procedure in the catheterization laboratory, as a complement to coronary angiography. In the era of widely available noninvasive aortic imaging (magnetic resonance angiography [MRA], spiral computed tomography [CT], transesophageal echocardiography [TEE]), the absolute need for aortography is decreasing. The one clinical setting in which aortography remains the gold standard is aortic transection, especially in centers where magnetic resonance imaging (MRI) is not readily available.

2. What important information regarding aortic aneurysms is typically *not* provided by aortography?

Although aortography can visualize aortic aneurysms easily, as areas of localized dilation of the aorta (Fig. 1), it is generally unable to show thrombus harbored by the aneurysm cavity. In the presence of a known aortic aneurysm, aortography generally is not indicated because of the risk of dislodging a blood clot from the aneurysm cavity resulting in thromboembolic complications.

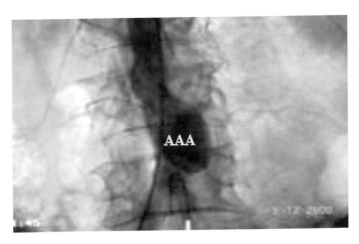

FIGURE 1. Abdominal aortic aneurysm (AAA). The ratio between the greatest diameter of the aneurysm and the diameter of the apparently healthy adjacent segment of the aorta exceeds 1.5. Note that the actual diameter of the aneurysmal region could be even greater than demonstrated by aortography (mural thrombus is undetectable by this method).

3. Describe the typical aortographic findings in aortic dissection.

Aortography can show the presence of an intimal flap, separating the true and the false lumen. The entry site of the dissection into a medial hematoma also can be identified (Fig. 2).

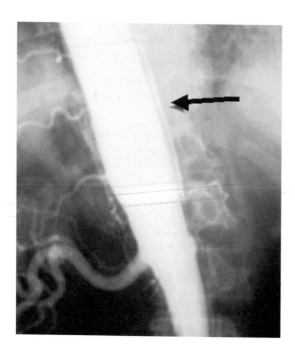

FIGURE 2. Aortic dissection. Note the thin linear structure running parallel to the aortic wall, representing the protrusion of cleaved endothelium into the vessel lumen (*arrow*).

4. Which important finding related to aortic dissection is typically *not* identified by aortography?

Approximately 10–15% of cases of aortic dissection do not have an associated intimal flap identified because the false lumen has been "thrombosed" into an intramural hematoma (thrombus accumulation in the media) without any communication with the aortic lumen. This condition involves the aortic wall only and as such is not shown by aortography.

5. What is the sensitivity and specificity of aortography for the diagnosis of aortic dissection?

Even assuming a high sensitivity and specificity of this procedure for *classic* aortic dissection, if one considers that 10–15% of the *total* number of dissections consists of intramural hematoma, the sensitivity and specificity of aortography for diagnosis of *any* type of aortic dissection are < 85–90% compared with ≥ 90% for some noninvasive imaging modalities (MRI).

6. Describe the typical aortographic findings in aortic transection.

Aortic transection is synonymous with aortic rupture and causes a typical pattern of contrast material extravasation from the aortic lumen. In many centers, aortography is the diagnostic procedure of choice for this condition. Newer techniques, such as spiral CT or MRA, are also excellent tools for diagnosing aortic transection and have the additional advantage of being noninvasive.

7. Discuss the role of aortography for identification of the implantation sites of coronary artery bypass grafts.

Although coronary artery bypass grafts usually are relatively easy to cannulate, these grafts may not be readily located in some patients. Before concluding that this problem is due to ostial occlusion of the grafts, it is useful to inject contrast material into the aortic root. This simple procedure may help localize the grafts, which, for technical reasons, occasionally may have "atypical" aortic implantation sites. In this setting, aortography is a form of "nonselective" graft visualization.

8. What is the role of aortography in the diagnosis of aortic regurgitation?

By injecting contrast material into the aortic root, aortic regurgitation can be identified and semiquantitatively graded. For a discussion of aortic regurgitation assessment by this method, see Chapter 6.

9. State the main indication of pulmonary angiography in adult patients.

Pulmonary angiography (arteriography) is the gold standard for the diagnosis of pulmonary thromboembolism and is indicated in patients in whom there is high clinical suspicion of pulmonary embolism and the results of noninvasive testing (nuclear ventilation-perfusion scan or CT) are inconclusive.

10. What is the role of pulmonary angiography in pediatric patients?

Children with pulmonary stenosis, whether isolated or as part of a more complex syndrome (e.g., tetralogy of Fallot), often have different degrees of main pulmonary artery and pulmonary artery branch stenosis. These can be delineated by pulmonary angiography and hemodynamic recordings. Identification of a pulmonary artery stenosis is important in establishing the surgical therapeutic approach.

11. What are the findings on pulmonary angiography in patients with pulmonary embolism?

The angiographic diagnosis of pulmonary embolism is based on the identification of an obstructed ("severed") pulmonary vessel or of an intraluminal filling defect in the pulmonary artery or one of its branches (Fig. 3).

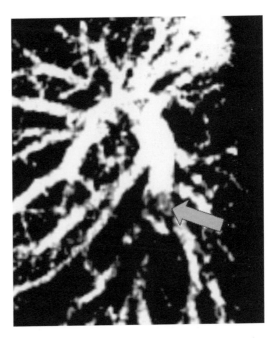

FIGURE 3. Pulmonary embolism. Note the nonhomogenous filling defect (*arrow*) in one of the large branches of the pulmonary artery, which appears "severed."

12. A patient was admitted for acute-onset shortness of breath and underwent pulmonary angiography to rule out pulmonary embolism after a ventilation-perfusion nuclear scan yielded inconclusive results. The pulmonary angiogram was interpreted as "negative for pulmonary embolism." What should be the next step in the management of this patient?

This patient probably does not have pulmonary embolism. In a large-scale study, pulmonary angiography was found to have a negative predictive value $> 99\%$ for this diagnosis. The most logical next step in the management of this patient is a systematic assessment for other causes of dyspnea.

13. Can cardiac catheterization assist in the selection of the best therapeutic strategy in a patient with pulmonary embolism?

One of the main questions arising in connection with the treatment of pulmonary embolism is when to use thrombolytic therapy. The main indications for thrombolysis in these patients include hemodynamic instability and significant, new-onset RV hypokinesis, in the appropriate clinical setting.

14. What are the angiographic findings in aortic coarctation?

Aortography can show the characteristic aortic narrowing and may be used for assessment of transstenotic gradients; however, angiography is being superceded by MRI or MRA for the diagnosis of aortic coarctation. (Fig. 4).

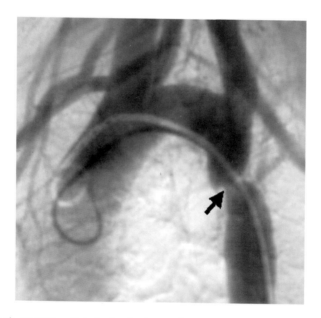

FIGURE 4. Aortic coarctation. Note the localized narrowing at the junction of the aortic arch and the descending aorta (*arrow*).

ECHOCARDIOGRAPHY

Steven A. Goldstein, M.D., Neil J. Weissman, M.D., Gabriel Adelmann, M.D., and Joseph Lindsay, M.D.

15. Define aortic dissection.

Aortic dissection is a life-threatening condition, characterized by a break in the integrity of the aortic wall, resulting in the presence of an *additional lumen*, also called *false lumen*, separated from the true lumen of the aorta by an intima-media partition termed the *dissection flap*. A variant of aortic dissection, called *intramural hematoma*, is not associated with a dissection flap.

16. Name the main classifications of aortic dissection.
The Stanford classification and the DeBakey classification (Fig. 5).

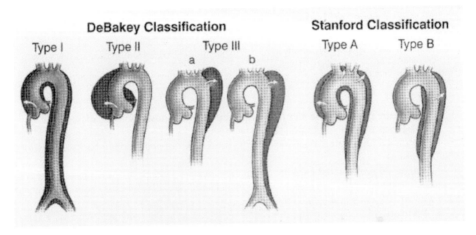

DeBakey Classification

Type I   Type II   Type III
                      a   b

Stanford Classification

Type A   Type B

FIGURE 5. The two most widely used classifications of aortic dissection. See questions 18 and 19 for further explanation. (From Kouchoukos NT, Dougenis D: Surgery of the thoracic aorta. N Engl J Med 336:1876–1888, 1997, with permission.)

17. Which characteristic of aortic dissection are the Stanford and the DeBakey classifications based on, and why is this important?
The *location* of aortic dissection. Aortic dissection location is one of the main determinants of prognosis and management (ascending aortic dissections are life-threatening, and emergent surgery is required).

18. Describe the Stanford classification of aortic dissection.
- **Type A:** The ascending aorta is involved. The dissection usually begins in the proximal ascending aorta and extends antegrade (downstream) toward (and sometimes involving) the descending aorta.
- **Type B:** The dissection begins in the descending thoracic aorta, beyond the level of the left subclavian artery, and extends distally.

19. Describe the DeBakey classification of aortic dissection.
- **Type I:** Originating in the ascending aorta and extending into the descending aorta (Stanford type A dissections).
- **Type II:** Originating in the ascending aorta but limited to the ascending aorta and arch (also Stanford type A dissections, but without distal extension).
- **Type III:** Limited to the descending aorta (Stanford type B).

20. Name the echocardiographic hallmark of aortic dissection.
The hallmark of *classic* aortic dissection (i.e., *not* intramural hematoma) is the **dissection flap,** appearing as a thin, distinct, mobile membrane within the aortic lumen, which oscillates with the cardiac cycle (see Figure 6A and B).

21. Does the absence of a dissection flap rule out aortic dissection?
No, because the dissection flap may be localized to a small area and missed by echocardiography, or the patient could have an intramural hematoma (a variant of aortic dissection discussed subsequently) that is not associated with a dissection flap.

22. Summarize the other echocardiographic findings of aortic dissection, besides the dissection flap.

Echocardiographic Findings Associated with Aortic Dissection

COMPONENTS OF AORTIC DISSECTION	COMPLICATIONS OF AORTIC DISSECTION
Dissection flap Aortic dilation that may cause left atrium (LA) compression Aortic wall thickening	Aortic regurgitation Pericardial effusion Pleural effusion Coronary artery dissection

23. What are the *clinical principles* that help guide the diagnosis of aortic dissection?
The diagnosis of aortic dissection should be:

1. Based on a **high index of suspicion** (e.g., acute onset of chest pain or back pain, history of hypertension).

2. **Diagnosed and treated rapidly**. When the diagnosis is suspected, a diagnostic imaging procedure should be carried out rapidly. There is increased mortality for every hour of treatment delay with an ascending aortic dissection.

3. **Accurate.** Missing an aortic dissection may lead to a fatal outcome, whereas a false-positive diagnosis may expose the patient to unnecessary surgery.

24. Name the noninvasive imaging modalities used for the diagnosis of aortic dissection.
CT, MRI, and TEE

25. Summarize the advantages and disadvantages of CT, MRI, and TEE for diagnosis of aortic dissection.

MODALITY	ADVANTAGES	DISADVANTAGES
TEE	Excellent sensitivity and specificity Rapid Portable (can be performed at the bedside) Safely performed on critically ill patients (e.g., patients on ventilators) Can detect, quantify, and define mechanism of aortic insufficiency Can detect involvement of coronary ostia Can detect pericardial effusion Can assess left ventricular (LV) function Can detect intramural hematoma	Can miss localized dissection of upper ascending aorta or arch May not define branch vessel involvement Semi-invasive, with a small potential for morbidity
CT	Rapid, noninvasive, immediately available Excellent sensitivity and specificity (spiral CT scan) Widely available Ability to diagnose other potentially important thoracic pathology that can mimic aortic dissection (pulmonary embolism, pneumothorax, pneumonia) Superior to TEE for diagnosis of neck vessel involvement in the dissection process	Radiographic contrast media required Does not detect aortic insufficiency Contraindicated in patients with pre existing renal impairment
MRI	Excellent sensitivity and specificity Produces transverse, sagittal, and coronal views	Time delay in obtaining a study if MRI not immediately available Difficult in critically ill patients (e.g., patients on ventilators)

(continued)

(Continued)

MODALITY	ADVANTAGES	DISADVANTAGES
	Does not require contrast enhancement Can detect pericardial effusion Can detect aortic regurgitation	Contraindicated in patients with pacemakers or intracranial aneurysm clips Expensive

26. What is the imaging method of choice for diagnosis of aortic dissection?

TEE, CT, and MRI have roughly the same sensitivity for diagnosis of aortic dissection (95–100%). There is no "procedure of choice," and hospitals generally use the diagnostic modality for which there is local experience. Because of its ready availability, TEE and CT tend to be the preferred methods in most centers.

27. Define the "blind spot" of TEE for visualization of the aorta.

A portion of the ascending aorta may not be seen adequately by TEE because of interposition of the trachea or right mainstem bronchus or both between the esophagus (TEE probe) and the ascending aorta. A dissection limited to this area may be missed.

28. What is the key to a successful CT diagnosis of aortic dissection?

It is essential to use spiral or helical CT scan for the diagnosis of aortic dissection because these technologies reduce artifact and allow one to collect more images during peak levels of contrast enhancement. Spiral CT also significantly reduces scan time. Newer scanners can image the entire aorta within seconds and can display three-dimensional images.

29. What is the role of aortography in the diagnosis of aortic dissection?

Long considered the gold standard in this setting, aortography is more time-consuming and may be less sensitive than the newer noninvasive techniques because it may miss an intramural hematoma. In addition, aortography is invasive, is costly, and exposes the patient to potentially nephrotoxic contrast media.

30. Why does aortography fail to detect intramural hematoma?

An aortogram is a luminogram (i.e., shows the aortic lumen, but is unable to visualize pathologic changes in the aortic wall). Aortography typically misses the diagnosis of intramural hematoma, which accounts for approximately 10–15% of all aortic dissections.

31. State the sensitivity of aortography for the detection of aortic dissection.

85–90%.

32. Are there situations in which more than one imaging test is required to confirm or exclude the diagnosis of aortic dissection?

Whenever an imaging test is insufficient to confirm or exclude confidently the diagnosis of aortic dissection, a second test is indicated. This is especially important in patients in whom there is a strong clinical suspicion for the diagnosis of dissection.

32. Can the true and false lumens be differentiated by TEE?

Yes.

1. The dissection flap moves toward the false lumen in systole and toward the true lumen in diastole, reflecting the pressure changes throughout the heart cycle (Fig.6A and B)

2. The sluggish blood flow in the false lumen results in spontaneous echo contrast ("smoke") on the two-dimensional study; color Doppler may reveal which lumen has the greatest amount of flow (Fig. 6C).

3. The false lumen may contain variable amounts of thrombus, mobile "strands" or "accessory flaps."

4. Occasionally the entry site of the aortic dissection may be seen, and flow often can be observed moving from the true lumen toward the false lumen in systole. (Fig. 6D).

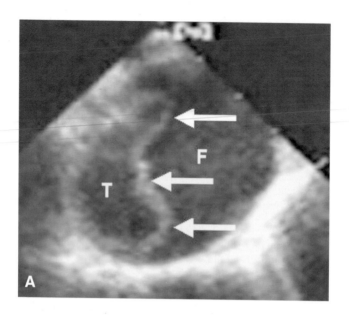

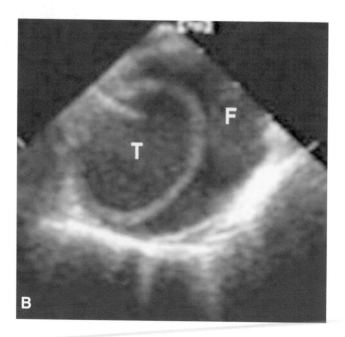

FIGURE 6. Dissection flap in diastole (*arrows*). Occasionally, the true (T) and false (F) lumens can be distinguished based on flap motion during systole and diastole. *A,* Diastolic still-frame bowing towards true lumen in diastole. *B,* Dissection flap in systole, bowing towards the false lumen. (*continued*)

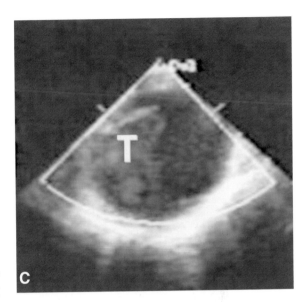

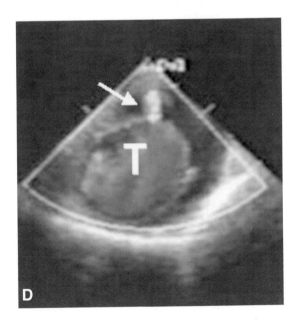

FIGURE 6. (*continued*) *C,* Dissection flap in diastole with flow in true lumen only. Occasionally, the two lumens can be distinguished based on blood flow. Dissection with flow in the true lumen only (T). (See also Color Plates, Figure 22.) *D,* Dissection flap in systole with flow in true lumen only and entry site visible. The "entry site" is a visualized (*arrow*), pointing toward the transducer (i.e., false lumen). (See also Color Plates, Figure 23.)

34. Is TEE useful for detecting involvement of the coronary arteries in patients with aortic dissection?

Yes. Using TEE, the coronary arteries can be imaged just above the level of the aortic valve. The left main coronary artery is nearly perpendicular to the echo beam and is imaged easily in most patients. The proximal right coronary artery, located farther from the TEE transducer, is more difficult to image. Nevertheless, it usually can be imaged for a stretch of several centimeters. In aortic dissection, several mechanisms may cause compromised coronary flow and myocardial ischemia. The dissection itself may extend into the coronary ostium (Fig. 7). Alternately the dissection flap may prolapse and obstruct the coronary orifice. Both of these situations can be detected by TEE. New segmental wall motion abnormalities are an indirect sign of coronary artery involvement.

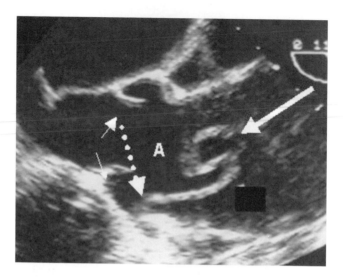

FIGURE 7. Dissection flap (*solid arrow*) extending into the sinus of Valsalva (*dashed arrow*). Note the complex ("spiral") course of the flap. A = aorta, small arrows = aortic valve leaflets.

35. What are the mechanisms of aortic regurgitation in patients with aortic dissection?

1. Dilation of the aortic root interfering with leaflet coaptation (this is the most common mechanism)

2. Leaflet prolapse resulting from impingement of the false lumen on the aortic annulus (Fig. 8)

Echocardiographic evaluation of aortic regurgitation mechanism and severity assists surgical decision making, determining whether the aortic valve can be left intact or needs to be reconstructed or replaced.

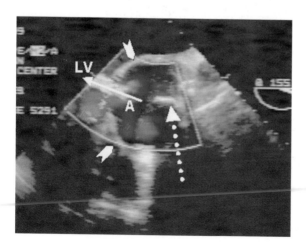

FIGURE 8. Aortic dissection (*dashed arrow*) can cause AI (*thin arrow*) because of dilation of the aortic root (*arrowheads*) or leaflet prolapse (not illustrated). Note the "ballooned" shape of the sinuses of Valsalva. (See also Color Plates, Figure 24.)

36. List the main pitfalls in the TEE evaluation of aortic dissection.

A **false-positive** diagnosis of dissection on TEE may result from:

1. Inadequate operator technique.
2. Foreshortened views of the aorta.
3. Reverberation and other artifacts (Fig. 9A), especially in the ascending aorta, mimicking a dissection flap. Reverberations can be due to:
   a. Right heart catheters; moving the catheter usually eliminates the reverberations.
   b. Aortic calcification, resulting in artifactual arc-like echodensities within the lumen.
4. The hemizygous sheath, which can mimic an intramural hematoma (Fig. 9B).

A **false-negative** TEE diagnosis of dissection is usually limited to type II aortic dissection in the blind spot of the arch (see question 27).

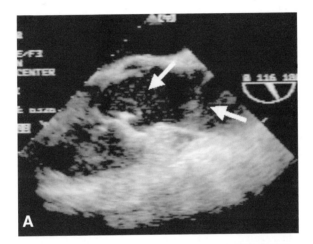

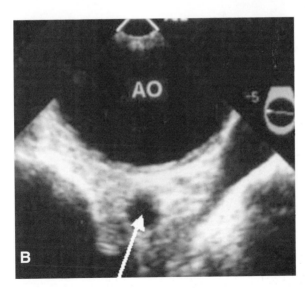

FIGURE 9. *A,* Pseudodissection. Foreshortened views of the aorta, as well as artifacts, can create the false impression of a dissection lumen (*arrows*). Imaging from multiple planes is essential. *B,* Hemiazygous sheath (*arrow*) masquerading as an aortic dissection. AO = aorta.

37. Do patients need serial follow-up after successful surgical repair of a dissection?
Yes. Postoperative follow-up by means of TEE, CT, or MRI is indicated for early detection of disease progression, recurrence, or complications. These examinations should:
- Measure the aortic diameter at various levels (with careful attention to progressive dilation)
- Detect aneurysm (including aneurysmal dilation of the sinuses of Valsalva) or pseudoaneurysm formation
- Assess the competence of the native or prosthetic aortic valve after surgical interventions

38. What is an intramural hematoma?
This is an atypical variant of aortic dissection. Intramural hematoma does not have a detectable dissection flap. Instead, there is accumulation of blood within the aortic media, despite the absence of a visible entry site. The hallmark of intramural hematoma is an abnormal thickening of the aortic wall that can be detected by TEE, CT, or MRI. Intramural hematomas often appear eccentric (crescent-shaped) in cross section (Fig. 10).

39. Define aortic aneurysm.
Aneurysms are dilated segments of a blood vessel. Aortic aneurysms can differ in:
- Location (ascending or descending aorta, aortic arch)
- Shape (fusiform versus saccular) (Fig. 11)
- Dimensions (length)

40. How is aortic aneurysm different from aortic dissection?
Aortic aneurysm is a dilation of the aorta involving all the layers of the aortic wall (intima, media, and adventitia). Most aortic aneurysms do not have a dissection complicating their course.

Aortic dissection is a cleavage of the aortic wall and may or may not occur in the setting of a preexisting aneurysm. (See Figures 6 and 11.)

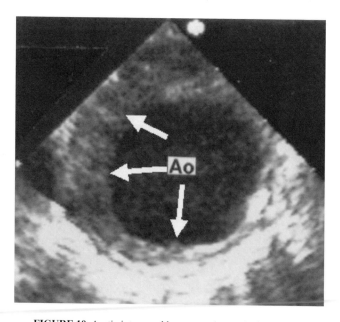

FIGURE 10. Aortic intramural hematoma (*arrows*). Ao = aorta.

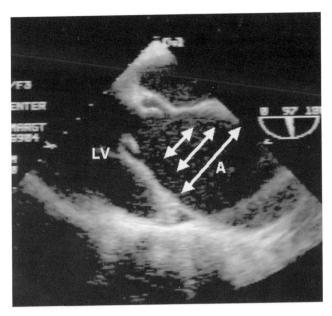

FIGURE 11. Fusiform aortic aneurysm (*double arrows*) are aortic dilations gradually increasing in diameter. A = aorta, LV = left ventricle.

41. Name the most frequent causes of aortic aneurysm and aortic dissection.
Aortic atherosclerosis and hypertension.

42. Although aortic aneurysm and aortic dissection are two separate entities, there is an important congenital condition in which an aneurysm may be complicated by dissection. Name this condition.
Marfan's syndrome (annuloaortic ectasia).

43. What is the pathogenesis of aortic rupture in patients with annuloaortic ectasia?
Dilation of the ascending aorta may lead to intimal tears that trigger dissection.

44. What are *dissecting aneurysms*?
This term occasionally has been used to designate *aortic dissection*. Its use is discouraged, however, because it may generate confusion between the two distinct entities of dissection and aneurysm.

45. Explain the difference between fusiform and saccular aneurysms.
These terms describe the shape of an aneurysm. **Fusiform** aneurysms have a stellate shape, gradually increasing and decreasing in size (see Figure 11). They are more common than saccular aneurysm. Atherosclerotic aneurysms are usually fusiform. **Saccular** aneurysms are usually balloon-shaped, focal dilations (**local** outpouchings) that communicate with the aortic lumen by either large or small openings. Syphilitic and mycotic aneurysms are most often saccular.

46. List the complications of thoracic aortic aneurysm.
- Aortic insufficiency
- Rupture of pericardium or left pleural space
- Compression of adjacent structures
- Thromboembolism

Echocardiography is an excellent technique to detect most of these complications.

47. What is the pathogenesis of aortic regurgitation in patients with thoracic aortic aneurysm?

Aortic regurgitation usually results from dilation of the aortic root, with failure of proper leaflet coaptation. Aortic regurgitation almost always is present when the aortic root diameter is > 5 cm. These aortic regurgitation jets are usually central.

48. How does rupture of an aortic aneurysm present?

Aortic aneurysms that rupture may have an **acute course,** complicated by catastrophic bleeding and death, or a **subacute course,** when the bleeding initially is contained by surrounding tissues. The manifestations depend on the involved portion of the aorta:

1. Rupture of the **ascending aorta** leads to hemopericardium (Fig. 12) and cardiac tamponade because this portion of the aorta is surrounded by pericardium throughout its course.

2. The aortic **arch** may rupture into the mediastinum (causing mediastinal hematoma), pleural space (hemothorax), tracheobronchial tree (hemoptysis), or esophagus (hematemesis).

3. The **descending** thoracic aorta may rupture into the mediastinum or left pleural space.

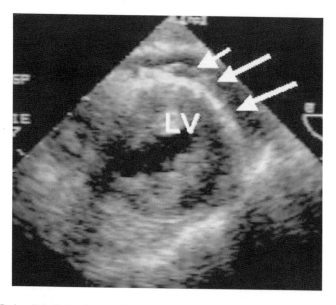

FIGURE 12. Pericardial effusion (*arrows*) in a patient with aortic dissection (not visualized from this plane). Note the pericardial clot (*arrows*).

49. Describe the echocardiographic appearance of hemothorax.

The diagnosis of hemothorax may be based on:
- Echo-free space adjacent to the involved segment of the thoracic aorta (aortic arch or descending aorta)
- The presence of atelectatic lung, appearing as a solid, echo-dense structure projecting into and out of the pleural fluid during respiration

It is usually not possible to differentiate hemothorax from a pleural effusion by echocardiography.

50. What mediastinal structures may be compressed by an aortic aneurysm?

1. Aneurysms of the **ascending aorta** may compress the coronary arteries, right ventricular (RV) outflow tract, pulmonary artery, and superior vena cava.

2. Aneurysms of the **aortic arch,** often asymptomatic, may produce dyspnea or cough from compression of the trachea or mainstem bronchi, dysphagia from compression of the esophagus, or hoarseness from left vocal cord paralysis secondary to compression of the left laryngeal nerve.

3. Aneurysms of the **descending aorta** infrequently produce compression symptoms.

51. What is the pathogenesis of thromboembolism in patients with aortic aneurysm?

Aortic aneurysm may harbor thrombus that can embolize to the systemic circulation. TEE often can identify thrombus within an aortic aneurysm.

52. What are the main forms of aortic trauma?

Trauma to the aorta occurs in <1% of motor vehicle accidents. Aortic trauma can result in a spectrum of lesions, ranging from minor to life-threatening:

- Aortic **laceration,** ranging from small **intimal tears** to frank rupture (transection) (Fig. 13), which may produce catastrophic bleeding and death or may be walled off to form a **pseudoaneurysm**
- Intramural hematoma
- Formation of intramural thrombi.

Classic aortic dissection is a rare complication of aortic trauma. Aortic dissection is generally a consequence of disease in the aortic media.

53. What is the role of TEE in evaluating patients with aortic trauma?

Although all of the complications of aortic trauma can be detected by TEE, aortography remains the gold standard.

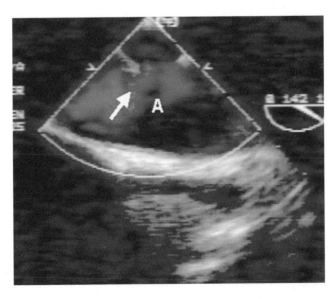

FIGURE 13. Aortic transection (rupture). Notice the blood flow toward the transducer, with a perpendicular orientation in respect to the long axis of the aorta (*arrow*). A = aorta. (See also Color Plates, Figure 25.)

54. What is the best technique for detecting thoracic aortic atherosclerosis?

TEE because of its proximity to the thoracic aorta and the high image resolution it provides. Until the advent of this imaging modality, the aorta was an underrecognized source of systemic embolism. TEE is useful in assessing the extent of atherosclerosis, its complications, therapeutic options, and response to therapy (plaque regression).

55. Describe the appearance of atherosclerotic disease on TEE images.

1. **Early atherosclerosis** appears as a flat (nonprotruding) intimal thickening ($<$ 3 mm thick).

2. An **intermediate** degree of atherosclerosis appears as diffuse thickening that may protrude $<$ 5 mm into the aortic lumen.

3. **Advanced** atherosclerosis appears as "complex" plaque, protruding $>$ 5 mm into the lumen and often mobile.

This arbitrary classification is simple, practical, and of prognostic value. An alternative method is to use planimetry in multiple sections to calculate atherosclerotic plaque volume as *aortic atherosclerotic plaque burden*. Although feasible, this alternative is time-consuming, requires meticulous technique, and is reserved for research purposes.

56. Does aortic atherosclerotic plaque have embolic potential?

Numerous studies have shown a correlation between "aortic debris" (atherosclerotic plaque) detected by TEE and embolic events.

57. Summarize the echocardiographic features of aortic atherosclerotic plaques with high embolic potential.

- The **size and degree of protrusion** of the plaque ($>$ 5 mm protrusion is considered high risk) (Fig. 14)
- **Mobility**—most mobile components of atherosclerotic plaque are likely blood clots
- **Ulceration** of the plaque (irregular surface)

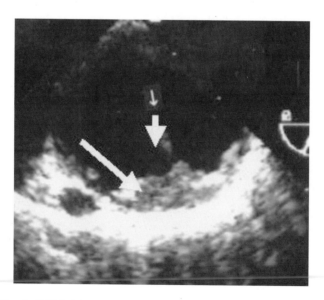

FIGURE 14. "Complex" (high-risk) aortic atherosclerotic plaque (*long arrow*) with a small, mobile component (*short arrow*) that has a very high embolic potential.

58. Can echocardiography detect aortic calcification?

Calcification is highly reflective and can be detected as bright echoes within the aortic walls and associated acoustic shadowing behind the calcium (Fig. 15)

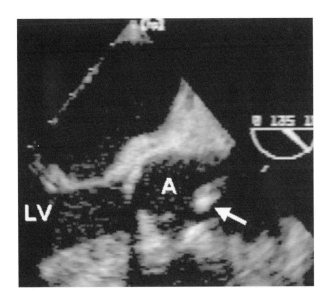

FIGURE 15. Calcified aortic atheroma (*arrow*). A = aorta, LV = left ventricle.

59. Is the degree of atherosclerosis homogeneous throughout the aorta?

No. In order of frequency, atherosclerosis affects:

- The abdominal aorta, particularly inferarenal
- The aortic arch at the distal portion near the left subclavian artery
- The ascending aorta

60. Is there an association between aortic plaque and the presence of atherosclerosis in other vessels?

Yes. Numerous studies have documented an association between aortic atherosclerosis detected by TEE or at autopsy and coronary and carotid atherosclerosis. In some studies, the presence of aortic plaque on TEE had a sensitivity of 90% and a specificity of 90% for angiographically proven significant obstructive coronary artery disease. These authors found that the presence of aortic atherosclerosis was a better predictor for coronary artery disease than hypertension, hypercholesterolemia, or positive family history.

61. What is the role of TEE in predicting the embolic complications of invasive procedures (cardiac catheterization, intra-aortic balloon pump insertion, cardiac surgery)?

TEE is ideally suited for identification of aortic atherosclerosis and sometimes helps to select the type and technique of invasive procedures. The radial approach may be selected for catheterization in a patient with substantial aortic atherosclerosis detected by TEE.

62. What is the best transthoracic view to detect coarctation of the aorta in adults?

Coarctation is seen best from the suprasternal notch using **two-dimensional** imaging to visualize the narrowing and **color Doppler** to show flow turbulence distal to the coarctation.

63. How can the severity of coarctation be determined echocardiographically?
- Increased systolic velocity, corresponding to a high peak systolic pressure gradient through the coarctation
- Persistence of the gradient (i.e., high velocity) throughout the cardiac cycle

64. Should the suprasternal notch view be obtained routinely?

Yes. This view shows the ascending aorta, the aortic arch, the proximal descending thoracic aorta, and the right pulmonary artery in some patients. This view is helpful in diagnosing patient ductus arteriosus, coarctation of the aorta, aortic dissection, and complex aortic atheroma. It is a useful adjunct to assess the severity of aortic regurgitation (flow reversal).

65. Define pulmonary hypertension.

Pulmonary artery hypertension is present when:
- The mean pressure > 20 mmHg at rest
- The systolic pulmonary artery pressure > 30 mmHg at rest

Echocardiography may overestimate the true pulmonary artery pressure if the right atrium (RA) pressure is assumed to be 10 mmHg and is actually less. Because of this, many consider an echocardiographic estimate of pulmonary artery pressure > 40 mmHg to represent pulmonary artery hypertension.

66. Why is echocardiography of pulmonary artery pressure important?

Pulmonary artery hypertension has nonspecific symptoms and electrocardiographic findings. The availability of Doppler echocardiography in this setting is of great clinical utility.

67. What are the echocardiographic features of pulmonary hypertension?

Doppler findings include a high-velocity tricuspid regurgitation jet and a decreased pulmonary acceleration time. **Two-dimensional signs** of ventricular pressure or volume overload or both include RV hypertrophy; dilation of the RV, RA, and pulmonary artery; and flattening of the interventricular septum in short-axis views ("D-shape") (Fig. 16).

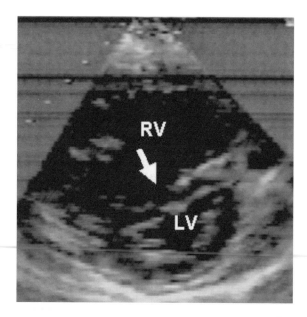

FIGURE 16. Right ventricular volume pressure overload (systolic frame). Note the compressed intraventricular septum, resulting in a D-shaped left ventricle (*arrow*).

68. Discuss the most widely used and reliable Doppler echocardiography method to quantitate pulmonary artery pressure.

Estimation of peak pulmonary artery pressure using the velocity of the tricuspid regurgitant jet is the most frequently used method because of its reliability and ease of use. This method uses the modified Bernoulli equation, which calculates the pressure gradient between two chambers based on the velocity of blood between the chambers. With pulmonary artery pressure, the two chambers are the RA and the RV (assuming the RV in systole is the same as the pulmonary artery in systole), and the blood flow between these chambers in systole is tricuspid regurgitation:

$$PAP(s) = RVP(s), and$$

$$RVP - RAP = \Delta p = 4v^2$$

where PAP(s) = systolic pulmonary artery pressure; RVP(s) = systolic RV pressure; RAP = RA pressure; Δp = pressure gradient between the RV and the RA; and v = the peak velocity of tricuspid regurgitation jet.

This method is applied easily in practice because:

1. Most patients with pulmonary hypertension have tricuspid regurgitation.
2. The RA pressure usually is estimated as 5–15 mmHg.

69. What is the echocardiographic method of estimation of the RA pressure?

If a predefined RA estimation (10 mmHg) is not used, the RA pressure can be based on observation of the inferior vena cava (IVC):

1. A normal RA pressure (approximately 5 mmHg) is associated with a normal IVC size and an inspiratory collapse > 50%.
2. A mildly to moderately increased RA pressure (approximately 10 mmHg) is associated with a normal size of the IVC and an inspiratory collapse < 50%.
3. A severely increased RA pressure (approximately 15 mmHg) is associated with a dilated IVC that lacks inspiratory collapse.

70. Give some technical tips for obtaining the maximum tricuspid regurgitation jet velocity.

To determine accurately the peak pulmonary artery systolic pressure, it is imperative to obtain the maximal tricuspid regurgitation jet velocity by using multiple views:

- Parasternal RV inflow view
- Short-axis view at the level of the aortic valve
- Apical four-chamber view
- Subcostal four-chamber view

Occasionally, echocardiographic contrast material (agitated saline injections or the newer contrast agents) may be necessary to enhance the intensity of a Doppler tricuspid regurgitation jet.

71. Are there any limitations to the tricuspid regurgitation jet method of estimating pulmonary artery pressure?

Yes.

- Absence of detectable tricuspid regurgitation; this is a relatively rare occurrence, especially in patients with a pulmonary artery pressure > 40 mmHg
- Difficult visualization of the tricuspid regurgitation jet
- Inadequate recording of the tricuspid regurgitation jet
- Misidentification of the jet signal (confusion with aortic stenosis or mitral regurgitation)
- Presence of pulmonary stenosis (which disqualifies the assumption that the RV and pulmonary artery systolic pressures are equal)

72. Are there any other methods for estimating pulmonary artery pressure?

Yes.

1. The RV isovolumic relaxation time is prolonged in patients with pulmonary hypertension (this method is technically demanding and seldom used in clinical practice).

2. The end-diastolic gradient between the pulmonary artery and the RV using the modified Bernoulli equation is based on a pulmonary regurgitation jet and an estimate of RV diastolic pressure, provided by the IVC size and collapsibility.

3. Pulmonary acceleration time (i.e., the interval between the opening of the pulmonary valve and the time of peak transvalvular flow velocity), is measured on a Doppler recording the flow through the pulmonary valve (shortened in patients with pulmonary hypertension). This method cannot distinguish normals reliably from patients with mild pulmonary hypertension (Fig. 17).

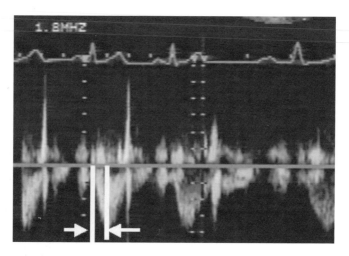

FIGURE 17. The pulmonary flow acceleration time (*between arrows*) represents the time interval between onset of flow through the pulmonic valve and the moment when peak velocity is reached (*thick vertical lines*).

73. Describe the M-mode echocardiographic features of pulmonary hypertension.

Several M-mode echocardiographic patterns of pulmonary valve motion have been described. These are indirect, low-sensitivity signs that do not allow quantitative assessments and seldom are used in contemporary practice.

74. Does echocardiography help determine the cause of pulmonary hypertension?

In addition to detecting and quantifying pulmonary hypertension, echocardiography may provide insight into the cause. Conditions that cause pulmonary hypertension include:

- Left heart failure (the most frequent cause of pulmonary hypertension), which can be idiopathic or secondary to valvular disease, coronary disease, or toxic drugs
- Large left-to-right intracardiac shunts (e.g., atrial septal defect), leading to pulmonary hypertension
- Diastolic dysfunction

The absence of these findings on echocardiography should raise the suspicion of a noncardiac cause of pulmonary hypertension, including:

- Pulmonary parenchymal disease (chronic obstructive pulmonary disease, interstitial lung disease)
- Pulmonary vascular disease (acute or chronic pulmonary embolism)
- Primary (idiopathic) pulmonary hypertension

75. List the echocardiographic findings associated with pulmonary embolism.

1. Thrombi in transit through the RA or RV, which are seen rarely (1–4% of all patients with pulmonary embolism) and appear as mobile, long, "snakelike" masses, usually unattached and appearing to "somersault."

2. RV dilation and dysfunction, often present but nonspecific. These findings may be due to other cardiopulmonary conditions common in patients in whom the diagnosis of pulmonary embolism is considered (e.g., chronic obstructive pulmonary disease, adult respiratory distress syndrome).

3. Normal or hyperdynamic LV function, in the absence of preexisting LV pathology.

4. Systolic and diastolic flattening of the ventricular septum ("D-shaped" ventricle), seen best in the short-axis view (see Figure 16).

5. Direct visualization of thrombi in the pulmonary artery (Fig. 18).

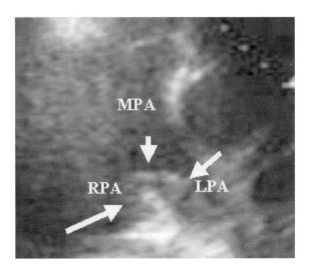

FIGURE 18. Pulmonary embolus (*arrows*) astride on the bifurcation of the main pulmonary artery (MPA) into the left and right branches (LPA, RPA) in a patient with pulmonary embolism.

76. What is the mechanism of RV dilation and dysfunction in patients with pulmonary embolism?

Obstruction of the pulmonary arteries and vasoconstriction results in an increased pulmonary vascular resistance. The RV has a narrow range over which it can handle acute afterload increases. The typical RV response to increased pulmonary vascular resistance is an elevated wall tension, which causes ventricular dilation and hypokinesis.

77. How can echocardiography assist in the differential diagnosis of pulmonary embolism?

Echocardiography is ideally suited for diagnosis of several conditions causing shortness of breath and hemodynamic instability that could be mistaken for pulmonary embolism, including:
- LV failure
- Pericardial pathology, such as constrictive pericarditis, cardiac tamponade
- Aortic dissection

78. How can echocardiography assist in the selection of optimal therapy in patients with pulmonary embolism?

Echocardiography can show:
- RV hypokinesis and dilation, which are an indication for thrombolytic therapy or thrombectomy

- A large clot in the right heart cavities or the pulmonary artery, which may be amenable to mechanical thrombectomy using specialized catheters

79. What is the difference between RV pressure overload and RV volume overload?
- **RV pressure overload** is synonymous with an increased RV systolic pressure (pulmonary hypertension).
- **RV volume overload** is overfilling of the RV, as in the case of atrial septal defect or significant tricuspid regurgitation.

The two conditions often are associated (e.g., an atrial septal defect resulting in pulmonary hypertension or pulmonary hypertension caused by lung disease that ultimately results in significant tricuspid regurgitation and volume overload of the RV).

80. How can RV pressure overload and RV volume overload be distinguished by echocardiography?
The normal LV cavity, as viewed from the parasternal short-axis view, has a circular shape in diastole and systole. With RV overload, the interventricular septum is flattened, and the LV assumes a characteristic *D* shape. The timing of this change in LV shape has diagnostic importance.
- In **RV volume overload,** the abnormal shape is present in diastole.
- In **RV pressure overload,** the abnormal shape is present in systole and often persists throughout the cardiac cycle (see Figure 16).

MAGNETIC RESONANCE IMAGING

Gabriel Adelmann, M.D., and Anthon R. Fuisz, M.D.

81. What is magnetic resonance angiography (MRA)?
MRA is a technique of blood vessel visualization. This chapter focuses on the use of MRI for the purpose of MRA.

82. Explain the role of contrast agents in the practice of MRA?
MRI is ideally suited to differentiate the flowing blood from the vessel wall, based on the different electromagnetic properties of the tissues. In principle, the use of contrast agents is not necessary in this setting. Contrast agents are useful, however, for:
- Improving the signal of flowing blood
- Facilitating faster MRI studies
- Visualizing smaller vessels

83. What are the advantages of MRA for visualization of the aorta compared with echocardiography?
1. It visualizes the entire thoracic aorta and can be extended easily to the abdominal aorta.
2. It visualizes the superior border of the aortic arch and the origin of the neck vessels.

84. What are the advantages of MRA for visualization of the aorta compared with CT?
1. It does not use ionizing radiation.
2. It does not use nephrotoxic contrast agents.
3. It is able to provide sections in any plane, as opposed to classic CT imaging systems, which provide only transversal sections (latest generation CT machines, using electron-beam technology, are able to provide accurate three-dimensional reconstruction of the heart and vessels).

85. List the elements of information regarding aortic blood flow that can be obtained by MRA.
- Aortic flow velocity
- Stroke volume

- The different characteristics of aortic blood flow in systole and diastole
- Information regarding the complex three-dimensional aortic blood flow hemodynamics

The normal aortic blood flow is helical, and the generated currents propagate blood flow through the coronary sinuses into the coronary arteries. These complex characteristics can be assessed by MRA.

86. What is the role of MRI in the diagnosis of aortic dissection?

Advantages

MRI can show:

- The true and the false lumen (Fig. 19)
- The entry and exit flap
- Involvement of the pericardium
- Progression of the dissection into the neck vessels or into the renal or other abdominal arteries
- Aortic regurgitation associated with the dissection

Disadvantages

- A longer study duration
- The inability of the test to be performed in the emergency department or operating room, which makes MRI impractical in patients with severe hemodynamic instability
- The necessity for significant patient cooperation, which may not be available in unstable patients (patient motion can generate significant artifact)
- The potential issue of claustrophobia

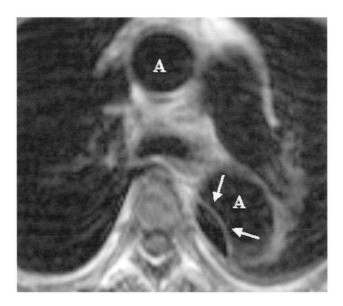

FIGURE 19. Dissection flap (*arrows*) seen in the descending thoracic aorta (A).

87. What is the role of MRI in the diagnosis of aortic aneurysm?

MRI can provide adequate visualization of aortic aneurysm (Fig. 20) and is helpful for serial follow-up of patients. Because nephrotoxic agents are not used, MRI is ideal in patients with coexisting kidney disease. Compared with CT, MRI is not able to visualize focal aortic wall calcification, however, an issue of potential significance in planning surgical intervention in these patients.

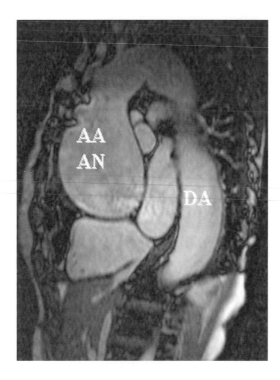

FIGURE 20. Aneurysm of the ascending aorta (AA AN). DA = descending aorta.

88. Identify the two congenital aortic diseases for which MRI is especially helpful.
1. Aortic coarctation (see Chapter 9)
2. Marfan's disease (MRI is an important alternative to TEE and CT in the initial diagnosis and serial follow-up of patients)

89. List the main challenges of MRI visualization of the pulmonary vasculature.
- The frequent occurrence of motion artifact caused by breathing
- The three-dimensional complexity of the pulmonary vasculature
- Diminished signal intensity at the interface with intrapulmonary air, owing to the substantially different electromagnetic properties of air compared with blood and pulmonary tissue

90. Name the main indication of MRI in the context of pulmonary vasculature pathology.
Pulmonary embolism.

91. What information is provided by MRI in patients with pulmonary embolism?
- Visualization of the thrombus, as an abrupt interruption of the lumen of the occluded pulmonary artery
- Assessment of the RV function, which is an important determinant of therapy (RV dysfunction is an indication for thrombolysis in eligible patients)

92. How does MRA compare with other modalities in the diagnosis of pulmonary embolism?
Compared with x-ray pulmonary angiography, MRI has the advantages of being noninvasive and not requiring nephrotoxic contrast agents or of ionizing radiation.

Compared with nuclear ventilation-perfusion scan, MRI has a higher sensitivity and specificity (in some laboratories, 40% of nuclear ventilation-perfusion scans have "indeterminate" results).

93. Identify additional congenital or acquired vascular conditions in which MRI may play an important diagnostic role.

1. Pulmonary arteriovenous malformation, a potential cause of high-output cardiac failure.

2. Superior vena cava syndrome, in which MRI can provide direct visualization of the venous obstruction and important information concerning the underlying condition.

3. Partial or complete anomalous pulmonary venous return (direct visualization of the pulmonary veins, identification of a dilated coronary sinus in patients in whom one of the pulmonary veins is draining into this vascular structure, or in patients with complete anomalous venous return, the failure to identify any pulmonary vein draining into the LA).

CHEST X-RAY

Matthew R. Brewer, M.D., Gabriel Adelmann, M.D., and Curtis E. Green, M.D.

94. What is pulmonary trunk enlargement?

The pulmonary trunk is seen on a frontal x-ray as the upper portion of the middle arch, belonging to the left cardiac border (the lower portion of this arch is represented by the LA appendage). In normal adults, the pulmonary trunk is usually concave, but occasionally it may be rectilinear or slightly convex. Marked convexity is considered to represent pulmonary trunk enlargement.

95. What is the differential diagnosis of pulmonary trunk enlargement?

It is important to distinguish **true** pulmonary trunk enlargement from **apparent** enlargement, because of **technical factors** (patient malpositioning) or **skeletal abnormalities,** including pectus excavatum, straight back syndrome, and scoliosis with a narrowed anteroposterior diameter of the chest. These conditions cause heart compression, displacement, and leftward rotation, giving the false impression of a dilated pulmonary trunk.

96. List the most frequent causes of true pulmonary trunk enlargement.

Pulmonary trunk enlargement can be **idiopathic** or **secondary** to
- RV dilation (the most frequent cause)
- Extracardiac shunt, such as patent ductus arteriosus (see Chapter 9)
- Congenital pericardial defect (see Chapter 7)

97. What are the radiographic findings in pulmonary hypertension?

- Enlarged pulmonary artery trunk and right pulmonary artery (normally the diameter of the right pulmonary artery is < 15 mm; a diameter > 17 mm, in the absence of shunt lesions, suggests pulmonary hypertension)
- Rapid tapering and narrowing of the pulmonary artery branches toward the periphery of the lung (peripheral oligemia, or "vessel pruning")

98. Can a chest x-ray provide information regarding the cause of pulmonary hypertension?

The pattern of oligemia (decreased vascular markings) can suggest the underlying condition:

1. **Patchy oligemia,** interspersed with **areas of increased perfusion,** suggests underlying lung disease or chronic pulmonary thromboembolism.

2. **Oligemia uniformly distributed** over both lung fields suggests the possibility of primary pulmonary hypertension. Occasional patients present with extreme bulging of one or both pulmonary arteries (Fig. 21).

99. How can pulmonary artery and venous hypertension be distinguished by chest radiography?

Pulmonary artery hypertension (precapillary hypertension) is characterized by a dilated pulmonary artery and by different patterns of oligemia. **Pulmonary venous hypertension** (postcapillary hypertension, pulmonary congestion) is characterized by different patterns of pulmonary *hyper*emia.

100. Describe the radiographic findings in systemic hypertension.

The radiographic findings in hypertension are nonspecific and consist mainly of tortuosity of the ascending and descending portions of the aorta. Additional findings may point to the underlying disease (e.g., aortic calcification, as a sign of atherosclerosis) or to the physiologic consequences of long-standing hypertension (LV dilation, pulmonary congestion). Hypertension typically causes LV hypertrophy, which is not detected by chest radiography (Fig. 22).

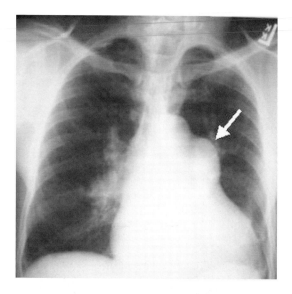

FIGURE 21. Primary pulmonary hypertension. Extreme bulging of the pulmonary artery (*arrow*) in a patient with primary pulmonary hypertension.

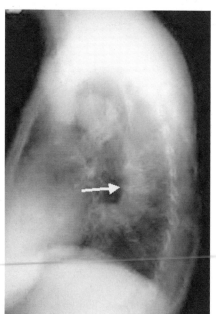

FIGURE 22. Tortuous aorta (*arrow*) in a patient with long-standing systemic hypertension.

101. Describe the radiographic findings in aortic atherosclerosis.

Aortic atherosclerosis generally is associated with calcification visible on chest x-ray as linear, "bright" ("white") densities running parallel to the aortic wall. These calcifications can be located at any level in the thoracic aorta but most commonly are seen at the junction between the aortic arch and the descending aorta ("aortic knob").

102. Describe the radiographic findings in aortic aneurysm.

Aortic aneurysms are areas of segmental dilation of the aorta, with a maximum diameter > 1.5 times that of the healthy adjacent segments. Aortic aneurysms can be fusiform (gradual increase and tapering of the vessel segment) or saccular ("abrupt" change in vessel diameter). Aortic aneurysms most often involve the ascending aorta and are seen on frontal and lateral chest x-rays as areas of localized dilation.

103. List the radiographic findings in aortic dissection.
- Mediastinal widening (Fig. 23)
- Enlargement of the cardiac shadow owing to progression of the dissection and bleeding into the pericardium (hemopericardium)
- New pleural effusion
- Extrapleural fluid collections (e.g., at the level of the pulmonary apices), which may represent progression of the dissection
- Changes regarding the presence or extent or both of any of the above-listed findings on serial chest x-rays

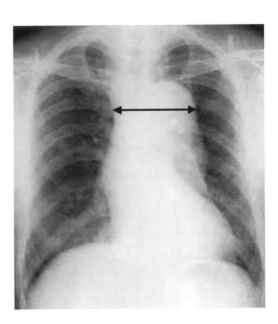

FIGURE 23. Widened mediastinum (*double-headed arrow*) in a patient with aortic dissection.

104. Discuss the diagnostic importance of mediastinal widening in patients with aortic dissection.

The presence of mediastinal widening is probably one of the most frequently raised questions in common practice when assessing a chest x-ray. This finding is thought to reflect accumulation of hematoma under the aortic intima or hemorrhage into the mediastinum. *This sign is neither sensitive, nor specific,* however, for aortic dissection, being absent in most cases of dissection and present in other conditions (aortic atherosclerosis, aortic aneurysm, and pulmonary atelectasis).

It is especially important to be aware of the limitations of chest radiography in the diagnosis of aortic dissection, such as:

1. The risk factors for aortic dissection (i.e., old age, hypertension, hypercholesterolemia) are the same as those of "simple" atherosclerosis, which has a much higher prevalence.

2. Aortic dissection can be difficult to distinguish from aortic atherosclerosis based on chest x-ray alone (both conditions may cause mediastinal "widening").

3. The pretest probability for aortic dissection may be lower in patients having chest x-rays than in patients undergoing more sophisticated (and more costly) imaging procedures. This is due to the low threshold for obtaining a chest x-ray in clinical practice. Judicious interpretation of the x-ray findings in the context of the clinical picture and specific risk factors is essential.

105. What is the diagnostic importance of a pericardial or pleural effusion in a patient with aortic dissection?

These findings are important red flags, indicating progression of the dissection and impending aortic rupture. **Emergent** surgery is lifesaving in this situation. Progression of these findings on serial chest x-rays is especially ominous.

106. I have been contacted by the attending physician from the radiology department about a patient in whom I have clinical concern for aortic dissection. She has just read my patient's chest x-ray, which was remarkable for significant mediastinal widening and a grossly enlarged cardiac shadow. What do I do next?

The findings described by the radiologist are highly suggestive of **proximal** aortic dissection that has progressed to the pericardial space. The clinician is faced with two important questions:

1. "Should I obtain an additional, confirmatory TEE, spiral CT scan, or MRI study, or can I confidently base my diagnosis on chest x-ray findings alone?"

2. "Should I contact the surgeon about a possible emergent intervention in this patient?"

The answer to the second question is probably *yes*. It is always a good idea to alert the surgeon about the possibility of an emergent intervention. This allows the surgeon to become acquainted with the specific medical problems of the patient and to make the practical arrangements for a possible surgical procedure.

Although there is no uniform answer to the first question, another imaging modality probably is necessary. On one hand, the chest x-ray has a relatively low sensitivity and specificity for the diagnosis of aortic dissection, and one always should try to avoid unnecessary surgery. On the other hand, aortic dissection extending to the pericardium is a deadly condition if left untreated. The following actions are essential:

- **Monitor the patient** (vital signs); based on the degree of hemodynamic stability and on the index of suspicion for aortic dissection, there may or may not be time for an additional, confirmatory study.
- **Consider the possibility of obtaining a confirmatory TEE in the operating room.**
- **Always involve the attending physician** in any decision making; however, **act rapidly** because any delay in diagnosis or therapy may be fatal.

107. What are the radiographic signs of aortic coarctation?

- The *3 sign*, in which the "waist" of the numeral 3 indicates the site of the coarctation, on the left mediastinal border
- *Rib notching*, representing the indentations produced by the anastomoses between vessels originating above and under the side of coarctation

11. INNOVATIVE TECHNIQUES AND FUTURE DIRECTIONS

CARDIAC CATHETERIZATION

Gabriel Adelmann, M.D., and Shmuel Fuchs, M.D.

1. Define coronary angioscopy.

Coronary angioscopy uses fiberoptics for direct visualization of the coronary lumen. The images are displayed in color on a television monitor, allowing visualization of:
- Atherosclerotic plaque and its complications, such as rupture or hemorrhage
- Coronary dissection after percutaneous interventions
- Intraluminal thrombus (platelet-rich thrombus versus fibrin-rich clot)

2. List the limitations of coronary angioscopy.

1. It cannot see through the blood unless the blood is "flushed" away or blood flow is occluded temporarily.

2. It shows only the surface of atherosclerotic plaque but cannot assess the underlying atheroma morphology.

3. It is limited to the proximal and mid portions of relatively straight, large epicardial coronary arteries.

4. It cannot visualize ostial or proximal lesions.

5. It can cause significant ischemia because of the bulky equipment and size of the angioscope catheter.

3. What is the clinical role of coronary angioscopy?

Coronary angioscopy is currently a research tool only, without established clinical indications.

4. What is intracoronary Doppler ultrasound?

The severity of a coronary stenosis can be assessed based on the changes in coronary blood flow velocity. This is performed by means of a Doppler flow wire inserted into the coronary artery. The use of blood velocity for the assessment of coronary stenosis severity is based on the assumption that coronary blood flow velocity is directly proportional with the volume of blood crossing the stenotic segment:

$$Q = k \times A \times v$$

where Q = the volume of blood per unit of time (mL/sec); k = a constant; A = is the cross-sectional area of the blood vessel (mm^2); and v = is the velocity of blood flowing through the coronary artery (m/sec).

5. What are the characteristics of normal coronary blood flow, as assessed by the Doppler flow wire method?

1. Flow in the left coronary system (left main coronary artery, left anterior descending, left circumflex) occurs mainly in diastole.

2. Flow in the right coronary artery (RCA) is almost equal in systole and diastole.

3. Average flow velocity is 9 to 70 cm/sec (although the range of normal velocities is broad, in an individual subject the blood flow velocity is usually similar in the three major epicardial coronary arteries).

6. Describe the pathologic changes in coronary blood flow that are detected by the Doppler flow wire.

In patients with significant coronary stenosis, the Doppler flow wire may show:

1. A blunting of the diastolic component of blood flow in the left coronary system, with a decreased *diastolic-to-systolic ratio* (< 1.7 in the left coronary artery) indicating a hemodynamically significant coronary stenosis. This method is not applicable in the RCA because of the uniform nature of RCA blood flow.

2. An increase in blood flow proximal to the stenosis, with a decrease distal to it, resulting in an increase in the *proximal-to-distal* flow velocity ratio > 1.7 indicates hemodynamically significant stenosis).

3. A diminished capacity of the coronary artery to increase its blood flow with pharmacologic vasodilation and hyperemia (e.g., using adenosine). This parameter is termed *coronary flow reserve*. A coronary flow reserve < 2.0 indicates hemodynamically significant coronary stenosis.

7. What is the main limitation of Doppler flow wire assessment of coronary blood flow?

Its strong dependence on the positioning of the catheter tip relative to the direction of blood flow (a limitation common to all the Doppler methods); if the tip of the Doppler wire is pointing toward the wall, the true blood flow velocity is underestimated.

8. What are the indications for coronary blood flow assessment by means of the Doppler flow wire?

Currently, there are no class I indications for this method, but there is a class IIa indication (no consensus, but the existing data favor the method) for assessment of the hemodynamic significance of coronary artery lesions that by angiography are *intermediate* (30–70%). It is occasionally unclear whether such an intermediate lesion causes any significant decrease in the blood flow. The blood flow depends directly on the blood velocity distal to the epicardial coronary artery stenosis, which can be assessed by the Doppler flow wire.

9. What is NOGA mapping?

NOGA is a diagnostic system that simultaneously records electrical activation and the local mechanical response of the heart. This method assesses the electromechanical coupling at different levels in the heart muscle. NOGA also provides information regarding end-diastolic and end-systolic volumes, ejection fraction, and regional myocardial shortening in systole.

Practically, a NOGA study consists of two parallel images, one depicting the voltage in different segments of the left ventricle (LV) and the other showing the local shortening. The voltage and the mechanical activity (shortening) are depicted in conventional colors (Fig. 1).

10. List some potential clinical applications of the NOGA mapping method.

NOGA has been used for assessing:
- The area of myocardium in jeopardy (i.e., that might become infarcted in case of an acute coronary event) in patients with coronary stenosis
- Detection of myocardial viability (no movement but electrically active)
- The presence of LV aneurysm and its role in the genesis of ventricular arrhythmia
- The presence and pathologic significance of other arrhythmogenic lesions, such as bypass tracts

11. What is the role of NOGA in current practice?

NOGA is currently an investigational device. It is a time-intensive procedure, which is being applied slowly.

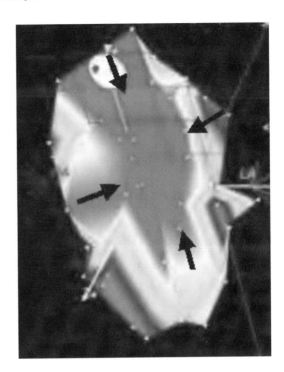

FIGURE 1. NOGA mapping. The area between the arrows (depicted in the red in the original image) corresponds to extensive anterior myocardial hypokinesis. (See also Color Plates, Figure 26.)

ECHOCARDIOGRAPHY

Gabriel Adelmann, M.D., Neil J. Weissman, M.D., and Steven A. Goldstein, M.D.

Contrast Echocardiography

12. Define contrast echocardiography.

Echocardiographic visualization of the heart walls is based on the different echogenicity of the myocardium and of the surrounding tissues. The myocardium is depicted in shades of gray, in contrast to the intracardiac blood, which appears black. In certain patients with poor acoustic windows, however, there is "noise" everywhere so that the difference in echogenicity between the heart walls and intracardiac blood is not sufficient to allow clear delineation of the endocardial border. This makes the assessment of the LV thickness and function difficult.

Contrast echocardiography uses special diagnostic agents, called *echo contrast agents*, which dramatically enhance the echogenicity of the blood and make it possible to assess the endocardial border of the heart. As an analogy, imagine you are looking at a cup made of clear glass and filled with water. It may be difficult to distinguish clearly the inner surface of the glass, but if one introduces a drop of ink in the water, this task becomes simple.

13. How does contrast echocardiography work?

The current echo contrast agents are microscopic gas bubbles. Gases are strong reflectors of ultrasound. As a result of their interaction with ultrasound, microbubbles reflect more ultrasound than blood cells. This causes the contrast-filled blood pool to be displayed in white rather than in black. The microbubbles function as "markers" for the blood in the heart chambers and in the myocardial microcirculation: Wherever there is blood, there are microbubbles, and conversely, wherever microbubbles are detected, there is blood flow.

14. What is the nature of the interaction between ultrasound and the microbubbles in the echo contrast agents?

When ultrasound "hits" the microbubbles in the echo contrast agents, the bubbles either start resonating (i.e., expanding and contracting in a cyclical fashion similar to a bell ringing after being struck) or are destroyed, depending on the power of the ultrasound beam. The gas bubbles resonate in a nonlinear fashion so that they emit several multiples of the ultrasound frequency that was sent out by the transducer (fundamental frequency). These frequencies are called *harmonics*. Recording some of the harmonics makes it possible to identify the contrast with a higher sensitivity than just using the fundamental frequency.

15. List the characteristics of an ideal contrast bubble.
- Be nontoxic
- Be reasonably inexpensive
- Have a radius as close as possible to the size of red blood cells (the larger the bubble, the greater its ability to produce contrast and to persist in the circulation, but bubbles > 5–8 μ may not cross the pulmonary circulation)
- Have an outer wall that does not allow rapid diffusion of the inner gas contents because that would make the bubbles shrink and not make it to the left heart chambers

16. What types of bubbles are used in current clinical practice?

For visualization of the right heart chambers and evaluation of intracardiac shunts, a suspension of air in normal saline is adequate (i.e., agitated saline). These "simple" air bubbles cannot cross the pulmonary circulation, however, and are not able to "survive" to reach the left atrium (LA) and LV. They are not useful for producing opacification of the left cardiac chambers in the normal subject.

For visualization of the blood pool in the left heart chambers and myocardial microcirculation, special microbubbles are required. These generally are composed of an outer shell (human albumin, a synthetic polymer, a phospholipid, a sugar, or a combination) enclosing an inert gas. Because of the increased resistance of the outer shell and the low diffusibility of the gases used, these bubbles are able to cross the pulmonary circulation and opacify the LA and the LV.

17. What are the current main indications for contrast echocardiography?

Endocardial border delineation and LV opacification. At this time, detection of myocardial blood flow and perfusion (myocardial contrast echocardiography) is an evolving technology with the potential of becoming a viable alternative to nuclear studies.

18. What percentage of echocardiographic studies need contrast for endocardial border delineation?

Approximately 3–10% of all standard echocardiographic studies and 15–20% of stress studies are technically suboptimal and can be salvaged by the use of an echocardiographic contrast agent.

19. What is the role of contrast echocardiography in the visualization of intracardiac shunts?

Contrast echocardiography is extremely useful in the detection of intracardiac shunts (patent foramen ovale, atrial septal defect) and has a greater sensitivity than color Doppler in this setting. Practically, both modalities (color Doppler and contrast echocardiography) generally are used whenever the clinical question of a shunt arises. If the shunt is seen by color Doppler, contrast echocardiography is not necessary. For the detection of shunts, the "contrast agent" is just agitated saline, which should not cross the pulmonary circulation and reach the left heart *unless* there is a shunt.

20. Can contrast echocardiography be used for Doppler studies?

Yes. Contrast material enhances Doppler tracings and was one of the original indications for which these agents were approved. Because of the strong reflective properties of echo contrast agents, technically suboptimal Doppler studies (which are rare) can be "rescued."

21. How can contrast material help in the evaluation of ischemic heart disease?

Contrast echocardiography often is used to improve endocardial border delineation and allows better assessment of wall motion abnormalities (at rest or during a stress echocardiogram) and ejection fraction. As mentioned earlier, echocardiographic contrast agents track with the blood flow. Using harmonic imaging and special echocardiography machine settings, it is possible to see the bubbles crossing the coronary microcirculation. If there is a coronary stenosis, the blood flow to the corresponding myocardial segment is reduced, resulting in a smaller number of bubbles being delivered to that segment. These perfusion defects can be evident under resting conditions or under physical exercise or pharmacologic stimulation (e.g., dobutamine, adenosine, dipyridamole). Myocardial perfusion is assessed by using low-intensity ultrasound (low mechanical index), which causes bubble resonation without significant destruction. Contrast echocardiography has been used for:

- Diagnosis of ischemic heart disease (Fig. 2)
- Assessment of myocardial viability
- Assessment of infarct size early after reperfusion therapy

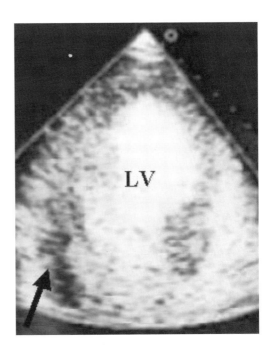

FIGURE 2. Myocardial contrast echocardiography (MCE). Note the "sparkling white" aspect of all the LV segments, except for the basal inferior-posterior wall (*arrow*). This patient had a critical stenosis of the RCA that did not allow the contrast material to penetrate the microcirculation of the inferior segment. Also note the white display color of the interventricular blood pool. LV = left ventricle, RV = right ventricle.

22. Why is echocardiographic assessment of myocardial microcirculation appealing?

The interest in this potential application is fueled by the wide availability and comparatively low cost of echocardiography compared with nuclear studies. In addition, there is a wealth of supplementary information obtained by echocardiography. Echocardiography is portable and can be done at the bedside, in the emergency department, or in the intensive care unit. Because of all these advantages, echocardiography theoretically seems an ideal modality for a complete diagnosis of ischemic heart disease.

23. What is the current role of myocardial contrast echocardiography for perfusion studies in clinical practice?

Despite the extensive research work accomplished to date in this field, myocardial contrast echocardiography has not been definitely proven to be able to replace nuclear studies in clinical practice. This is an area of intense research and rapid development.

24. Myocardium is *usually* visualized in white on classic two-dimensional echocardiography studies. How can further opacification by contrast agents be visualized?

Although "regular" two-dimensional echocardiography uses a high mechanical index, which results in myocardial display in white, the low mechanical index used on contrast studies results in the myocardium being shown in black. This makes it possible to visualize the endocardial border (when the heart chambers are replenished by contrast material) and the myocardium (when the contrast material crosses the microcirculation).

25. What are the main artifacts seen with myocardial contrast echocardiography?

As mentioned earlier, reduced coronary perfusion to a segment of the myocardium is seen as a decrease in opacification. The main artifacts seen with myocardial contrast echocardiography can be classified into two groups:

1. Decreased opacification of normally perfused myocardial segments (false-positive studies), usually caused by:
   a. **Inadequate myocardial contrast administration** (too few bubbles in the microcirculation, not because of vessel narrowing, but because too few were injected).
   b. **Shadowing (attenuation),** which is severe ultrasound attenuation by the near-field bubbles, so that there is little ultrasound at greater depths. This is the most frequent cause for nondiagnostic myocardial contrast opacification studies.
2. Normal or increased opacification of ischemic segments (false-negative studies), usually caused by:
   a. **Blooming** (spreading of contrast signals from a myocardial segment to the adjacent ones).
   b. **Wall motion artifact,** when heart motion in the chest cavity briefly brings into the imaging plane adequately perfused myocardial segments from the vicinity.

26. The principles of myocardial contrast echocardiography are straightforward, and the appeal of performing these studies in any setting (from outpatient office to intensive care unit) is great. Can I start performing these studies on my patients?

Myocardial contrast echocardiography has not yet been approved as a routine diagnostic method to assess perfusion. Intensive training in a qualified center is necessary for mastering this technique. At present, this technique is confined to a few select tertiary centers.

27. Compare myocardial contrast echocardiography with other myocardial imaging technologies (nuclear scan, positron emission tomography [PET], magnetic resonance imaging [MRI]).

	INTRA CELLULAR CONTRAST UPTAKE	PERFUSION TRACER	SPATIAL RESOLUTION (MM)	AVAILABLE AT THE BEDSIDE	MAIN CLINICAL APPLICATIONS
MCE	No	Yes	1–2	Yes	Evaluation of chest pain Myocardial viability Assessment of perfusion after myocardial infarction
SPECT	Yes (active uptake for thallium, passive diffusion for technetium)	No	12–20	No	Myocardial viability Assessment of perfusion after myocardial infarction Evaluation of chest pain Preoperative evaluation
PET	Some agents (e.g., FDG)	Some agents (e.g., 15O water, 13N ammonia)	6	No	Myocardial viability
MRI	Some agents	Some agents	Variable	No	Myocardial viability Direct visualization of coronary arteries

MCE = myocardial contrast echocardiography; SPECT = single-photon emission computed tomography; FDG = fluorodeoxyglucose.

28. Does contrast echocardiography have any therapeutic applications?

Microscopic bubbles filled with gas are administered intravenously and are carried by the systemic circulation. Their greatest disruption occurs only at the site of exposure to the diagnostic ultrasound waves, however. In a sense, microbubbles behave like magic bullets that can target a specific organ (that has ultrasound sent through it), despite systemic administration. This has led to the concept of local drug delivery by microbubbles that would carry the active substances to their intended site of action, where the contents are released from their envelope by means of ultrasound. In addition, certain types of bubbles have been shown to lyse blood clots under the influence of ultrasound, without producing systemic activation of the fibrinolytic system. The potential use of microbubbles for therapeutic purposes is under active investigation.

Three-Dimensional Echocardiography

29. Summarize the basic principles of three-dimensional imaging.

Three-dimensional echocardiography displays visual information recorded from all three planes in space. These images can be produced:

- **Sequentially,** as two-dimensional images that subsequently are reconstructed into a three-dimensional image. This is a currently available technique.
- **Real time or live three-dimensional** (a three-dimensional ultrasound wave is emitted toward the heart, and the resulting echoes are recorded in three-dimensions, in real time). This technique is under development and has recently become commercially available.

Three-dimensional images are displayed on two-dimensional screens. The impression of depth is created by gray shading (rendering) or by simultaneously displaying multiple two-dimensional sectors that are registered in space (with a known orientation between the two-dimensional sectors).

30. Direct visualization of an object in three-dimensional echocardiography seems more reasonable than recording a set of two-dimensional images then mentally reconstructing them into a three-dimensional concept. Why hasn't three-dimensional echocardiography replaced conventional two-dimensional echocardiography?

At present, three-dimensional echocardiography is an evolving technique that is just now becoming widely available.

31. Describe the applications of three-dimensional echocardiography in the diagnosis of valvular heart disease.

Because of the complex structure of heart valves, three-dimensional echocardiography is ideal for imaging the heart valves (Fig. 3). Valvular stenosis or incompetence and thickening of the valve leaflets can be seen clearly. It also is possible to reproduce the surgeon's view of the valve. Three-dimensional echocardiography also allows accurate planimetry (direct contour measurement) of the heart valve orifice areas. Regurgitation jets can be reconstructed in three-dimensions, displaying their origin and their course more accurately.

32. Describe the applications of three-dimensional echocardiography in the diagnosis of ischemic heart disease.

Because of its unique characteristics, three-dimensional echocardiography allows assessment of regional wall motion abnormalities and calculation of LV mass and volumes by spatial visualization of the ventricular walls, rather than by making geometric assumptions. Combining three-dimensional imaging with myocardial contrast echocardiography is an exciting potential development in the field of ischemic heart disease. Three-dimensional reconstruction of the proximal course of the coronary arteries also has been achieved.

33. Describe the applications of three-dimensional echocardiography in the diagnosis of congenital heart disease.

Three-dimensional echocardiography is ideally suited to visualize a wide variety of con-

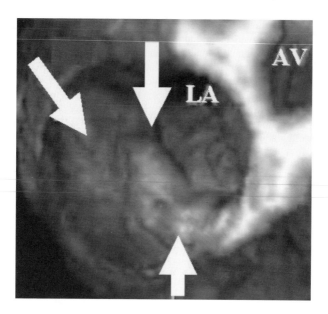

FIGURE 3. Three-dimensional echocardiogram of the mitral valve (short axis). The large white arrows are pointing at bulges in the surface of the valve leaflets. Although these bulges can be also identified by two-dimensional echo, three-dimensional echo reveals their true spatial complexity. This may substantially improve the anatomic definition of the mitral valve. LA = left atrium, AV = aortic valve.

genital heart defects, including atrial and ventricular septal defects, bicuspid aortic valves, Ebstein's anomaly, tetralogy of Fallot, and aortic coarctation. In addition, three-dimensional echocardiography seems ideally suited for guiding the delivery of percutaneous devices used in the treatment of certain congenital heart diseases (e.g., patent foramen ovale or atrial septal defect closure).

34. Compare three-dimensional echocardiography with other three-dimensional imaging technologies (computed tomography [CT], MRI).

As opposed to CT and MRI, which are well-established diagnostic procedures, three-dimensional echocardiography still is viewed as a technique under development. The prospect of a diagnostic method that would be rapid, feasible at the bedside, and offer a unique combination of functional and structural information is especially attractive.

Integrated Backscatter

35. What is integrated backscatter?

Ultrasound reflection can be unidirectional (specular reflection from a perfect ultrasound "mirror") or multidirectional (scattering). Backscattered ultrasound (ultrasound received back from bouncing off a tissue) can be used for characterizing the physical properties of the reflecting tissue. The properties of the backscatter may reflect the biologic characteristics of the tissue being imaged. In the case of the myocardium, the primary determinant of ultrasound scattering is the collagen in the extracellular matrix. Additional factors influencing myocardial backscatter include myocardial fiber orientation, myocardial blood flow, water content, and the different phases of the cardiac cycle. These tissue characteristics may be altered in the presence of disease.

36. What clinical applications have been proposed for integrated backscatter?
The integrated backscatter approach has been used to study a variety of cardiac conditions, including myocardial ischemia, cardiomyopathy, and changes in LV properties caused by arterial hypertension.

37. What is the current role of backscatter techniques in the diagnosis and management of heart disease?
Although the concept of integrated backscatter analysis is attractive, this technique has not yet found a routine clinical application and at this time is confined to research purposes only.

Tissue Doppler

38. What is tissue Doppler?
The classic ultrasound application of the Doppler principle is the assessment of blood flow in the heart chambers and in the great vessels. These are high velocities (on the order of m/sec). Usual ultrasound technology filters out lower velocities from the final display. Tissue Doppler is a Doppler ultrasound modality that selectively measures the velocities **within the myocardium** (which are considerably lower, on the order of cm/sec) (Figs. 4 and 5). This is achieved by conventional pulsed or color Doppler and by filtering out the higher velocity signals from blood.

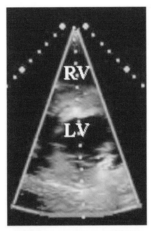

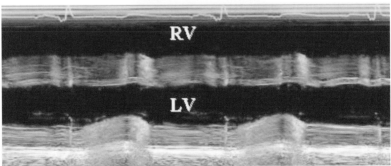

FIGURE 4. Tissue Doppler imaging (TDI). Two-dimensional imaging (*A*) and the color M mode image corresponding to the section axis (*B*). The red color indicates myocardial motion toward the transducer, whereas the blue color indicates motion away from the transducer. By simultaneously inscribing the ECG, it is possible to delineate the different phases of systole and diastole and pathologic changes in these phases. (See also Color Plates, Figure 27.)

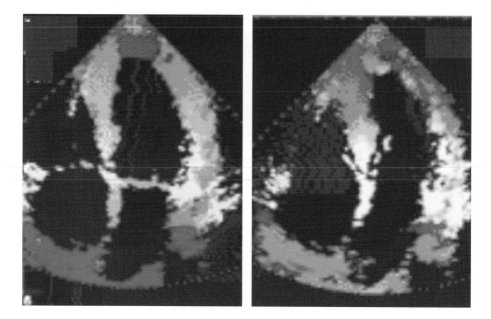

FIGURE 5. Tissue Doppler imaging, four-chamber view. *A,* Systole. *B,* Diastole. (See also Color Plates, Figure 28.)

39. Provide some synonyms for tissue Doppler.
Tissue Doppler imaging (TDI), Doppler tissue imaging (DTI), tissue velocity imaging (TVI), and Doppler myocardial imaging (DMI).

40. Does tissue Doppler require special equipment?
Yes. The echocardiography machine must have special software and filters. Filters are required to eliminate high-velocity blood flow and to allow detection and measurement of low-velocity signals from wall motion. The instruments must be modified to display these lower velocity signals from tissue (myocardium). Most current machines have the appropriate modifications as either standard technology or add-on options.

41. Describe some of the limitations of tissue Doppler.
Tissue Doppler is susceptible to the same limitations as all Doppler techniques, including angle dependence of the ultrasound beam, physiologic variations (beat-to-beat), and size and position of the sample volume. Tissue Doppler is affected by the motion of the heart as a whole (e.g., translation, rotation), and the effects of translation and rotation cannot be separated from those of myocardial contraction and relaxation, which are what one desires to determine. As an analogy, think of a person climbing an escalator that is moving upward; an external observer (i.e., at the street level) sees that person approaching at a speed that represents the sum of the escalator velocity and of the person's active motion; however, these two components cannot be distinguished easily.

42. List the clinical applications of tissue Doppler.
- Evaluation of systolic (global and regional) and diastolic function of the ventricles
- Distinguishing constrictive pericarditis from restrictive cardiomyopathy
- Distinguishing normal versus pseudonormal mitral inflow patterns
- Diagnosis of cardiomyopathies

- Detection of cardiac transplant rejection
- Detecting the earliest site of electrical activation in patients with the Wolff-Parkinson-White syndrome to help localize the bypass tract

43. What is the role of tissue Doppler in clinical practice?

Tissue Doppler appears to be gaining acceptance slowly in the United States, although its final role in clinical practice is yet to be determined.

NUCLEAR MEDICINE

Manuel D. Cerqueira, M.D., Gabriel Adelmann, M.D., and Benjamin Kleiber, M.D.

44. Is it possible to measure the LV ejection fraction under ambulatory conditions?

Yes. A new nuclear detector, which may be viewed as the nuclear counterpart of a Holter monitor, has been introduced. This device allows you to monitor patients with episodes of ischemia that are not detected on routine studies. In addition, it can be used in monitoring patients after myocardial infarction and in the evaluation of the LV ejection fraction response to physical exercise or therapeutic interventions.

45. What is the foreseeable future of first-pass studies?

This time-honored method has gained new popularity with the introduction of multidetector cameras (capable of the rapid acquisition inherently necessary for first-pass studies). A new generation of gamma cameras may be used at the bedside, with a tracer known as *tantalum-178*.

46. What is infarct-avid nuclear imaging?

Detection of acute myocardial necrosis (infarction) can be done with technetium-based tracers or using a special radiotracer/antibody compound, indium-antimyosin. These tests do not "turn positive," however, until 24–48 hours after the acute event, which, in the age of widespread availability of troponin assay, makes them practically clinically useless. An experimental agent (technetium-glucurate) may produce positive results within 1 hour after the acute event (infarction) and may have high utility in patients with chest pain, in the presence of nondiagnostic electrocardiographic or enzyme changes. This test also may help with the assessment of patient response to thrombolytic therapy.

47. What is MIBG imaging, and what is its clinical utility?

Ischemic damage to the cardiac nerves is believed to play a major role in the development of congestive heart failure and arrhythmia. This mechanism seems to be especially important in diabetics. Nuclear visualization of the myocardial innervation using special tracers (MIBG) allows assessment of the sympathetic innervation of the myocardium and may provide important prognostic information in patients with:

- Myocardial infarction
- Severe ventricular arrhythmia or cardiac arrest
- Heart failure

By performing parallel perfusion and innervation studies, a mismatch between the blood flow and the integrity of the sympathetic innervation may be shown (Fig. 6). It has been suggested that these patients are at higher risk for complications after myocardial infarction, including severe arrhythmia. Although still of research interest alone, MIBG imaging is envisioned by many to play an important role in the future.

48. Name some of the foreseeable future fields of application of nuclear cardiology.

- Imaging of atherosclerotic plaque
- Imaging of thrombus
- Platelet imaging

- Imaging in asymptomatic patients with siblings having premature ischemic heart disease
- Assessment of myocardial metabolism by free fatty acid imaging
- Detection of myocardial hypoxia

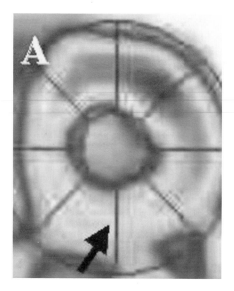 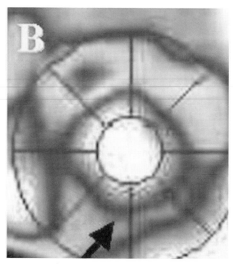

FIGURE 6. Perfusion/innervation mismatch in a patient after myocardial infarction treated by thrombolysis. *A,* Preserved myocardial blood flow. *B,* Decreased sympathetic innervation of the posterior wall. (See also Color Plates, Figure 29.)

49. What is the potential place of digitization in the future of nuclear cardiology?

The "digital revolution" is expected to influence nuclear cardiology by allowing more accurate analysis of the radioactive signal emitted by nuclear diagnostic agents and more effective storage and retrieval of information and integration of nuclear data into a database including all the clinical information available for a given patient.

50. Besides systolic and diastolic LV function, what other clinically relevant parameters may be calculated by gated SPECT, using modern technology?

Clinically relevant parameters that may be calculated using modern acquisition equipment and dedicated software include:

- LV cavity volumes
- LV mass
- Myocardial wall thickening
- The heart-to-lung ratio (the nuclear equivalent of the cardiothoracic index used in classic radiology)
- The percent hypoperfused myocardium (a global expression of the ischemic burden in a given patient)

Although some of these parameters already are used frequently in current practice, others, such as the heart-to-lung ratio or the percent hypoperfused myocardium, are still of research interest only.

51. What is fatty acid imaging, and what are its potential uses?

Normal myocardial cells use free fatty acids for their energy requirements and glucose under ischemic conditions. PET scan can detect myocardial ischemia based on this "metabolic switch."

Although the classic method to achieve this consists of demonstration of an increased cellular uptake of FDG glucose, it has been shown that ischemia also can be assessed by demonstration of a suppressed cellular metabolism of free fatty acids.

52. How is the myocardial energy metabolism assessed by free fatty acid imaging?

The uptake of free fatty acids, as shown by PET, is directly proportional to the concentration of myocardial adenosine triphosphate.

53. What is the current place of free fatty imaging in clinical practice?

This role remains to be defined and ultimately will depend on demonstration of the incremental value of this method over the existing techniques in a cost-effective fashion.

54. What is Tc-NOET, and what are its pinnacle applications?

Tc-NOET is a radiotracer used in clinical practice in Europe and under active investigation in the United States. The great advantage of this tracer is that it shows redistribution, similar to thallium. If this characteristic is validated by ongoing studies, Tc-NOET may prove to be a nearly ideal technique that combines the high image quality characteristic to technetium-based tracers with the viability assessment that has been for many years the distinctive characteristic of thallium imaging. Fig. 7 shows a NOET perfusion scan.

SHORT AXIS

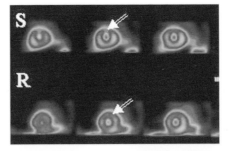

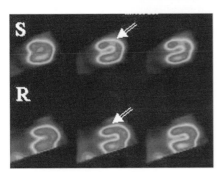

HORIZ. AXIS

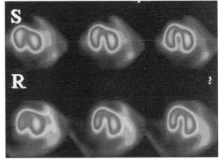

VERT. AXIS

FIGURE 7. Anterior ischemia demonstrated by technetium-NOET. (See also Color Plates, Figure 30.)

12. EPIDEMIOLOGIC CONCEPTS IN CARDIAC IMAGING

Gabriel Adelmann, M.D.

1. What is the sensitivity of a diagnostic test?

The sensitivity of a test reflects its ability to identify all the patients with the disease being investigated. The key concept is: If the patient has the disease, the test will pick it up. If the test is negative, the patient most probably does not have the disease. However, if the test is positive, the patient might or might not have the disease. If the test has a high sensitivity, it will not miss patients with the disease, although many other subjects without the disease may also test positive.

Sensitivity is defined by the mathematical formula:

$$S = \text{(number of true positives)} / \text{(total number of patients with the disease)}$$

or, equivalently,

$$S\,(\%) = \text{(number of true positives)} / \text{(true positives + false negatives)} \times 100$$

where true positives are the patients in whom the test is positive and who, indeed, suffer from the disease, and false negatives are the patients in whom the test is negative but who do suffer from the disease. The false negatives have been missed by the diagnostic test. Assuming an ideal test, which never misses the diagnosis, the sensitivity would be 100%.

2. Why is it important for a diagnostic test to have a high sensitivity?

The higher the sensitivity of a diagnostic test, the lower the probability of missing the presence of disease in a patient; missing the diagnosis would, of course, leave the patient untreated and exposed to complications.

3. What is the specificity of a diagnostic test?

The specificity of a test reflects its ability to identify patients without the disease. The key concept is: If the test is positive, the patient has the disease. Note that, if the test is negative, the patient might have the disease or not; with a high-specificity test, there will be very few people without the disease mislabeled as having it.

Specificity is defined as:

$$Sp\,(\%) = \text{(true negatives)} / \text{(total number of patients without the disease)} \times 100$$

or, equivalently,

$$Sp\,(\%) = \text{(true negatives)} / \text{(true negatives + false positives)} \times 100$$

where true negatives are patients in whom the test is negative and who, indeed, do not suffer from the disease, and false positives are those in whom the test is positive, despite the absence of disease.

In the case of an ideal test, which would never mislabel a healthy subject as having the disease, the false positives would be zero, and the specificity would be 100%.

4. Why is it important for a diagnostic test to have a high specificity?

High-specificity tests help prevent exposing healthy people to the risks, psychological distress, and financial strain of a treatment for a disease that they do not, in fact, have.

5. Despite the mathematical appeal of the explanations above, it seems to me that there shouldn't be more than one definition for a "good" test and that if a test has a high sensitivity, it should also have a high specificity. Right?

Wrong. Consider the basic logical equation underlying the definition of sensitivity:

1. The patient has the disease.
2. The test is positive.
3. The presence of (1) implies the presence of (2).

It is very tempting to conclude that, if the logic of the statements above is correct, the following statements will also be correct:

a. The patient does not have the disease.
b. The test is negative.
c. The presence of (a) implies the presence of (b).

However, this reasoning is totally wrong. For all we know, there may be a million healthy people who test positive for every one person who does indeed have the disease *and* tests positive. The only thing a high sensitivity tells us is that, if the test is negative, the patient does not have the disease.

Consider this analogy: a bank has been robbed, and the suspect has been reported to be a male in his 30s, of average height and weight, and wearing a brown suit. The police were on the scene immediately and have retained for questioning 20 young men matching the description. The chief inspector is confident that the true perpetrator is among these people. The problem is: what do you do next to pinpoint the real robber and let the innocent go home? The first strategy (of retaining everybody corresponding to the description) has a high sensitivity but a very low specificity for answering the question. What is needed now is a more *specific* technique, such as fingerprinting. It would have been practically impossible to fingerprint all the people who were around the bank at the time of the robbery, so that the initial selection approach, for all its low specificity, is extremely valuable.

Conversely, in the case of specificity, one may not infer that if the test is negative, the patient does not have the disease. Indeed, for all we know, there may be a million sick people who tested negative, in addition to the one healthy person who tested negative and really does not have the disease. The only thing a high specificity tells us is that, if the test is positive, the patient has the disease.

Consider this analogy: you want to know if it's cloudy outside, but you cannot see the sky from your window. You look out anyway. At this point, there are two possibilities. If it is raining outside, then you can be absolutely sure the sky is cloudy. In other words, the "rain test" is highly specific for a cloudy sky. If it is not raining outside, you cannot know for sure if it is cloudy or not. The "rain test" is not sensitive for a cloudy sky.

6. What is the relationship between sensitivity and specificity?

Generally, the higher the sensitivity of the test, the lower its specificity, and vice versa. Consider this analogy: in a museum there is a priceless statue that, because of its great age, has become very brittle. To insure the safety of the work of art, the museum manager has decided to install a device that detects vibration. If the detector is highly sensitive, one can be certain that no really significant vibration (such as might endanger the work of art) will pass unnoticed, but the highly sensitive detector also will generate a lot of false alarms from innocuous vibrations, such as that caused by a car driving by the museum building or a child stomping in one of the exhibit halls.

Conversely, if one installs a detector with high *specificity,* which will only start to beep at a higher level of vibration, there will not be a lot of false alarms, but, unfortunately, some potentially dangerous vibrations might go undetected.

The choice of the "beeping threshold" of the device is a complex decision, based on questions such as: How important is that statue really? If it breaks, can it be fixed? If it breaks and it's fixed, will one be able to tell the damage? What are the financial and technical resources available for the protection of this object? Would taking extra care of this one object imply that other works of art, which might be just as important (or even more so), would be unduly neglected?

The choice of a medical study to image the heart, with the attending decisions regarding the desired sensitivity, specificity, time, and financial expenditure, has to weigh the very same issues of how important is it to catch every patient with the disease versus potentially alarming several people without the disease by giving them the false-positive results.

7. What is the accuracy of a diagnostic test?

Accuracy is defined as the percentage of subjects in whom the test correctly establishes the presence or absence of disease.

Accuracy = (true positives + true negatives) / total number of patients who had the test

8. What is the positive predictive value (PPV) of a diagnostic test?

PPV represents the probability that a patient who tested positive should indeed have the disease.

PPV = (true positives) / (all positives) = (true-positives) / (true positives + false positives)

9. What is the negative predictive value (NPV) of a diagnostic test?

NPV represents the probability that a patient who tested negative should indeed be free of disease.

NPV = (true negatives) / (all negatives) = (true-negatives) / (true-negatives + false negatives)

10. What are the factors that determine the PPV or NPV of a medical test?

It is tempting to consider the NPV and PPV of a test as the ultimate, clinically relevant, quality-control characteristic of the test. However, it must be realized that the PPV and NPV also depend on the probability of the disease in the population that is being studied. Thus, a 1-mm ST segment depression on a treadmill test in an otherwise healthy young woman will be viewed quite differently than the very same electrocardiogram (ECG) finding in a middle-age male with risk factors and chest pain. In other words, the same test (ECG) and the exact same finding (1-mm ST segment depression) will have a widely different PPV for coronary artery disease in these two patients, because the prevalence of that type of disease is widely different in the two age and gender groups.

11. What is Bayes' theorem, and how does it apply to imaging tests?

Bayes' theorem is fundamental to the pertinent interpretation of any diagnostic test. Suppose we're screening people for coronary ischemia, using a very accurate test (such as a myocardial perfusion scan) that will give a positive result 90% of the time when ischemia is present. What is the probability that a person who tests positive has coronary ischemia? If your answer is 90%, you are wrong; read the last sentence again. The test is positive in 90% of *patients with ischemic heart disease*, not in 90% of *people being tested!* Thus, the probability that a positive study should really indicate the presence of disease in a testee is:

90% × the probability that that specific patient should have the disease (based on epidemiological data such as age, gender, risk factors) × the probability of testing positive (i.e., the probability of having a true-positive test + that of having a false-positive test)

In a patient with a very low pretest probability of disease, the product above will be very low, regardless of the accuracy of the test. Similarly, it will be high if the pretest probability of disease is high. A positive test result does not, in itself, indicate the presence of disease in a testee; rather, the probability of disease is dictated by the probability of disease in the population that the testee belongs to. An astute physician will be as unimpressed by a normal perfusion scan in a 70-year-old diabetic, hypertensive smoker with typical resting chest pain as he will be by an abnormal result in a 20-year old woman with stabbing, brief chest pain. Despite the test results, the former patient will be sent to coronary angiography, whereas the latter will be reassured. In fact, an astute physician will not obtain nuclear scans in these patients in the first place but will reserve this diagnostic modality to intermediate-probability patients. It is in these patients, and in them only, that the result of a nuclear perfusion scan will influence further management (a 40-year-old patient with one risk factor and with effort-induced chest discomfort will receive therapy and possible referral for coronary angiogram if the nuclear scan is positive, and just follow-up and risk factor management if the test is negative.)

12. What is the threshold model of clinical decision analysis?

The threshold model basically answers the question: Is it worthwhile applying *this* strategy (test, treatment, etc.) in *this* patient? (i.e., what is the threshold for performing/not performing the test?). The decision depends on the type of disease, the availability and risk/benefit ratio of the suggested medical strategy, and the patient's own wishes. Some of the questions to be answered in this setting include:

1. **Is the disease important enough to warrant a medical test in the first place?** Should one perform expensive and time-consuming viral cultures for a common cold in an otherwise healthy person? Should one perform an extensive virologic and bacteriologic work-up in a febrile HIV-positive patient?

2. **Would the results of the test change the management of the disease?** What, beside the obvious aspirin or Tylenol, would one do anyway if the viral cultures came back positive for common cold? Would one necessarily treat the HIV patient according to the microbiological results, or would one prefer wide-spectrum antibiotics anyway?

3. **Is the risk of that test greater than the risk of not treating the patient?** Imagine a patient with gout who has severely painful, yet not very frequent, attacks and to whom a new medicine is proposed. The medicine is highly effective against gouty arthritis but may have unforeseen adverse effects. Should the patient take the medicine or not? Obviously, it all depends on how incapacitated he or she is by the attacks, and how frequent and how severe the adverse effects of the medicine are. Now apply this analogy to a patient with terminal HIV disease to whom a new therapeutic cocktail is being proposed.

13. What is referral bias?

Referral bias refers to the fact that the results of a medical activity (diagnostic method, therapeutic strategy) are conditioned not only by the skills and technical endowment of those performing the activity, but also by the type of patients being subjected to that medical activity.

Consider an analogy. Suppose there are two surgeons, A and B. The mortality in the patient population treated by surgeon A is 20%, whereas the mortality of those treated by surgeon B is only 2%. Who is the better surgeon? The correct answer to this question is: I don't know, because, there may be two scenarios:

- Surgeon A has significantly poorer skills than surgeon B.
- Surgeon A is a top-of-the-range specialist working in a tertiary center who only accepts "desperate" cases, that are beyond the skills of surgeon B. Perhaps, if surgeon B were to treat the same patient population, the mortality in his hands would be 50%, but, surgeon B works in a general surgical practice and takes only "healthy" patients, which makes him "look better.")

In other words, two important factors determine the answer to the original question: the skills of the surgeon and the degree of complexity of the patient's disease. The fact that only very sick patients are *referred* to the care of surgeon A introduces a *bias* in the assessment of *surgeon A's* skills.

Note that, in this analogy, one may also identify a referral bias regarding *surgeon B's* skills. Indeed, surgeon A was heard exclaiming his disappointment at the skills of surgeon B ("My colleague, surgeon B, cannot take care of his own patients, and he always refers them to me!"). This is a very unfair statement because surgeon A only sees a minority of his colleague's patients (i.e., the very complicated ones). He is not aware of the innumerable additional patients competently treated by surgeon B. In this respect, surgeon A is *biased* in his assessment of his colleague's skills, because of the patients *referred* to him.

14. How does this apply to cardiologic imaging techniques?

Suppose that 20% of patients sent for cardiac catheterization because of a positive nuclear scan are found to have normal coronaries. Does this mean that nuclear testing is an unreliable diagnostic method? Indeed, what does this figure (i.e., 20%) tell us about the sensitivity and specificity of nuclear scan as a diagnostic method? The answer is, it tells us very little. To understand this apparently surprising statement, let's consider the definitions of sensitivity and specificity.

Sensitivity = true positives / all patients with the disease

Specificity = true negatives / patients without the disease

Neither of these parameters can be calculated by looking at the patients sent to the cath lab because the doctors in the cath lab do not know the denominator in either of the equations but only see the false positives. Indeed, "negatives" (whether true or false) are generally not sent to cardiac catheterization (gatekeeping from unnecessary invasive procedures is what nuclear perfusion studies are all about!).

15. So how does one establish who is a capable physician or not? How does one decide if the medical test is a "good" test or not?

By comparing the results of that physician's activity (or diagnostic tests' accuracy) to what might be expected based on the risk factor profile of the population being treated. Let us consider an area where smoking and consumption of saturated animal fat are highly prevalent. Let us now suppose that the risk for coronary artery disease in this population is 20% in people older than 50 years. If the test finds a prevalence of ischemic heart disease in only 10% or in over 40%, there is a significant problem.

This concept has been termed *normalcy rate*. In the case of nuclear cardiology, this is the percentage of patients with a low pretest probability of disease (as assessed based on risk-factor profiles) who are indeed found to have a normal nuclear perfusion scan.

13. COST-EFFECTIVENESS ISSUES IN CARDIAC IMAGING

Gabriel Adelmann, M.D.

1. What is cost-effectiveness in medical care?

The concept of cost-effectiveness in medical care is based on choosing an optimal diagnostic and therapeutic strategy, based on available evidence (evidence-based medical practice), and achieving this at the lowest possible cost in comparison with other possible or competing strategies.

2. What are the main factors driving cost-effectiveness in the setting of medical care?

Some of the important determinants of cost-effectiveness in medical care are the adoption of clear and universally accepted practice guidelines, individualization of a medical treatment according to the needs of the specific patient, but using evidence-based medicine the adoption of clear and universally accepted criteria by which to judge the results of a medical strategy understanding that "cheap it is not necessarily bad " and "expensive is not necessarily good." For instance, *not* performing a secondary, confirmatory imaging study (e.g., TEE or MRI) in a patient with suspected aortic dissection from an initial diagnostic test (e.g., spiral CT) can be both cost-effective and the best medical care (because it helps avoid time delays till the establishment of appropriate therapy).

3. Describe some of the new trends in diagnostic imaging that affect the delivery of optimal medical care.

- The need to digitally store images centrally, with remote access at the point of care
- An increase in the role of specialized diagnostic imaging units, which may lead to shorter hospital stays and an increased cost-effectiveness of medical care
- Consolidation of practice into larger systems (i.e., single or multiple-specialty groups or hospitals) with access to a variety of state-of-the-art imaging techniques
- The increasing role of the noninvasive imaging cardiologist as a "gate-keeper" for interventional procedures
- The increasing role of preventive medicine (e.g., dobutamine stress testing in patients without a history or symptoms of ischemic heart disease, before a major noncardiac surgical procedure)
- The need to analyze outcome data and the yield of different imaging strategies

4. What is the influence of new computer technologies on the practice of cardiac imaging?

The explosive development of information processing and storage technology has already started to change the practice of medicine profoundly. Two of the novel approaches made possible by modern information processing technology are *electronic storage* and *transmission of medical records and images,* which greatly facilitate data transmission for initial interpretation or for obtaining a second opinion. Mobile technician-operated diagnostic units will be able to collect patient information in a variety of sites (ranging from busy urban or suburban locations, to remote rural areas) and to transmit the patient information over the Internet to expert readers—the advent of the virtual office (e.g., access to images, patient information, scheduling, refills).

5. What is the difference between credentialing and accreditation in the practice of cardiac imaging?

Credentialing refers to the process the physician must go through to become certified as an individual to perform and interpret the imaging procedure. For many of the cardiac imaging procedures, a physician is required to undergo a training process and to pass a special examination.

Accreditation refers to the certification process of a laboratory to perform a certain imaging procedure. The accreditation is based on assessment of:

Physical facilities of the laboratory
Personnel qualifications
Nonimaging medical capabilities of the laboratory
Quality of image interpretation and reporting
Degree of safety of the laboratory
Degree of confidentiality provided
Patient satisfaction

6. What is the role of credentialing and certification in the practice of cardiac imaging?

The certification examinations for different imaging modalities (e.g., echo) have just recently been introduced; consequently, most physicians currently performing these diagnostic studies are not formally certified. However, with the increased importance of health care standardization, it is expected that in the near future physicians who perform and interpret imaging procedures will be certified to do so.

7. Who are the current "gate-keepers" for cardiac imaging?

In general, primary care physicians order the majority of cardiac imaging procedures. In doing so, they may or may not be required to ask for the input of a cardiologist or of a third-party payer.

8. Where are most cardiac imaging services rendered?

The outpatient setting is where most cardiac imaging is delivered.

9. What is the meaning of *appropriateness of testing* when discussing quality assessment?

This concept refers to the selection of a test that would:

- Be appropriate to the patient's condition (e.g., pharmacologic rather than exercise cardiac imaging in a patient with orthopedic problems)
- Yield all the necessary information for optimal therapeutic decisions (e.g., intravascular ultrasound in the setting of a coronary stenosis of unclear significance by angiography)
- Avoid costly and extraneous imaging tests, yielding information that would not change the patient's treatment (e.g., transthoracic rather than transesophageal echocardiography for the diagnosis of suspected pericardial effusion)

10. What is meant by the *outcome* of an imaging laboratory?

The primary *outcome* of a diagnostic facility refers to that facility's track record for false-positive and false-negative studies, for predictive accuracy, and for quality and consistency of study interpretation.

11. What are the factors that determine whether a new technology will gain widespread application and will ultimately "survive" in the competitive market of cardiac imaging?

A new imaging technology will gain widespread acceptance if it provides information that cannot be obtained by means of established technologies or if it provides information in a more cost-effective fashion than the established technologies.

BIBLIOGRAPHY

GENERAL TEXTS ABOUT CARDIAC IMAGING

1. Lee RT, Braunwald E (eds): Atlas of Cardiac Imaging. Philadelphia, Current Medicine, 1998.
2. Watt I: Cardiac imaging cost and benefit. In Halley Project 1998–2000, 2nd Refresher Course Series. Milan, Springer, 1998.

ECHOCARDIOGRAPHY

3. Asher CR, Klein AL: Diastolic heart failure: Restrictive cardiomyopathy, constrictive pericarditis, and cardiac tamponade: Clinical and echocardiographic evaluation. Cardiol Rev 10:218–229, 2002.
4. Breen JF: Imaging of the pericardium. J Thorac Imaging 16:47–54, 2001.
5. Feigenbaum H: Echocardiography. Philadelphia, Lea & Febiger, 1994.
6. Goldman JH, Foster E: Transesophageal echocardiographic (TEE) evaluation of intracardiac and pericardial masses. Cardiol Clin 18:849–860, 2000.
7. Karia DH, Xing YQ, Kuvin JT, et al: Recent role of imaging in the diagnosis of pericardial disease. Curr Cardiol Rep 4:33–40, 2002.
8. Lang RM, Mor-Avi V, Zoghbi WA, et al: The role of contrast enhancement in echocardiographic assessment of left ventricular function. Am J Cardiol 90(suppl 10A):28J-34J, 2002.
9. Marwick TH: Stress echocardiography. Heart 89:113–118, 2003.
10. Mochizuki Y, Patel AK, Banerjee A, et al: Intraoperative transesophageal echocardiography: Correlation of echocardiographic findings and surgical pathology. Cardiol Rev 7:270–276, 1999.
11. Oh JK, Seward JB, Tajik JA: The Echo Manual, 2nd ed. Philadelphia, Lippincott Williams & Wilkins, 1999.
12. Otto C: Textbook of Clinical Echocardiography. Philadelphia, W.B. Saunders, 2000.
13. Schaff H (ed): Mayo Clinic Practice of Cardiology, 3rd ed. St. Louis, Mosby, 1996.
14. Weyman AE (ed): Principles and Practices of Echocardiography, 2nd ed. Philadelphia, Lea & Febiger, 1994.
15. Zoghbi WA: Evaluation of myocardial viability with contrast echocardiography. Am J Cardiol 90(suppl 10A):65J-71J, 2002.

IVUS

16. Dijkstra J, Koning G, Reiber JH: Quantitative measurements in IVUS images. Int J Card Imaging 15:513–522, 1999.
17. Jimenez J, Escaned J: Intracoronary ultrasound in acute coronary syndromes: From characterization of vulnerable plaques to guidance of percutaneous treatment of complex stenoses. J Interv Cardiol 15:447–459, 2002.
18. Mintz GS, Nissen SE, Anderson WD, et al: American College of Cardiology Clinical Expert Consensus Document on Standards for Acquisition, Measurement and Reporting of Intravascular Ultrasound Studies (IVUS). A report of the American College of Cardiology Task Force on Clinical Expert Consensus Documents. J Am Coll Cardiol 37:1478–1492, 2001.
19. Nissen SE: Who is at risk for atherosclerotic disease? Lessons from intravascular ultrasound. Am J Med 112(suppl 8A):27S-33S, 2002.
20. Nissen SE: Application of intravascular ultrasound to characterize coronary artery disease and assess the progression or regression of atherosclerosis. Am J Cardiol 89(4A):24B-31B, 2002.

CARDIAC CATHETERIZATION

21. Baim DS, Grossman W: Grossman's Cardiac Catheterization: Angiography and Intervention, 6th ed. Philadelphia, Lippincott Williams & Wilkins, 2000.
22. Corti R, Farkouh ME, Badimon JJ: The vulnerable plaque and acute coronary syndromes. Am J Med 113:668–680, 2002.
23. Kern MJ: The Cardiac Catheterization Handbook, 3rd ed. St. Louis, Mosby International, 1998.
24. Raff GL, O'Neill WW: Interventional therapy of the acute coronary syndromes. Prog Cardiovasc Dis 44:455–468, 2002.
25. Schwartz RS, Henry TD: Pathophysiology of coronary artery restenosis. Rev Cardiovasc Med 3(suppl):S4-S9, 2002.
26. Storger H: Incidence, prevention, and treatment of vascular perforations complicating coronary interventions. J Interv Cardiol 15:505–510, 2002.
27. Uretsky BF: Cardiac Catheterization: Concepts, Techniques, and Applications. Boston, Blackwell Science, 1997.

NUCLEAR MEDICINE

28. Cerqueira MD (ed): Nuclear Cardiology. Boston, Blackwell Scientific, 1994.
29. Cerqueira MD, Lawrence A: Nuclear cardiology update. Radiol Clin North Am 39:931–946, vii-viii, 2001.
30. Cerqueira MD, Weissman NJ, Dilsizian V, et al: Standardized myocardial segmentation and nomenclature for tomographic imaging of the heart: A statement for healthcare professionals from the Cardiac Imaging Committee of the Council on Clinical Cardiology of the American Heart Association. J Nucl Cardiol 9:240–245, 2002.
31. Chamuleau SA, Van Eck-Smit BL, Meuwissen M, Piek JJ: Adequate patient selection for coronary revascularization: An overview of current methods used in daily clinical practice. Int J Cardiovasc Imaging 18:5–15, 2002.
32. Depuey G, Garcia E, Berman DS: Cardiac SPECT Imaging. Philadelphia, Lippincott Williams & Wilkins, 2001.
33. Dilsizian V, Narula J (eds): Atlas of Nuclear Cardiology. Philadelphia, Current Medicine, 2003.
34. Elhendy A, Bax JJ, Poldermans D: Dobutamine stress myocardial perfusion imaging in coronary artery disease. J Nucl Med 43:1634–1646, 2002.
35. Garcia EV, et al: Physical and Technical Aspects of Nuclear Cardiology. Reston, VA, Society of Nuclear Medicine, 1997.
36. Gewirtz H, Tawakol A, Bacharach SL: Heterogeneity of myocardial blood flow and metabolism: Review of physiologic principles and implications for radionuclide imaging of the heart. J Nucl Cardiol 9:534–541, 2002.
37. Iskandrian AE, Verani MS (eds): Nuclear Cardiac Imaging: Principles and Applications, 3rd ed. Oxford; Oxford University Press, 2003.
38. Langer O, Halldin C: PET and SPET tracers for mapping the cardiac nervous system. Eur J Nucl Med Mol Imaging 29:416–434, 2002.
39. Murphy K (ed): Nuclear Cardiology/PET. Reston, VA, Society of Nuclear Medicine, 2001.
40. Taillefer R, Tamaki N: New Radiotracers in Cardiac Imaging: Principles and Applications. Stamford, CT, Appleton & Lange, 1999.

CARDIAC CT

41. Chen JTT: Essentials of cardiac roentgenology. In Coleman R, Edward R (eds): Essentials of Cardiac Imaging. Philadelphia, Lippincott-Raven, 1997.
42. Chiles C, Putman CE (eds): Pulmonary and Cardiac Imaging. New York, Marcel Dekker, 1997.
43. Greenberg SB: Assessment of cardiac function: Magnetic resonance and computed tomography. J Thorac Imaging 15:243–251, 2000.
44. Khan IA, Nair CK: Clinical, diagnostic, and management perspectives of aortic dissection. Chest 122:311–328, 2002.
45. Miller SW: Cardiac Radiology. St. Louis, Mosby, 1996.
46. Müller NL,Grist TM (eds): Radiological Society of North America: Scientific Assembly: Categorical Course in Diagnostic Radiology: Thoracic Imaging-Chest and Cardiac. Oak Brook, IL, Radiological Society of North America, 2001.
47. Ohnesorge BM, et al: Multi-slice CT in cardiac imaging: Technical principles, clinical application, and future developments. Berlin, Springer, 2002.
48. Zaret BL, Beller G (eds): Nuclear Cardiology: State of the Art and Future Directions, 2nd ed. St. Louis, Mosby, 1999.

CARDIAC MRI

49. Duerinckx AJ: Cardiac MRI for clinicians: An overview. Int J Cardiovasc Imaging 17:437–443, 2001.
50. Paelinck BP, Lamb HJ, Bax JJ, et al: Assessment of diastolic function by cardiovascular magnetic resonance. Am Heart J 144:198–205, 2002.
51. Pons-Lladó G, et al: Atlas of Practical Cardiac Applications of MRI. Dordrecht, Kluwer Academic Publishers, 1999.
52. Van Der Wall: Nuclear cardiology and cardiac magnetic resonance: Physiology, techniques, and applications Weesp, Netherlands, H. Soto Productions, 1992.

INDEX

Page numbers in **boldface type** indicate complete chapters.

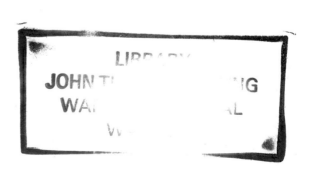